AF810462

Stress and Orality

Francis Hartmann • Gérard Cucchi

Stress and Orality

New Data About Teeth Clenching & Outcomes, Migraine, Fibromyalgia, Fatigue

With contribution by Jacques Orofino

Our warmest thanks to Françoise GILLESPIE and Jean-Pierre BOUVILLE for their valuable contributions

Springer

Francis Hartmann
Université de la Méditerranée
Aix-Marseille (France)

Gérard Cucchi
Université de la Méditerranée
Aix-Marseille (France)

ISBN 978-2-8178-0270-1 ISBN 978-2-8178-0271-8 (eBook)
DOI 10.1007/978-2-8178-0271-8
Springer Paris Heidelberg New York Dordrecht London

Library of Congress Control Number: 2013944579

© Springer-Verlag France 2014
This work is subject to copyright. All rights are reserved by the Publisher, whether the whole or part of the material is concerned, specifically the rights of translation, reprinting, reuse of illustrations, recitation, broadcasting, reproduction on microfilms or in any other physical way, and transmission or information storage and retrieval, electronic adaptation, computer software, or by similar or dissimilar methodology now known or hereafter developed. Exempted from this legal reservation are brief excerpts in connection with reviews or scholarly analysis or material supplied specifically for the purpose of being entered and executed on a computer system, for exclusive use by the purchaser of the work. Duplication of this publication or parts thereof is permitted only under the provisions of the Copyright Law of the Publisher's location, in its current version, and permission for use must always be obtained from Springer. Permissions for use may be obtained through RightsLink at the Copyright Clearance Center. Violations are liable to prosecution under the respective Copyright Law.
The use of general descriptive names, registered names, trademarks, service marks, etc. in this publication does not imply, even in the absence of a specific statement, that such names are exempt from the relevant protective laws and regulations and therefore free for general use.
While the advice and information in this book are believed to be true and accurate at the date of publication, neither the authors nor the editors nor the publisher can accept any legal responsibility for any errors or omissions that may be made. The publisher makes no warranty, express or implied, with respect to the material contained herein.

Printed on acid-free paper

Springer is part of Springer Science+Business Media (www.springer.com)

Foreword

The original approach of our work is the combined result of a 25-year-long personal clinical evaluation of the problem and a long study of Anglo-Saxon renowned literature about **temporomandibular disorders** (TMD). The current work claims to pay tribute to all of these authors. This data is supported by fundamental research in neuroscience, especially relating to the *various* and *numerous connections between trigeminal and non-trigeminal nervous structures*. Clinically, it must be considered under stressful conditions leading to sensitization. The purpose of this book is not to explain the mechanisms of stress which are largely described and updated in worldwide literature. Therefore, current data on the hypothalamic-pituitary-adrenal axis (HPAA) will only be mentioned to enlighten some little known effects of stress, especially in the *oral sphere*. The relation between the **TMD mechanisms** and some clinical forms of **migraine**, **fibromyalgia**, and **chronic fatigue** will be suggested as they all appear as disadaptive phenomena. The following research only deals with clinical forms in stressed and introverted patients who **severely clench their teeth**. Those patients led their general physician to focus on their deleterious oral parafunctional habit. Such disclosure proved highly useful in providing an accurate diagnosis and well-oriented therapeutical protocols.

General Introduction

Practitioners are often confronted to patients who complain about pain and/or discomforts and who have been diagnosed with *migraine* or *fibromyalgia* or *chronic fatigue*. For some – particularly those stressed and introverted – classical medical treatments do not yield satisfactory results. Perplexed clinicians frequently speak of *atypical* ailments. For many years, dentists and stomatologists' research interests have focused on temporomandibular joint dysfunctions. This disease of the stomatognathic system is known as *temporomandibular disorders* (TMD). TMD are no longer considered as a real syndrome but rather as a plurifactorial disease of the oral sphere, caused by socio-psycho-emotional and/or acute or chronic peripheral stressors (occlusion[1] disturbances, lingual dysfunctions, physical traumatisms, postural troubles, etc.). Various clinical forms are generally classified as *myogenous*, *arthrogenous*, and *mixed*. But it is still a maze and a permanent cause of debate among specialists, even considered by some as the *great impostor*. The Part I of our book deals with a number of clinical investigations into a possible diagnosis of TMD. When dealing with trigeminal nerves (V), mouth, and teeth, physicians are often concerned primarily with acute pain or infection. Why would non-dental practitioners also show a clinical interest in TMD? In some cases symptoms go well beyond the sole oral sphere and stomatognathic functions – for example, various aches (neck, shoulders, arms, back, loins, etc.) dizziness, tinnitus, fever, or sleeping disorders – which may result from stressful conditions (maladaptation), as well as some predisposed psychological profiles which lead to certain behavioral habits.

The purpose of our book is to call the attention of practitioners to an unexplored deceptive oral habit that is frequently part of TMD: **severe parafunctional teeth clenching**. Indeed, neuroscience contributes some precious data on the relation between *trigeminal* and *non-trigeminal nervous centers*. Under persisting stressful conditions, **sensory overstimulation and nociception can spread out from V to non-V nerve areas**. Specialists sometimes speak of *sensitization*. These neural

[1]Dental occlusion – static and dynamic relation between upper and lower dental arches.

phenomena often cause or exacerbate various functional disturbances. Intense, durable strange symptoms may appear even in *areas quite distant from the mouth*. No clinician can be logically expected to associate the trigeminal sphere and parafunctional clenching to pathological mechanisms. Yet, we should keep in mind that the trigeminal territory is involved in various essential physiological functions, that is, *eating, breathing, speaking, hearing, standing, etc*. Therefore, the oral sphere has a major role in human adaptation.

Illness is a rupture in this permanent psychosomatic adaptation to stressors. What's more, depending on one's own biotype, illnesses can differ, as well as clinical signs and symptoms. It has been said that the rupture affects primarily the most tired organs or systems not the weakest. In case of maladaptation, can the highly affected trigeminal territory be responsible for initiating or emphasizing pathological disorders? Our book is a search for an answer to this key question. Under these conditions, how and why does one tend to experience parafunctional clenching? Some theories are offered here taking into account the psychological profiles of *clenchers*. Some symptoms may be common to both TMD and some forms of clinical disorders – such as migraine or fibromyalgia or chronic fatigue – in patients with severe clenching. The issue of accurate diagnosis and choice of effective therapeutic strategies must then be addressed. This book does not pretend to provide a panacea or comprehensive protocol for treating TMD, let alone atypical forms of migraine, fibromyalgia, or chronic fatigue. It only aspires to contribute to helping clinicians unmask the *great impostor* through an improved early diagnosis of the deleterious parafunctional habit of severe clenching. Because spasticity is responsible for severe clenching, therapeutics (Part III) only focuses on anti-spasticity treatments,[2] that is, **relaxing and moderating treatments** (RMT). It represents the first phase of the treatment and allows a clearer evaluation of some etiological factors. Furthermore, reduced symptomatology and increased patient's awareness of the parafunction contribute to raising his spirits. Part IV deals with some atypical forms of migraine, fibromyalgia, chronic fatigue, etc. in stressed and introverted patients who experience severe clenching. Some of these disorders may be better explained if clinicians considered the possible pathophysiological role played by the paired V in patients with introverted psychological backgrounds living under stress conditions. Our final purpose is to inspire clinicians to check patients methodically for **parafunctional teeth clenching** and help them recover fully from this dreadfully deleterious oral habit.

[2]Methods for rehabilitation of physiological conditions (dental, postural, or others) are not dealt with here.

Contents

Part I Diagnosis

Introduction 3
References 4

Symptoms 5
1 Pain 5
1.1 Location 6
1.2 Nature and Aggravating or Relieving Factors 20
1.3 Resistance to Drugs 21
2 Discomforts 22
2.1 Auditory Problems 22
2.2 Problems with Swallowing and Phonation 22
2.3 Problems with Posture and Vision 23
2.4 Fatigue and Sleeping Disorders 24
2.5 Psychological Mood Disorders 25
2.6 Prolonged Unexplained Fever 25
2.7 Immunodeficiency Disorders 26
2.8 Autonomic Problems 26
2.9 Problems with Nutrition 26
References 26

Objective Signs 35
1 Examination 35
1.1 Extraoral Examination 35
1.2 Intraoral Examination 35
2 Palpation 42
2.1 Extraoral Palpation 42
2.2 Intraoral Palpation 50

3 Listening ... 55
3.1 Acute Factors ... 55
3.2 Chronic Factors ... 57
4 Other Tests ... 58
References ... 58

Stomatognathic Parafunctions ... 65
References ... 69

In Conclusion ... 71

Part II Pathophysiology

Introduction ... 75
References ... 85

Characteristics of Periodontal Proprioception ... 87
1 Physiological Receptors ... 89
2 Nociceptive Receptors ... 94
References ... 95

The Trigeminal Nerve Pathways and Their Central Projections ... 97
References ... 107

Useful Physiological Reminders ... 113
1 The Rest Position of the Jaw ... 115
2 Inhibition Reflex of the Jaw-Closing Muscles Originating in the Periodontium (IRJCMOP) ... 116
3 Phasic Activity of the Stomatognathic Muscles ... 116
4 The Brain Control on Muscular Activities ... 117
5 Other Implicated Nervous Centres ... 118
References ... 119

Pathophysiological Conditions ... 121
Foreword ... 121
1 Skeletal Muscular Spasticity ... 122
2 Stomatognathic Muscular Spasticity ... 124
3 Oral Parafunctions ... 128
3.1 Familiar Grinding ... 128
3.2 Clenching: A Misunderstood Condition ... 129
4 Theory of Sensitization of the Low Neural Pathways ... 132
5 Theory of the *High Association Pathways* ... 140
References ... 147

The Behavioral Side of Clenching ... 151
1 Biochemical Data ... 162
1.1 Serotonin ... 162

1.2 Dopamine 164
1.3 Substance P 165
1.4 Acetylcholine 165
1.5 Others 165
References 165

Painful Outcomes of Parafunctional Clenching 169
References 178

Discomfort as the Outcome of Parafunctional Clenching 183
1 Auditory Problems 183
2 Problems with Swallowing and Phonation 190
3 Problems with Posture and Vision 193
4 Fatigue 198
5 Sleep Disturbances 200
6 Prolonged Unexplained Fever 202
6.1 Physiological Reminders 202
7 Immunodeficiency Problems 204
8 Autonomic Problems 206
9 Problems with Memory 209
10 Problems with Nutrition 212
References 215

In Conclusion 221

Part III Therapeutics

Introduction 225
Alternative Methods 228
References 228

Objectives 233
References 239

The Relaxing and Moderating Treatment (RMT) 241
1 Local Procedures 241
1.1 Technical Methods 244
1.2 Possible Actions 247
2 Functional Exercises 252
3 Clenching Self-Control: The *Lips Technique* 255
4 Drug Prescription 260
5 General Relaxation and Psychotherapy 261
References 264

In Conclusion 271

Part IV Medical Prospects

Medical Prospects 275
1 The Trigeminal Nerve Is Wellknown For Its "Tic douloureux" But Largely Underestimated For Its Non-algic Sensory Role 275
2 Migraine 279
3 Fibromyalgia 282
4 Chronic Fatigue 284
References 290

General Synthesis 297

Part I
Diagnosis

Introduction

Chapters "Symptoms" and "Objective Signs" both present clinical investigations of TMD patients. However, any practitioner should be able to compare our examples to the signs and symptoms he or she encounters daily, particularly in patients with obvious *migraine* or *fibromyalgia* or *chronic fatigue* disorders. Chapter "Stomatognathic Parafunctions" focuses on **oral parafunctional habits**. This data is important to discussions about differential TMD diagnoses or possible links to clinical forms of the three conditions noted above. There are few epidemiologic studies about the long-term clinical evolution of TMD signs and symptoms. In young adults, persisting symptoms tend to be more frequent in women (92 %) than in men (29 %) [10]. A number of studies [7, 8] confirmed that TMD signs and symptoms reduce with age. Because of the multiplicity of signs and symptoms, examining TMD patients is like going through a maze. A definite diagnosis may be difficult to establish. Patients themselves may find it difficult to accept possible links between some of their symptoms and masticating. According to experts, the patient's history together with accurate clinical records is the key to a comprehensive patient-centered diagnosis [1–6, 9]. Early diagnosis helps the clinician begin therapeutic treatment sooner. Therefore, it may have a rapid and sometimes spectacular beneficial effect on the signs and symptoms. It also reduces the risk of long-term complications and psychological disturbance (hopelessness, depression, etc.). Such diagnosis may be first established on the basis of confusing early signs. More conclusive elements later emerge following meticulous clinical examination. Otherwise, patients may suffer for a long time from well-diagnosed symptoms that persist because of inadequate treatment. In such cases it appears more important to evoke a possible stomatognathic origin of the illness. In Part II we will present a number of theoretical pathophysiological mechanisms. The purpose of anamnesis is to connect the various symptoms felt by the patient: pain, discomfort, and associated events. The purpose of the clinical examination is to reveal objective factors in concrete terms. But special efforts are made to reveal parafunctional oral habits. Some of those habits, such as dental or masticatory signs, belong to the field of dental surgery. They are also of great interest to other clinicians because they may explain the possible involvement of the oral sphere in uncommon clinical forms of

F. Hartmann, G. Cucchi, *Stress and Orality*,
DOI 10.1007/978-2-8178-0271-8_1, © Springer-Verlag France 2014

migraine, fibromyalgia, chronic fatigue, etc. in stressed introverted patients with severe jaw-clenching problems.

References

1. Auvenshine RC (2007) Temporomandibular disorders: associated features. Dent Clin North Am 51(1):105–127
2. Clark GT, Delcanho RE, Goulet JP (1993) The utility and validity of current diagnostic procedures for defining temporomandibular disorder patients. Adv Dent Res 7(2):97–112
3. De Wijer A, Lobbezoo-Scholte AM, Steenks MH, Bosman F (1995) Reliability of clinical findings in temporomandibular disorders. J Orofac Pain 9:181–191
4. Lobbezoo-Scholte AM, De Wijer A, Steenks MH, Bosman F (1994) Interexaminer reliability of six orthopedic tests in diagnostic subgroups of craniomandibular disorders. J Oral Rehabil 21:273–285
5. Mc Neill CH (1993) Temporomandibular disorders. Guidelines for classification. Assessment and management, 2nd edn. Quintessence, Chicago
6. Okeson JP (1995) Bell's orofacial pain, 5th edn. Quintes (ed), Chicago
7. Österberg T, Carlsson GE, Wedel A, Johansson U (1992) A cross-sectional and longitudinal study of craniomandibular dysfunction in an elderly population. J Craniomandib Disord Facial Oral Pain 6:237–246
8. Ow RKK, Loh T, Neo J, Khoo J (1995) Symptoms of craniomandibular disorder among elderly people. J Oral Rehabil 22(6):413–419
9. Von Korff M (1995) Health services research and temporomandibular pain. In: Sessle BJ, Bryant PS, Dionne RA (eds) Temporomandibular disorders and pain related conditions. IASP Press, Seattle
10. Wänman A (1995) The relationship between muscle tenderness and craniomandibular disorders: a study of 35-years old from the general population. J Orofac Pain 9(3):235–243

Symptoms

1 Pain

Craniofacial pain (CFP), particularly in case of TMD, is a major reason for consulting, [2, 3, 12, 13, 21, 22, 25, 32, 48, 52–54, 58, 59, 67, 70, 73, 80, 82, 89, 90, 97, 98, 108, 112, 114, 115, 132, 133, 141, 142, 153, 157] even among children [95]. Most people assume that the causal factors are related to cervicarthrosis or migraine. Such restrictive view should in fact be eclipsed by a wider notion of disorders of the stomatognathic system as a whole. It may even be necessary to consider the body's postural system and the individual's psychosocial dimension. In any case, the diagnosis must include the examination of orofacial tissues: stomatognathic muscles, TMJ, teeth, mucosa, ganglions, salivary glands, the ORL sphere [146], and the ophthalmic sphere.

The natural role of effectors (muscles and glands) consists in carrying out the orders of the brain as responses to stressors. Thus, the stomatognathic muscles can appear as elective targets [73, 83, 111, 142] for *peripheral* and *central stressing factors*. In that way, they can facilitate TMJ disorders [112, 142], **referred**[1] **pain** (CFP), and even unexplained pain spreading down to the neck, the nape, and the arm [5, 22, 135, 164].

The TMD "myogenous forms" are usually compared to myofascial pain dysfunction syndrome (MPDS). The CFP has many various possible causes and their diagnosis remains complex and disconcerting. A significant connection between TMD and headaches has been established [14, 38, 62, 66]. Stomatognathic muscle spasticity may or may not be associated with problems of dental occlusion. Yet, it frequently appears to be linked to psycho-emotional factors, while pain is often

[1]In a "referred pain," the topographic dissociation appears between two anatomical territories which are innervated by distinct nervous branches (for instance, cardiac trouble and referred pain in the arm or in the jaw). In a "reported pain," the topographic dissociation originates from nociceptive input begun somewhere on the peripheral or central sensitive ways; the pain is felt as coming from the corresponding peripheral field (for instance, leg scrotal pain from a radicular compression). The term "projected pain" involves the referred pain and the reported pain.

F. Hartmann, G. Cucchi, *Stress and Orality*,
DOI 10.1007/978-2-8178-0271-8_2, © Springer-Verlag France 2014

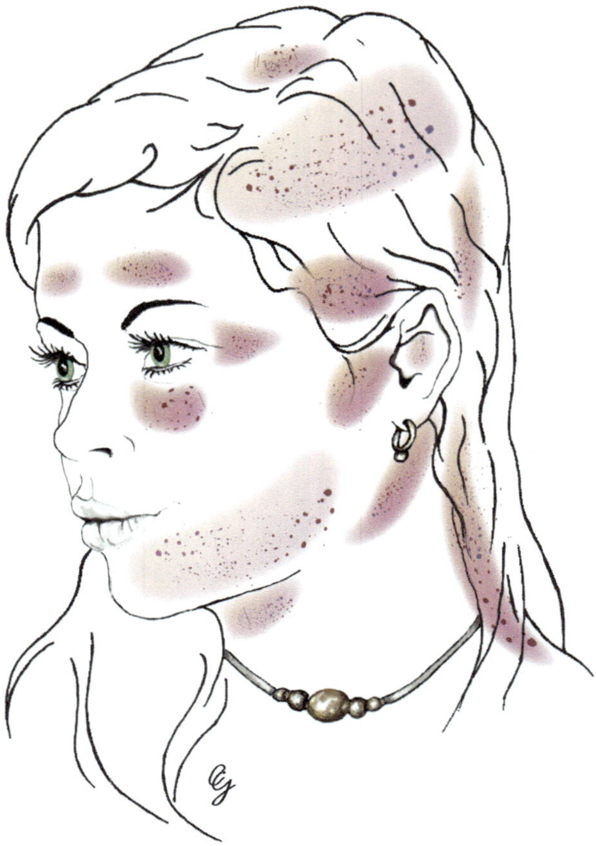

Fig. 1 Main areas of pain as observed in TMD

related to the psychosocial profile of the patient [151, 158]. The allowance made for pain repercussions on individual behavior is a prognosis element that must be evaluated [170]. Finally, rheumatoid arthritis has also been found to affect the TMJ [91] and generate severe pain in some TMD patients [9].

When questioning a patient about his or her pain, medical history should establish the *location* (Fig. 1), the *nature*, the *aggravating* or *relieving causes*, and finally the *resistance* to *drugs*.

1.1 Location

TMD patients often complain of cranial, facial, maxillary, and cervical pain, including pain in more specific zones such as temporal, retro-orbital, or nuchal areas. In their famous manual, Travell and Simons [153] presented the correlated referred pain between contractured stomatognathic muscles and head posture muscles. The following figures (Figs. 2, 3, 4, 5, 6, 7, 8, 9, 10, 11, 12, 13, 14, 15, 16, 17, 18, 19, 20, 21, 22, 23, 24, 25, 26, and 27) allow a better understanding of daily clinical observations, while an appropriate diagnosis remains difficult.

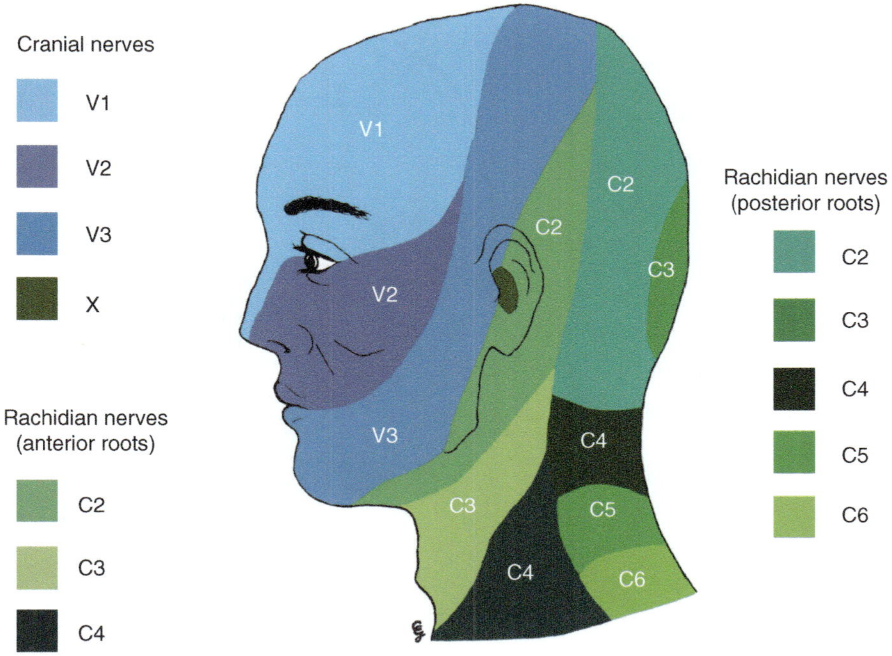

Fig. 2 Head and neck dermatomes (Modified from Bossy [19])

Part II defends the irrefutable value of connecting the frequency and durability of this type of pain with trigeminal involvement when **severe parafunctional habits** are present. So the projected pain may appear as "not corresponding" with the topographical distribution of nervous segments or peripheral nerves (Fig. 2). The pain may sometimes be caused by other factors[2]. Thus, TMD could be a major frequent cause of CFP and also of observed pain in **territories distant from the oral sphere** (Fig. 28) such as neck, shoulder, chest, back, and limbs [8, 22, 26, 28, 36, 42, 52, 65, 69, 70, 85, 89, 97, 101, 106, 116, 132, 135, 138, 153, 154, 163] with increased pain sensitivity in remote areas [86]. A rather high percentage (76 %) of TMD patients observed in a primary care clinic reported pain outside the stomatognathic system [82]. More rarely pain was reported in lower areas, for instance, in the pelvic region or inferior limbs. Such pain is frequently associated with feelings of "calf cramps." Clinicians should be interested in these remote painful symptoms which are likely to appear in other clinical sets, particularly by widespread pain in fibromyalgia.

[2]For instance, from ligament insertions [123]. About trigeminal neuropathic paroxysmal pain felt in gingiva and/or cheek, the cause can come from a compression of the buccal nerve in the temporalis [100]. In the same order, paresthesia of the tongue can be provoked by compression of lingual nerve in the lateral pterygoid muscle (LPMs) [79]. The spasticity of these two stomatognathic muscles can generate a nervous compression and must be relieved by the clinician. Otherwise, pain can rarely come from an osseous problem [125].

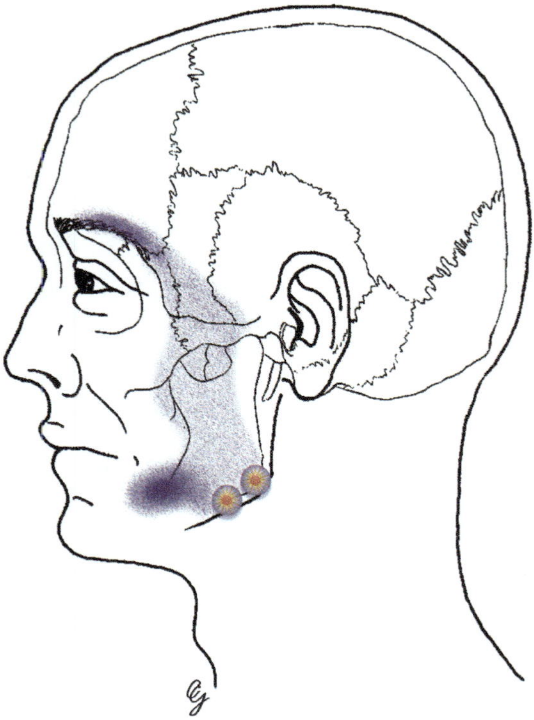

Fig. 3 Referred pain from the musculus masseter superficialis, lower fibers. In *purple* areas of pain, *little sun in circle* muscular trigger point (Modified from Travell and Simons [153])

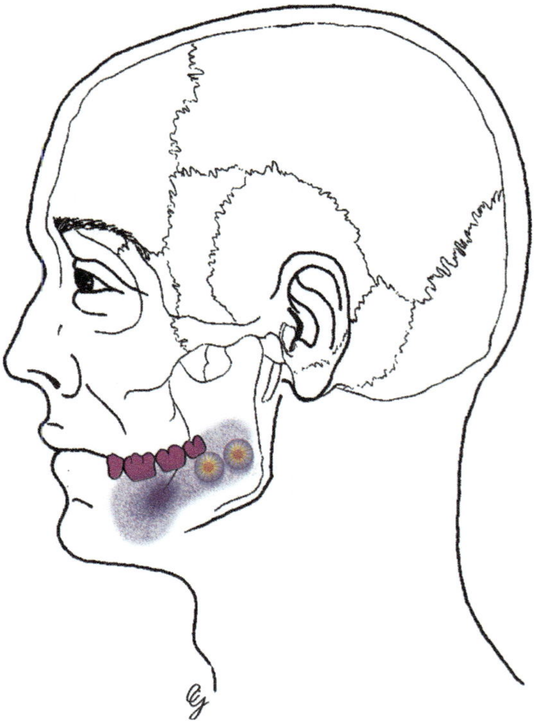

Fig. 4 Referred pain from the musculus masseter superficialis, medial fibers (Modified from Travell and Simons [153])

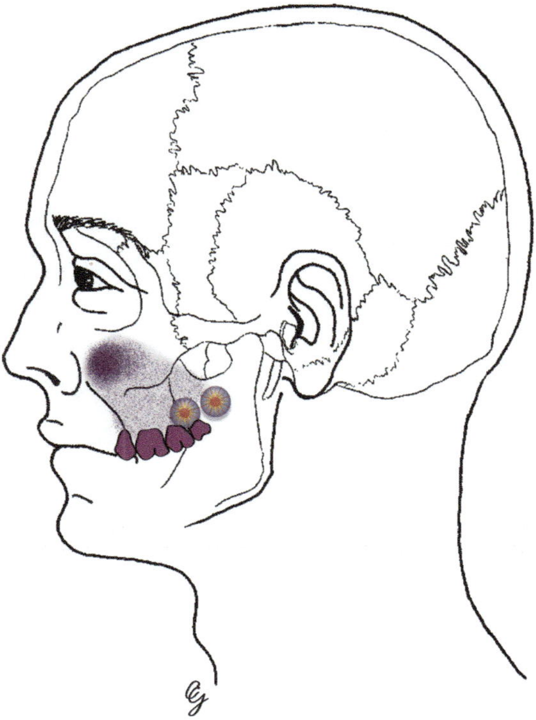

Fig. 5 Referred pain from the musculus masseter superficialis, upper fibers (Modified from Travell and Simons [153])

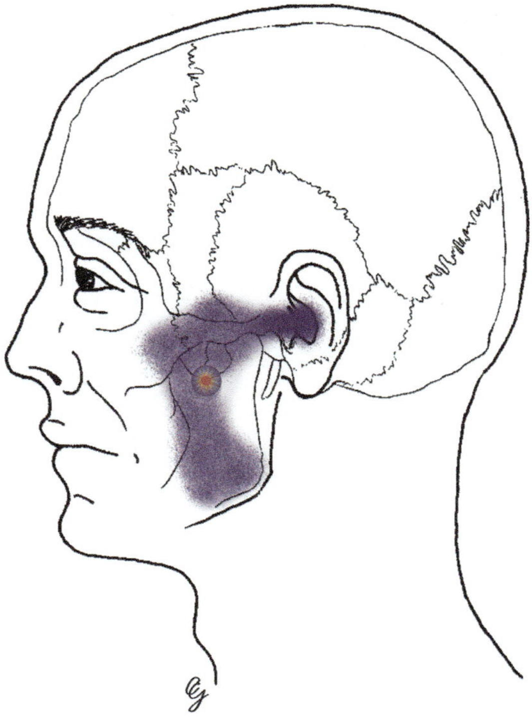

Fig. 6 Referred pain from the musculus masseter profundus (Modified from Travell and Simons [153])

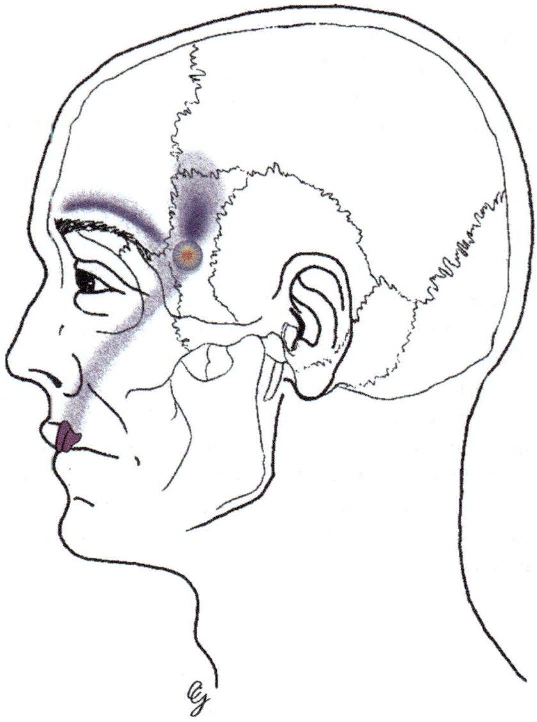

Fig. 7 Referred pain from the musculus temporalis, zone 1 (Modified from Travell and Simons [153])

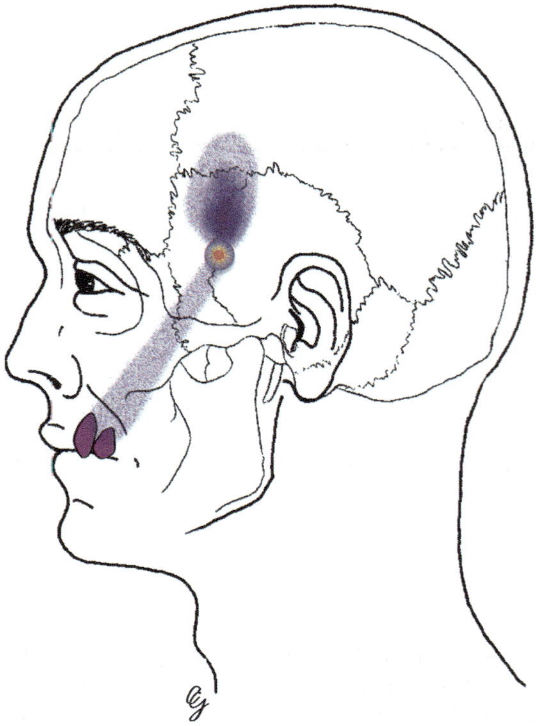

Fig. 8 Referred pain from the musculus temporalis, zone 2 (Modified from Travell and Simons [153])

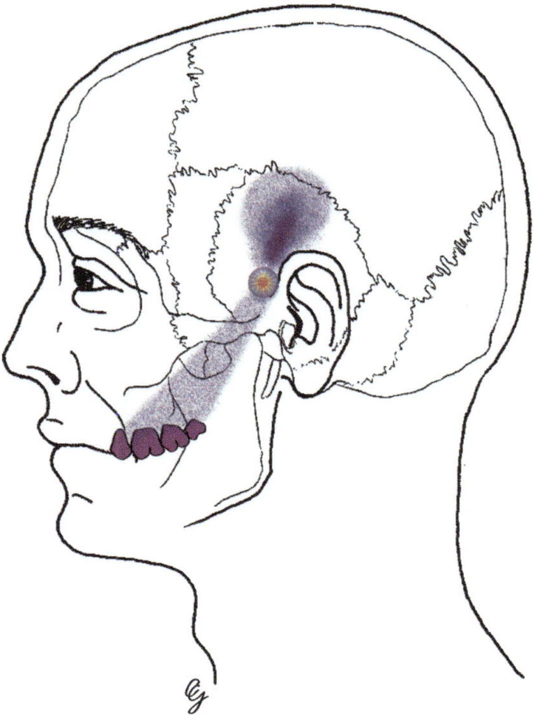

Fig. 9 Referred pain from the musculus temporalis, zone 3 (Modified from Travell and Simons [153])

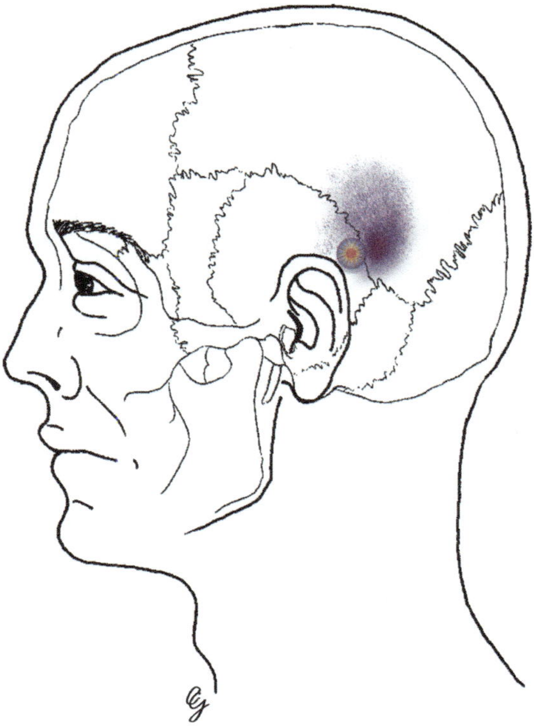

Fig. 10 Referred pain from the musculus temporalis, zone 4 (Modified from Travell and Simons [153])

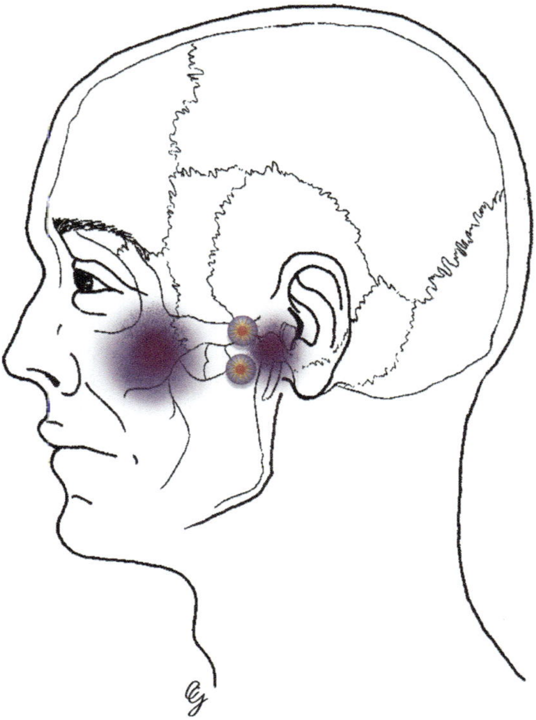

Fig. 11 Referred pain from the musculus pterygoideus lateralis (Modified from Travell and Simons [153])

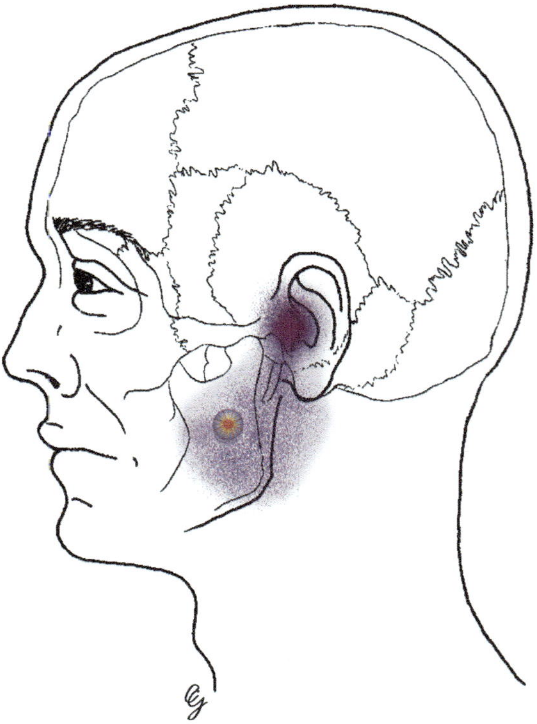

Fig. 12 Referred pain from the musculus pterygoideus medialis (Modified from Travell and Simons [153])

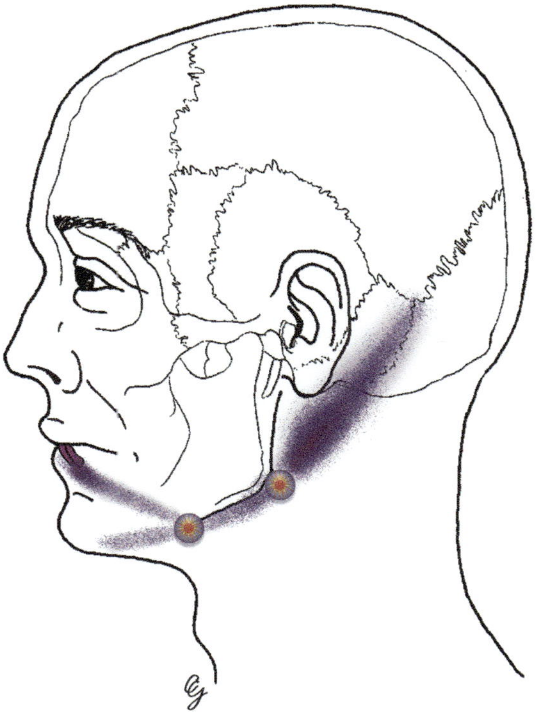

Fig. 13 Referred pain from the musculus digastricus (Modified from Travell and Simons [153])

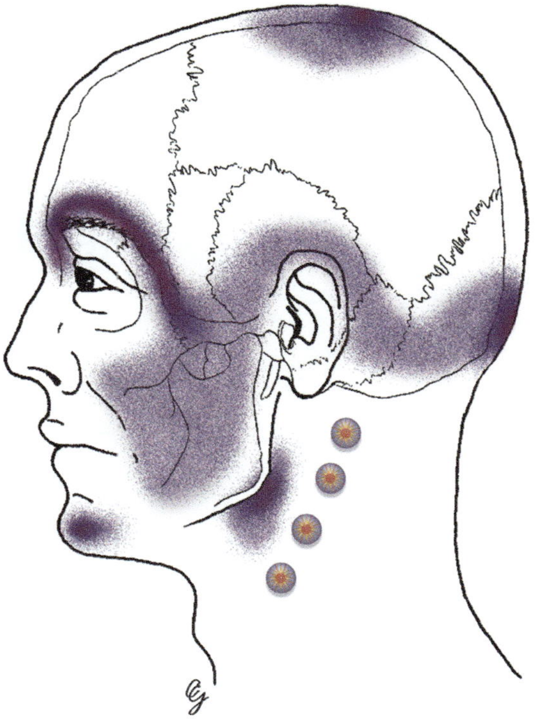

Fig. 14 Referred pain from the musculus sternocleidomastoideus, sternal belly (also involved in clenching [172]) (Modified from Travell and Simons [153])

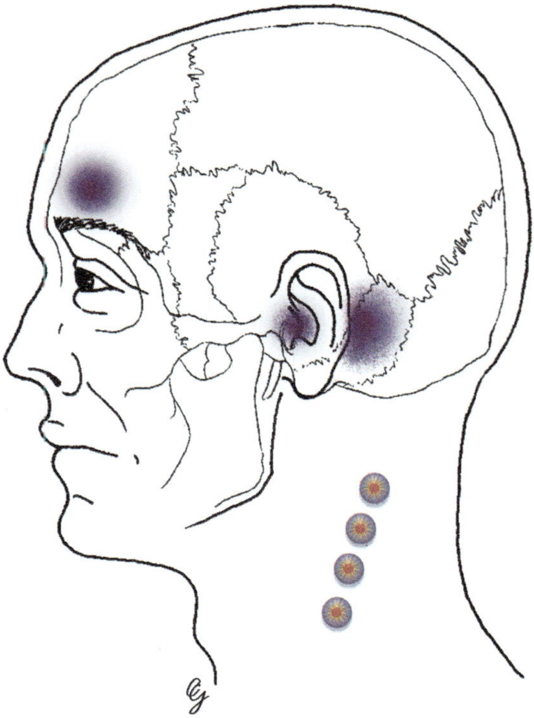

Fig. 15 Referred pain from the musculus sternocleidomastoideus, clavicular belly (also involved in clenching [172]) (Modified from Travell and Simons [153])

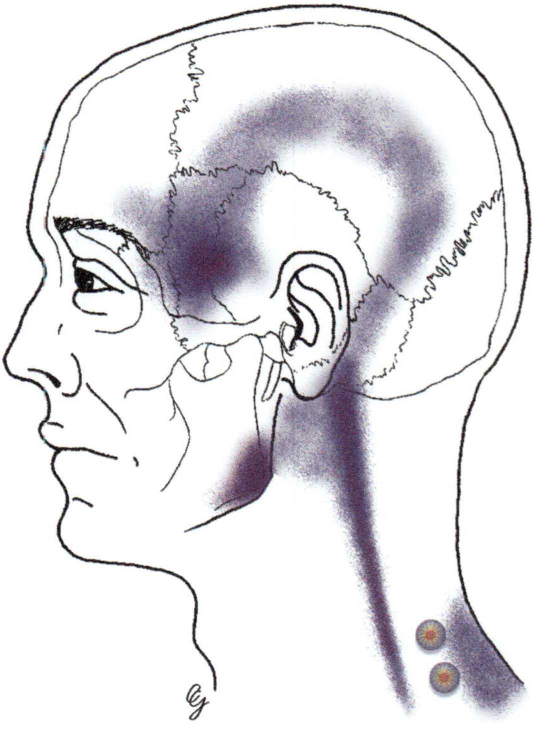

Fig. 16 Referred pain from the musculus trapezius (Modified from Travell and Simons [153])

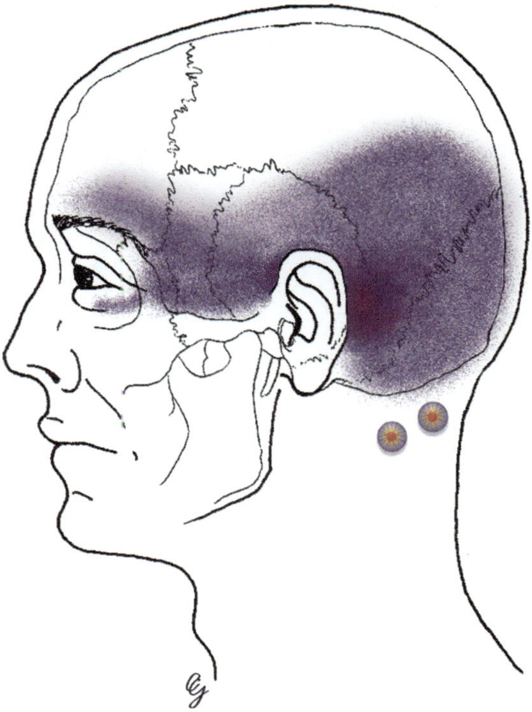

Fig. 17 Referred pain from the musculi suboccipitales: m. rectus capitis posterior major, m. rectus capitis posterior minor, m. obliquus capitis inferior, and m. obliquus capitis superior (involved in grinding) (Modified from Travell and Simons [153])

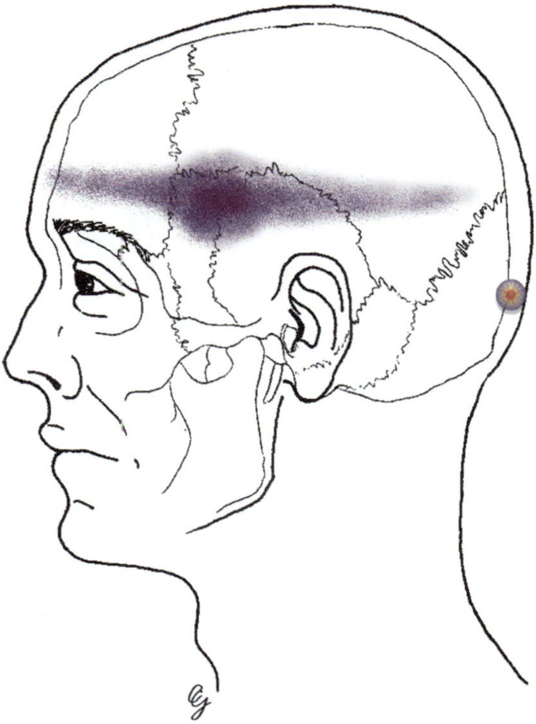

Fig. 18 Referred pain from the musculus semispinalis capitis (Modified from Travell and Simons [153])

Fig. 19 Referred pain from the musculus semispinalis cervicis (Modified from Travell and Simons [153])

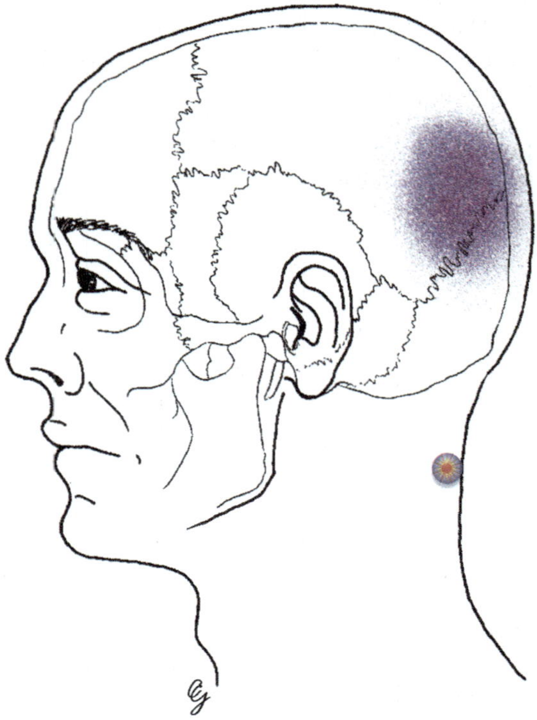

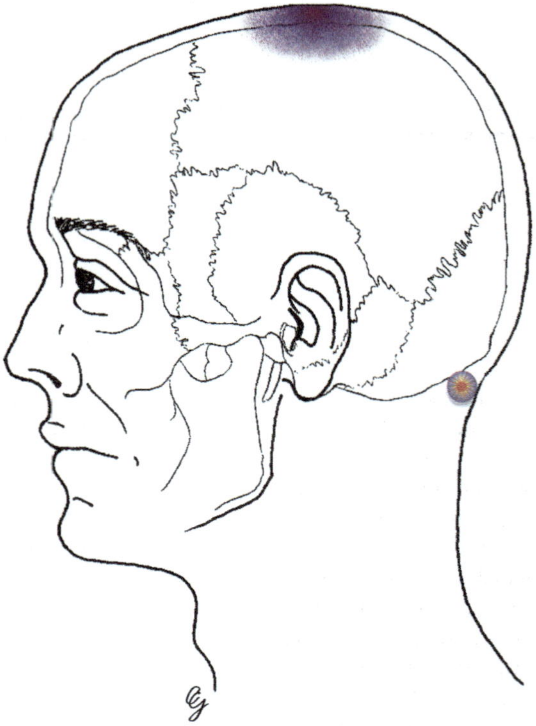

Fig. 20 Referred pain from the musculus splenius capitis (Modified from Travell and Simons [153])

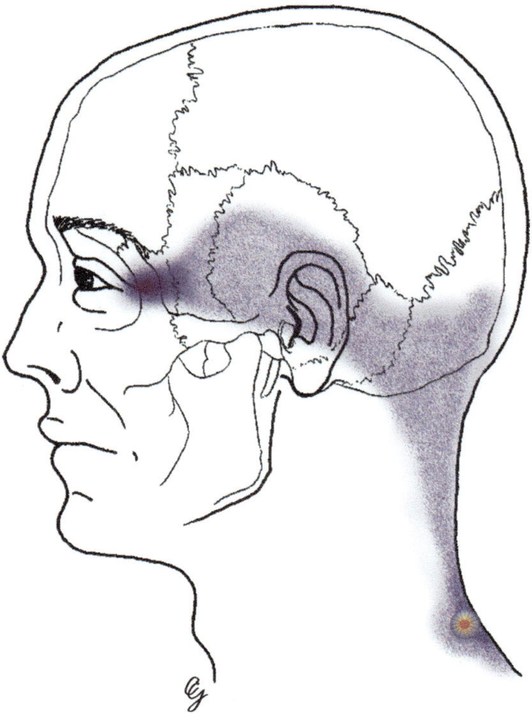

Fig. 21 Referred pain from the musculus splenius cervicis (Modified from Travell and Simons [153])

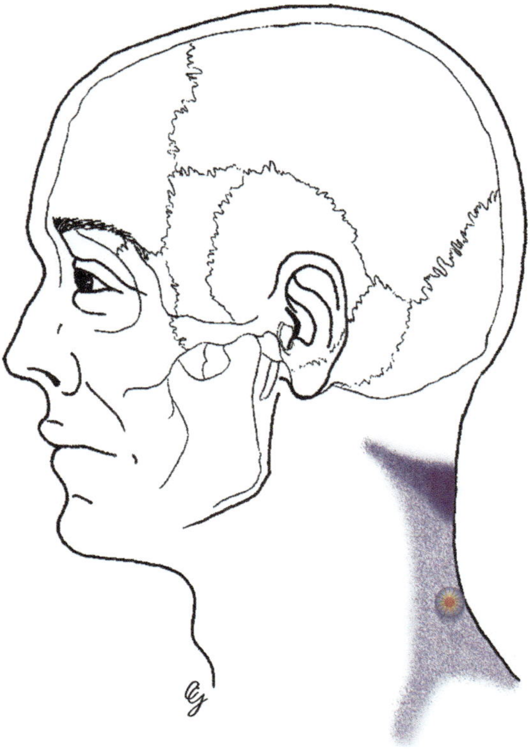

Fig. 22 Referred pain from the musculus multifidus (Modified from Travell and Simons [153])

Fig. 23 Referred pain from the musculus occipitofrontalis (anterior fibers) (Modified from Travell and Simons [153])

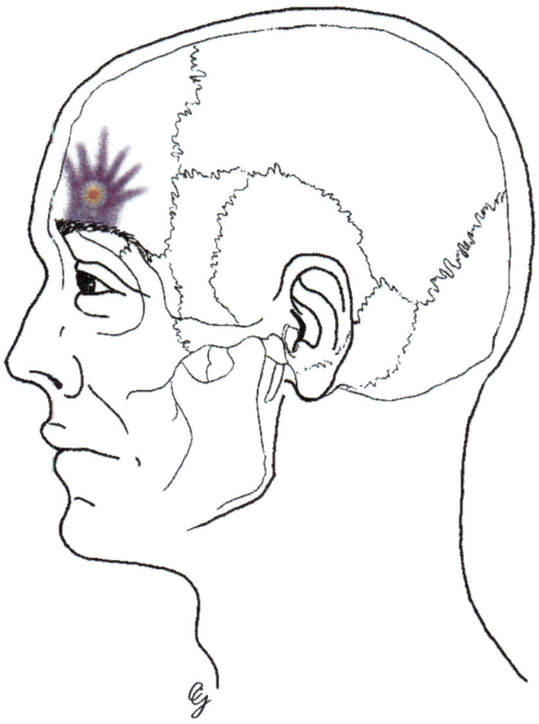

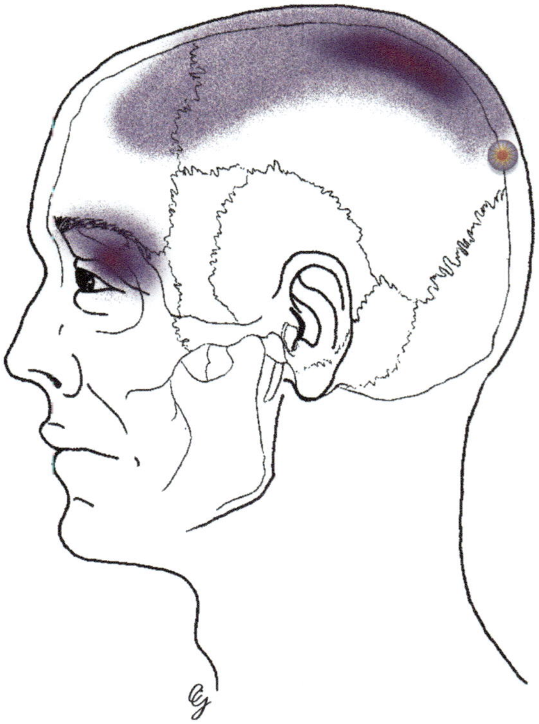

Fig. 24 Referred pain from the musculus occipitofrontalis (posterior fibers) (Modified from Travell and Simons [153])

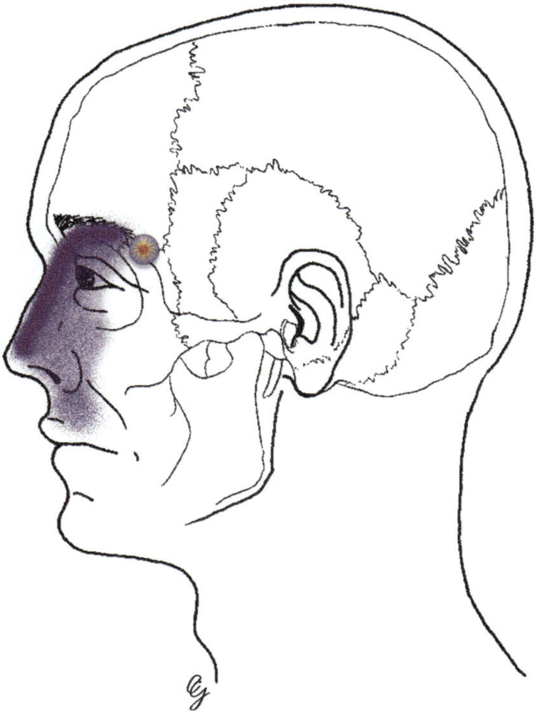

Fig. 25 Referred pain from the musculus orbicularis oculi (Modified from Travell and Simons [153])

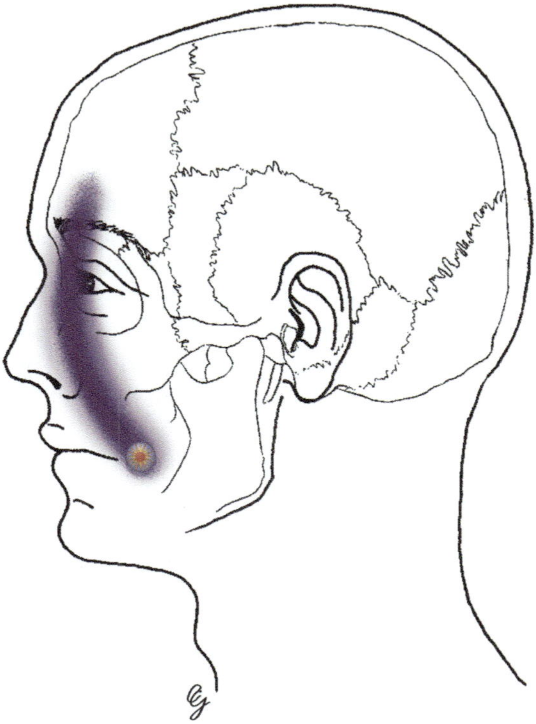

Fig. 26 Referred pain from the musculus zygomaticus major (Modified from Travell and Simons [153])

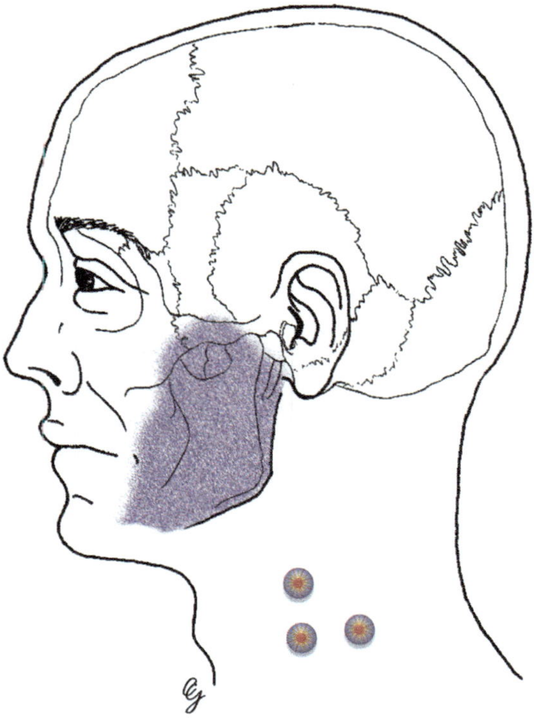

Fig. 27 Referred pain from the platysma muscle (Modified from Travell and Simons [153])

1.2 Nature and Aggravating or Relieving Factors

Most patients complain of severe, persistent, and invalidating pain that may reach a crisis level with some periods of remission. The descriptive terms used by the patient must be properly noted: pain may be sharp or a burning, or pulsing, or throbbing, or pounding feeling, etc. In fact, such pain is often uninterrupted and persistent with no typical aspect, no reproducible topography, and no known organic substratum.

The events which precede the onset of pain can be helpful in establishing an etiological diagnosis in that it may indicate initiating causes. The pain may have started after an episode of trauma (fall, blow to the jaw, road traffic accident, diving with a scuba etc.) [7, 64]. Sometimes it is triggered by certain forms of treatment (general anesthetic, fitting of dentures with the wrong occlusion, complex posterior dental extraction, etc.).

The time of pain during the day may be variable. It may be felt upon waking up, or after a meal, or at the end of the day, or after sustained physical or mental effort. Pain that begins or worsens in the evening could signal an etiology of joint disorders. Pain affecting the eyes, temporal area, ears, or shoulders is more likely to worsen in the morning [129]. However, several cases correspond to tension-type headaches. They are connected to stomatognathic, scalp, and nuchal muscular contractions and provoke chronic, persistent deep pain. Trigger points in these muscles may generate unilateral headaches which resemble *migraine* [51] (see Part IV).

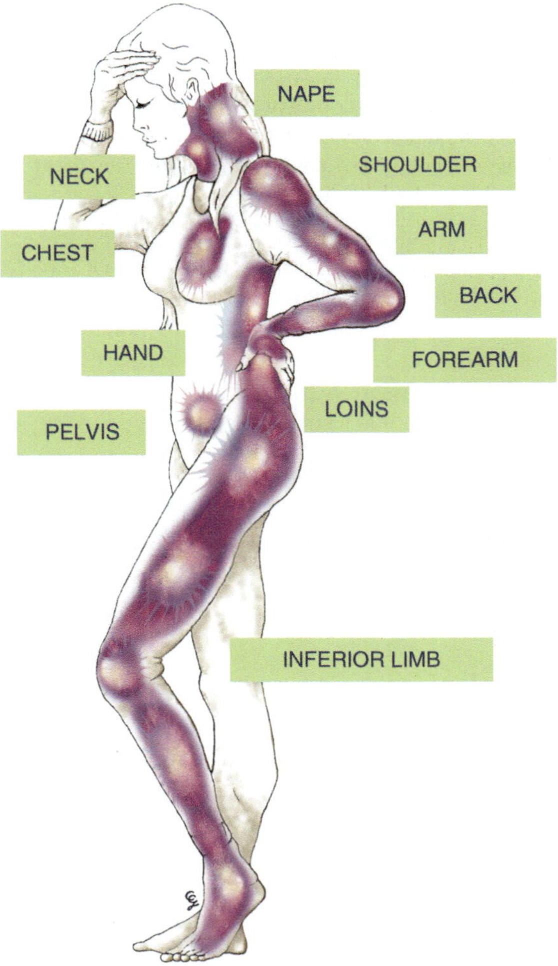

Fig. 28 Pain below the craniofacial area

Clinical reality reveals indurated fibrositic or myositic zones. A recent study has stressed the aggravating role of tobacco on pain intensity in TMD patients [110]. In some cases anxio-depressive factors are frequent trigger points. Such causes usually suggest psychalgia. In some cases the atypical clinical pain encourages the patient to express a feeling of muscular tension.

1.3 Resistance to Drugs

Such pain is generally partially resistant to common opiates, nonsteroidal anti-inflammatory drugs (NSAIDs), and neuroleptics. The sedative effects of myorelaxant drugs confirm the involvement of neuromuscular excitability in generating this type of pain (see Part III). Moreover, the oral parafunction definitely seems to be an aggravating factor in the resistance of severe pain to drug treatment [114]. In view of the neuromuscular hyperactivity involved in tension-type headaches, it seems inappropriate to underestimate psychological factors. Any functional pain could induce vascular reflexes [102]. Such association between spasms and vascular reflexes triggers most noninflammatory visceral pain. As they express functional disharmony, these reflexes often follow psychosomatic mechanisms and facilitate psychosomatic pain [131]. Yet CFP without obvious organic pathology should not be automatically diagnosed as psychalgia and treated with neuroleptics [4]. In cases of headaches, some simple clinical procedures (such as muscular palpation) may relieve neuromuscular disorders. A functional exploration (somesthetic evoked potentials and blink reflex) [124] can be helpful in confirming an opinion objectively and reassure a patient who was diagnosed too quickly as psychalgic by a puzzled practitioner [141, 173].

2 Discomforts

2.1 Auditory Problems

Tinnitus is "an auditory feeling which does not result from an external excitation of the ear." It is generally described as buzzing (low-pitched sounds), fluttering sounds, ringing sounds, and whistles (high-pitched sounds). The patient also complains about a feeling of filled ear(s), sometimes of reduced hearing, or itching in the external auditory meatus. Tinnitus has been suggested in cases of TMD for a long time [10, 17, 24, 43, 55, 60, 77, 126, 134]. Investigations revealed a high occurrence of ear symptoms in TMD patients [37, 92] or patients suffering from orofacial pain [45]. Frequent TMD signs and symptoms have also been observed in ORL populations [39, 137]. Tinnitus diagnoses in TMD patients are established under one essential condition: a negative ORL investigation. In such cases, patients can be referred to dental surgeons [165] for a diagnosis based on stomatognathic muscular palpation [92]. Painful palpation of the *medial pterygoid muscle* (MPMs) may confirm the stomatognathic origin of tinnitus [10].

2.2 Problems with Swallowing and Phonation

In their daily practice, some practitioners are faced with patients complaining of problems with phonation and/or swallowing: difficulties in pronouncing certain sounds, hoarse voice, irritating laryngeal coughing (without infection), feeling of persistent angina, sore throat [45], feeling of a hair stuck in the throat, feeling of a lump in the throat, feeling of anxiety in the back of the throat, feeling of tightness in the throat, and dysphagia. Sometimes these symptoms are accompanied by supra- and infrahyoid pain. An epidemiological correlation has been revealed in teachers between TMD and laryngeal and vocal dysfunctions [99]. Some patients undergo sophisticated ORL and gastroenterologic or neurologic examinations that show absolutely nothing. When they continue to complain, patients are referred to psychiatrists. When they encounter problems with phonation, dentists should also consider a differential diagnosis between unintentional prosthesis misfit and TMD. Medical history must also draw the practitioner's attention to certain particular sensitive troubles such as oral or tongue pricking or burning[3].

Nausea is a subjective feeling of sickness which reaches the cortical level[4]. It can be accompanied by inefficient gastric and parietal contractions [19].

Vomiting is a gastric protection reflex which can occur at different levels: bulbar, hypothalamic (supra-optical area), and cortical. In some cases, it follows nausea and can be accompanied by various vegetative symptoms: sweat, sickliness, salivation, diarrhea, hypotension, and tachycardia. In the TMD patients we observed, nausea and vomiting were events that forced them out of bed after they had clenched their teeth tightly, durably, and frequently in their sleep during the previous nights [72, 74].

2.3 *Problems with Posture and Vision*

Dizziness is characterized by various feelings described by patients as general instability, a feeling of sailing or spinning through the space around them. It is defined as a cerebral trouble, a sensation of error where the patient believes that he or she and his or her surroundings are stimulated by gyratory or oscillatory movements. The origin can be labyrinthic, vascular, cerebral, auditory, visual, toxemic, hysterical, tumorous, as well as neuromuscular [153]. Some patients may complain about dizziness, a feeling of ocular troubles, although ORL and ophthalmologic clinical investigations show nothing unusual. Some surveys have shown that dizziness is more frequent in TMD patients than in control subjects [74, 126]. Scientific research revealed the close link between the *trigeminal* and *oculocephalogyrus systems* (see Part II). A patient may complain about cervical problems. If an etiological diagnosis of some forms of dizziness proves difficult, the practitioner should also examine the articular and muscular structures of the stomatognathic system [16, 20, 33, 40, 46, 76, 81, 104, 145, 170].

When physical traumas such as *whiplash* occur, TMJ may be affected and cannot be ignored. Therefore, when post-traumatic complaints about recurrent dizziness

---

[3]In cases of tongue burning, the clinician should consider acoustic neuroma [50] and refer the patient to a specialist.

[4]The reflex trigger zones include the posterior dorso-lingual zones (innervated by the glossopharyngeal nerve = IX), the velopalatine regions (innervated by the maxillary nerve = V2), and the soft palate, the superior breathing ways, and posterior pharyngeal wall (innervated by the vagus nerve = X).

persist and all standard investigations show nothing unusual, secondary stomatognathic disorders [27, 75, 162] should definitely be considered. During the examination of the cervical posture, it is recommended to look for trigger points by palpating *sternocleidomastoid muscles* (SCM), particularly in the presence of chronic Meniere disease symptoms [15] or idiopathic dizziness [153]. Finally some ophthalmologic symptoms more rarely accompany retro-orbital referred pain. Like subjective phenomena, ophthalmic symptoms of asthenopia and latent anisocoria[5] may be present. Asthenopia (eye discomfort, eye ache) sometimes reveals strabismus (squint) that may have been latent since birth but only revealed by the development of TMD.

2.4 Fatigue and Sleeping Disorders

Fatigue is a kind of failure in the process that links action potential and activation of contraction. Patients often complain about persistent fatigue particularly when standing up. This kind of fatigue is sometimes accompanied by a feeling of painful tension in the stomatognathic muscles. It can even affect some muscles involved in head posture. Therefore, these clinical forms of self-diagnosed fatigue can be linked to TMD [44]. Proper investigations have revealed that sudden awakening may occur during the night when teeth are tightly clenched by spasmed stomatognathic muscles. The affected patients seem to be running a "*mandibular marathon*." The question of a possible link between TMD and some forms of chronic fatigue (CF) will be examined further (Part IV).

True insomnia and/or obstructive sleep apnea (OSA) are rather uncommon in TMD patients [35]. They usually complain of difficulties falling asleep, non-restorative sleep, restless sporadic sleep[6] (frequent movements, nightmares, etc.), and waking up too early. Sleep disorders and waking up tired are often related to professional stress [69], with frequent comorbidity of severe pain and psychological distress in TMD patients [171]. It is believed that nocturnal bruxism is a behavioral reaction to diurnal stress and that it evidences apprehension towards past, present, or future stressful situations [56]. Its repercussion on catecholamine has been evaluated in urinary rates [34]. A tightly correlated nocturnal grinding has been shown in children with parasomnia's signs (muscles cramps, bed-wetting, colic, drooling while sleeping, sleeptalking) [161]. Some female patients suffering from depression and mood disturbances complained about intense CFP and showed hyperactivity in the extensor muscles through inhibition of mouth-opening reflexes during REM phases [159]. Previous issues have connected concomitant nocturnal bruxism periods with several body movements [121, 155, 171]. These periods were preceded or

[5]Anisocoria is characterized by unequal pupil size. The inequality usually disappears with sympathicomimetic eye drops. The smaller pupil is generally on the affected side.

[6]The dopamine dysregulation is evoked in the restless legs syndrome (RLS). Now no any comorbidity has been yet searched with TMD, but fundamental data enlightened a strange correlation between occlusal disharmony and dopa disturbances in the rat [174].

followed by cardiovascular phenomena or tingling feelings in the superior limbs [167]. Nocturnal bruxism tends to perturb values that reflect cardiovascular autonomic functions [148]. A heart rate increase of 16.6 % in average has been observed during nocturnal bruxism episodes [120]. As a result most experts' investigations focused on nocturnal grinding though nocturnal clenching is a worse aggravating factor, even if logically more difficult to evaluate.

2.5 Psychological Mood Disorders

While some authors have reported cases of TMD among children [49], some symptoms may appear in teenagers, with [63, 94] or without [18] significant differences between genders. The incidence of chronic orofacial pain in *female patients* is frequently emphasized [71, 107, 108]. But the essential causes of this clinical fact are still subject to discussion [41]: (1) on the one hand, the cause may be psychosocial distress [119, 127, 149], and (2) on the other hand, central hypersensibility appears as a more accepted factor [140]. TMJ are known to be potential targets for female hormones (estrogen and progesterone) [1]. Otherwise, no differences based on race have been observed in TMD symptoms in young women [128]. A good number of studies [3, 97, 119, 130, 132, 139, 149] revealed that a typical psychological profile was often that of an *introverted*, *hyper-emotive*, and *perfectionist female*. Persistent symptoms despite treatment may bring on depressive tendencies, sometimes expressed as mood swings such as nervousness or aggressiveness [114, 122]. Objective clinical signs such as onychophagia may serve as an indicator of this type of profile. It is now more frequent to focus on evaluating the relation between a patient and his or her surroundings. Thus, the influence of *psycho-emotional* and *psychosocial factors* is more and more taken into account by experts [6, 11, 18, 29, 31, 57, 84, 88, 93, 96, 105, 117, 118, 136, 143, 144, 147, 150, 156, 160, 166, 168, 169].

Finally young adults may sometimes be affected by *anterograde amnesia.*

2.6 Prolonged Unexplained Fever

Prolonged unexplained fever (PUF) is described as fever that lasts for 2–3 weeks without a known cause [47]. Among non-pathological hyperthermia subjects, the presence of PUF has been noted in *parafunctional gumchewers* [23, 68, 78, 87]. For many years a number of TMD patients have shown signs of thermoregulation troubles. Most elaborate clinical and paraclinical investigations have failed to yield an explanation for PUF. This general problem was managed by trigeminal relaxing and moderating treatment (RMT) such as described in Part III, without having recourse to antipyretic drugs. The RMT must take account of the patient's behavior information in order to identify his or her *deleterious parafunctional oral habits*.

2.7 *Immunodeficiency Disorders*

In some patients, a weakened immune system [52, 153] has been associated with various conditions of stress, which justifies a better assessment of general factors [152]; indeed, the possible existence of general factors should be considered, including viral illnesses (common cold, herpes, etc.) in both the development of TMD and in cases of relapse or worsening of symptoms [153]. With reference to general factors, it is important to keep in mind the role of environmental stressors that may be involved in initiating or intensifying an overexcitable state. One typical example of such factors is noise.

2.8 *Autonomic Problems*

Some autonomic problems such as salivation disorders (too much, too little) or eye watering are local. But symptoms may be quite distant from the oral sphere. A study revealed that TMD patients had a much higher rate of *cardiac*, *respiratory*, *digestive*, and *neurological symptoms* than patients in the control group [145]. Therefore, TMD patients showed greater sensibility to noxious stimuli [103] with increased cardiovascular response to pain sensitivity [113]. Another study pointed out the relation between TMD and respiratory problems in asthmatic children [30]. Other cases observed include patients suffering from a burning sensation in the stomach, shortness of breath, urination disorder, irregular menstrual cycle, pain in the ovarian region, occasional or chronic constipation, persistent diarrhea, gastrointestinal disorders with no evidence of organic disease [45], etc. Patients may also suffer from neurovascular symptoms such as a feeling of cold hands particularly during sleep-related bruxism [167].

2.9 *Problems with Nutrition*

In some cases patients will admit to being preoccupied with their weight. Eating disorders such as *bulimia* or *lack of appetite* are not uncommon [61]. Although projections of dental inputs to the hypothalamus were poorly understood until 1965, the involvement of oropharyngeal afferents in hypothalamic hyperphagia has now been established [109].

References

1. Abubaker AO, Wassim FR, Raslan WF, Sotereanos GC (1993) Estrogen and progesterone receptors in temporomandibular joint discs of symptomatic and asymptomatic persons: a preliminary study. J Oral Maxillofac Surg 51(10):1095–1100

2. Agerberg G, Bergenholtz A (1989) Craniomandibular disorders in adult population of Bothnia, Sweden. Acta Odontol Scand 47:129–140
3. Agerberg G, Inkapööl L (1990) Craniomandibular disorders in an urban Swedish population. J Craniomandib Disord Facial Oral Pain 4:154–164
4. Ahles TA, Yunus MB, Gaulier B et al (1986) The use of contemporary MMPI norms in the study of chronic pain patients. Pain 24:159–163
5. Ahlin JH, Ramos-Gomez FJ (1982) Treatment of temporomandibular joint related headaches in the pedodontic patient: a preliminary report. J Pedod 6:164–175
6. Akhter R, Hassan NM, Aida J et al (2007) Association between experience of stressful life events and muscle-related temporomandibular disorders in patients seeking free treatment in a dental hospital. Eur J Med Res 12(11):535–540
7. Aldridge RD, Fenlon MR (2004) Prevalence of temporomandibular dysfunction in a group of scuba divers. Br J Sports Med 38:69–73
8. Andrade AV, Gomes PF, Teixeira-Salmela LF (2007) Cervical spine alignment and hyoid bone positioning with temporomandibular disorders. J Oral Rehabil 34(10):767–772
9. Ardic F, Gokharman D, Atsu S et al (2006) The comprehensive evaluation of temporomandibular disorders seen in rheumatoid arthritis. Aust Dent J 51(1):23–28
10. Arlen H (1977) The otomandibular syndrome: diagnosis. Ear Nose Throat J 57(12): 553–556
11. Auerbach SM, Laskin DM, Frantsve LM, Orr T (2001) Depression, pain, exposure to stressful life events, and long-term outcomes in temporomandibular disorder patients. J Oral Maxillofac Surg 59(6):628–633
12. Bell WH (1989) Orofacial pains: classification, diagnosis, management, 3rd edn. Year Book Medical Pub Inc (ed), Chicago, p 420
13. Bernhardt O, Gesch D, Schwahn C et al (2005) Risk factors for headache, including TMD signs and symptoms, and their impact on quality of life. Results of the Study of Health in Pomerania (SHIP). Quintessence Int 36(1):55–64
14. Bevilaqua-Grossi D, Lipton RB, Bigal ME (2009) Temporomandibular disorders and migraine chronification. Curr Pain Headache Rep 13(4):314–318
15. Bjorne A, Agerberg G (1996) Craniomandibular disorders in patients with Meniere's disease: a controlled study. J Orofac Pain 10(1):28–37
16. Bjorne A, Berven A, Agerberg G (1998) Cervical signs and symptoms in patients with Meniere's disease: a controlled study. Cranio 16(3):194–202
17. Block SL (1976) Possible etiology of ear stuffiness (barohypoacousis) in MPD syndrome TMJ and facial pain. J Dent Res Abstract 55, 752:B250
18. Bonjardim LR, Gaviao MB, Pereira LJ, Castelo PM (2005) Anxiety and depression in adolescents and their relationship with signs and symptoms of temporomandibular disorders. Int J Prosthodont 18(4):347–352
19. Bossy J (1990) Anatomie clinique: neuro-anatomie. Springer Verlag (éd), Paris
20. Boyd CH (1987) The effect of head position on EMG evaluations of representative mandibular positioning muscle groups. Cranio 5:51–53
21. Braun B, Shifman EL (1991) The validity and predictive value of four assessment instruments for evaluation of the cervical and stomatognathic systems. J Craniomandib Disord Oral Facial Pain 5:239–244
22. Brechner VL (1982) Myofascial pain syndrome of the lateral pterygoid muscle. Cranio 1(1):42–45
23. Brobeck JR (1960) Food and temperature. Rec Prog Horm Res 16:439–466
24. Brooks GB, Maw AR, Coleman J (1981) "Costen's syndrome" – correlation or coincidence: a review of 45 patients with TMJ dysfunction, otalgia and oral symptomes. Clin Otolaryngol 88:361–367
25. Budtz-Jorgensen E, Luan W, Holm-Pedersen P, Fejerskov O (1985) Mandibular dysfunction related to dental, occlusal and prosthetic conditions in a selected elderly population. Gerodontics 1:28–33
26. Burgess J (1991) Symptom characteristics in TMD patients reporting blunt trauma and/or whiplash injury. J Craniomandib Disord Facial Oral Pain 5:251–257

27. Carroll LJ, Ferrari R, Cassidy JD (2007) Reduced or painful jaw movement after collision-related injuries. A population-based study. J Am Dent Assoc 138(1):86–93
28. Catanzariti J-F, Debuse T, Duquesnoy B (2005) Cervicalgies chroniques et dysfonctionnement de l'appareil manducateur. Rev Rhum 72(12):1283–1287
29. Celic R, Panduric J, Dulcic N (2006) Psychologic status in patients with temporomandibular disorders. Int J Prosthodont 19(1):28–29
30. Chaves TC, Grossi DB, de Oliveira AS et al (2005) Correlation between signs of temporomandibular (TMD) and cervical spine (CSD) disorders in asthmatic children. J Clin Pediatr Dent 29(4):287–292
31. Chun D, Koskinen M, Moffett L (1990) Distress, jaw habits, and connective tissue laxity as predisposing factors to TMJ send in adolescent. J Craniomandib Disord Facial Oral Pain 4:165–167
32. Ciancaglini R, Radaelli G (2001) The relationship between headache and symptoms of temporomandibular disorder in the general population. J Dent 29(2):93–98
33. Clark RKF, Wyke BD (1974) Contributions of the temporomandibular articular mechanoreceptors to the control of mandibular posture: an experimental study. J Dent Res 2:121–129
34. Clark GT, Rugh JD, Handelman SL (1980) Nocturnal masseter muscle activity and urinary catecholamine levels in bruxers. J Dent Res 59:157–176
35. Collesano V, Segu M, Masseroli C, Manni R (2004) Temporomandibular disorders and sleep disorders: which relationship? Minerva Stomatol 53(11–12):661–668
36. Cook NR, Evans DA, Funkenstein HH et al (1989) Correlates of headache in a population-based cohort of elderly. Arch Neurol 46:1338–1344
37. Cooper BC, Cooper DL (1993) Recognizing otolaryngologic symptoms in patients with temporomandibular disorders. Cranio 11(4):260–267
38. Cooper BC, Kleinberg I (2009) Relationship of temporomandibular disorders to muscle tension-type headaches and a neuromuscular orthosis approach to treatment. Cranio 27(2):101–108
39. Cox KW (2008) Temporomandibular disorder and new aural symptoms. Arch Otolaryngol Head Neck Surg 134(4):389–393
40. Da Cunha MH, Da Silva A (1986) Le syndrome de déficience posturale. Son intérêt en ophtalmologie. J Franç Ophtalmol 9(II):747–755
41. Dao TT, LeResche L (2000) Gender differences in pain. J Orofac Pain 14:169–184
42. D'Attilio M, Epifania E, Ciuffolo F et al (2004) Cervical lordosis angle measured on lateral cephalograms; findings in skeletal class II female subjects with and without TMD: a cross sectional study. Cranio 22(1):27–44
43. De Felicio CM, De Oliveira Melchior M, Pimenta Ferreira CL et al (2008) Otologic symptoms of temporomandibular disorder and effect of orofacial myofunctional therapy. Cranio 26(2):118–124
44. De Leeuw R, Bertoli E, Schmidt JE, Carlson CR (2005) Prevalence of post-traumatic stress disorder symptoms in orofacial pain patients. Oral Surg Oral Med Oral Pathol Oral Radiol Endod 99(5):558–568
45. De Leeuw R, Klasser GD, Albuquerque RJC (2005) Are female patients with orofacial pain medically compromised? J Am Dent Assoc 136(4):459–468
46. De Wijer A, Lobbezoo-Scholte AM, Steenks MH, Bosman F (1995) Reliability of clinical findings in temporomandibular disorders. J Orofac Pain 9:181–191.
47. Dinarello CA, Wolff SM (1978) Pathogenesis of fever in man. N Engl J Med 298(11):607–612
48. Dworkin SF, Leresche L (1992) Research diagnostic criteria for temporomandibular disorders: review, criteria, examinations and specifications, critique. J Craniomandib Disord Facial Oral Pain 6:301–355
49. Egermark-Eriksson I, Carlsson GE, Magnusson T (1987) A long-term epidemiologic study of the relationship between occlusal factors and mandibular dysfunction in children and adolescents. J Dent Res 66(1):67–71

50. Ferguson JW, Burton JF (1990) Clinical presentation of acoustic nerve neuroma in the oral and maxillofacial region. Oral Surg Oral Med Oral Pathol 69:672–675
51. Fernandez-de-Las-Penas C, Cuadrado ML, Pareja JA (2006) Myofascial trigger points, neck mobility and forward head posture in unilateral migraine. Cephalalgia 26(9):1061–1070
52. Fonder AC (1988) The dental distress syndrome (quantified). Quant Med 1:1
53. Forssell H, Kangasniemi P (1984) Correlation of the frequency and intensity of headache to mandibular dysfunction in headache patients. Proc Finn Dent Soc 80:223–226
54. Forssell H, Kangasniemi P (1984) Mandibular dysfunction in patients with muscle contraction headache. Proc Finn Dent Soc 80:211–216
55. Franklin DJ, Smith RJ, Catlin FI, Helfrick JF (1986) Temporomandibular joint dysfunction in infancy. Int J Pediatr Otorhinolaryngol 12(1):99–104
56. Funch DP, Gale EN (1980) Factors associated with nocturnal bruxism and its treatment. J Behav Med 3:385–397
57. Gatchel RJ, Stowell AW, Buschang P (2006) The relationships among depression, pain, and masticatory functioning in temporomandibular disorder patients. J Orofac Pain 20(4):288–296
58. Gelb H (1985) Clinical management of head, neck and TMJ pain and dysfunction: a multi-disciplinary approach to diagnosis and treatment. WB Saunders Co (ed), Philadelphia/London/Toronto
59. Gelb H (1994) New concepts in craniomandibular and chronic pain management. Mosby Wolfe (ed), London
60. Gelb H, Gelb ML, Wagner ML (1997) The relationship of tinnitus to craniocervical mandibular disorders. J Cranio 15(2):136–143
61. Girod C (1987) Aspects endocriniens de l'obésité. Rev Franç Endocrinol Clin 28:9–15
62. Glaros AG, Owais Z, Lausten L (2007) Reduction in parafunctional activity: a potential mechanism for the effectiveness of splint therapy. J Oral Rehabil 34(2):97–104
63. Godoy F, Rosenblatt A, Godoy-Bezerra J (2007) Temporomandibular disorders and associated factors in Brazilian teenagers: a cross-sectional study. Int J Prosthodont 20(6):599–605
64. Goldberg MB (1999) Posttraumatic temporomandibular disorders. J Orofac Pain 13(4):291–294
65. Gole DR (1993) A clinical observation: a relationship of occlusal contacts to distal musculature. Cranio 11(1):55–61
66. Gonçalves DA, Bigal ME, Jales LC et al (2010) Headache and symptoms of temporomandibular disorder: an epidemiological study. Headache 50(2):231–241
67. Graff-Radford SB (2007) Temporomandibular disorders and headache. Dent Clin North Am 51(1):129–144
68. Grossman SP (1968) Hypothalamic and limbic influences on food intake. Fed Proc 27:1349–1360
69. Hagberg C, Hagberg M, Kopp S (1994) Musculoskeletal symptoms and psychosocial factors among patients with craniomandibular disorders. Acta Odontol Scand 52:170–177
70. Hall E, Terezhalmy GT, Pelleu GB, Bethesda PD (1986) A set of descriptors for the diagnosis of dental pain syndrome. Oral Surg Oral Med Oral Pathol 61:153–157
71. Halpern LR, Levine M, Dodson TB (2007) Sexual dimorphism and temporomandibular disorders (TMD). Oral Maxillofac Surg Clin North Am 19(2):267–277
72. Hartmann F (1992) Cranio-mandibular disorders inducing nausea and vomiting. In: Bianchi AL, Grélot AD, Miller GI, King GI (eds) Mechanisms and control of emesis. Colloque INSERM/John Libbey Eurotext Ltd C, Paris/Montrouge, pp 51–58
73. Hartmann F, Cucchi G (1987) Muscle ptérygoïdien et SADAM: diagnostic précoce et traitement. Rev Odont Stomatol 16(3):209–218
74. Hartmann F, Cucchi G (1993) Les dysfonctions cranio-mandibulaires (SADAM). Nouvelles perspectives médicales. Springer-Verlag (éd), Paris, 176p
75. Hartmann F, Sauget Y, Orofino J (1990) Incidences des chocs sur la posture et le mouvement de l'articulation temporo-maxillaire. Arch Inter Physiol Bioch 98(4):C16–C17

76. Huggare JA, Rausta AM (1992) Head posture and cervicovertebral and craniofacial morphology in patients with craniomandibular dysfunction. Cranio 10(3):173–177
77. Ioannides CA, Hoogland GA (1983) The disco-malleolar ligament: a possible cause of subjective hearing loss in patients with temporomandibular joint dysfunction. J Maxillofac Surg 2:227–231
78. Isaac N, Kernbaum S (1981) Prolonged fevers of unknown origin. Nouv Press Med 7(10):3311–3317
79. Isberg AM, Isacsson G, Williams WN, Loughner BA (1987) Lingual numbness and speech articulation deviation associated with temporomandibular joint disk displacement. Oral Surg Oral Med Oral Pathol 64:9–14
80. Jensen R, Rasmussen BK, Pedersen B et al (1993) Prevalence of oromandibular dysfunction in a general population. J Orofac Pain 7(2):175–182
81. Jensen R, Olesen J (1996) Initiating mechanisms of experimentally induced tension-type headache. Cephal 16(3):175–182
82. John MT, Miglioretti DL, LeResche L et al (2003) Widespread pain as a risk factor for dysfunctional temporomandibular disorder pain. Pain 102(3):257–263
83. Juniper RP (1984) Temporomandibular joint dysfunction: a theory based upon electromyographic studies of the lateral pterygoid muscle. Br J Oral Maxillofac Surg 22:1–8
84. Kafas P, Leeson R (2006) Assessment of pain in temporomandibular disorders: the bio-psychosocial complexity. Int J Oral Maxillofac Surg 35(2):145–149
85. Kampe T, Tagdae T, Tagdae G et al (1997) Reported symptoms and clinical findings in a group of subjects with long-standing bruxism. J Oral Rehabil 15:314–325
86. Kashima K, Rahman OI, Sakoda S, Shiba R (1999) Increased pain sensitivity of the upper extremities of TMD patients with myalgia to experimentally-evoked noxious stimulation: possibility of worsened endogenous opioid systems. Cranio 17(4):241–246
87. Kernbaum S (1990) Eléments de pathologie infectieuse 5ème éd. Simep/Specia
88. Kight M, Gatchel RJ, Wesley L (1999) Temporomandibular disorders: evidence for significant overlap with psychopathology. Health Psychol 18(2):177–182
89. Kleier DJ (1985) Referred pain from a myofascial trigger point mimicking pain of endodontic origin. J Endod 11(9):408–411
90. Knutsson K, Hassrelgren G, Nilner M, Petersson A (1989) Craniomandibular disorders in chronic orofacial pain patients. J Craniomandib Disord Facial Oral Pain 3(1):15–19
91. Koh ET, Yap AU, Koh CK et al (1999) Temporomandibular disorders in rheumatoid arthritis. J Rheumatol 26(9):1918–1922
92. Kuttila S, Kuttila M, Le Bell Y et al (1999) Aural symptoms and signs of temporomandibular disorder in association with treatment need and visits to a physician. Laryngo 109(10):1669–1673
93. Lautenbacher S, Spernal J, Schreiber W, Krieg JC (1999) Relationship between clinical pain complaints and pain sensitivity in patients with depression and panic disorders. Psychosom Med 61:822–827
94. LeResche L, Mancl LA, Drangsholt MT et al (2005) Relationship of pain and symptoms to pubertal development in adolescents. Pain 118(1–2):201–209
95. Liljestrom MR, Le Bell Y, Anttila P et al (2005) Headache children with temporomandibular disorders have several types of pain and other symptoms. Cephalalgia 25(11):1054–1060
96. Lindroth JE, Schmidt JE, Carlson CR (2002) A comparison between masticatory muscle pain patients and intracapsular pain patients on behavioral and psychosocial domains. J Orofac Pain 16(4):277–283
97. Lobbezoo-Scholte AM, De Leeuw JRJ, Steenks MH, Bosman F, Buchner R, Olthoff LW (1995) Diagnostic subgroups of craniomandibular disorders. J Orofac Pain 9(1):24–43
98. Lupoli TA, Lockey RF (2007) Temporomandibular dysfunction: an often overlooked cause of chronic headaches. Ann Allergy Asthma Immunol 99(4):314–318
99. Machado IM, Bianchini EMG, de Andrada E, Silva MA, Ferreira LP (2009) Voice and temporomandibular joint disorders in teachers. CEFAC Rev 11(4):630–643

100. Maeda S, Miyawaki T, Kuboki T, Shimada M (2000) A trigeminal neuralgia-like paroxysmal pain condition presumably due to buccal nerve compression in the temporalis muscle. Cranio 19(1):56–60
101. Magnusson T, Carlsson GE (1983) A 2 1/2 year follow up of changes in headache and mandibular dysfunction after stomatognathic treatment. J Prosthet Dent 49:398–402
102. Maixner W (1989) Autonomic and somatosensory interactions: physiological and pathophysiological implications. Proc Finn Dent Soc 85(4):395–407
103. Maixner W, Fillingim R, Kincaid S et al (1997) Relationship between pain sensitivity and resting arterial blood pressure in patients with painful temporomandibular disorders. Psychosom Med 59(5):503–511
104. Makofsky H, August B, Bellis J (1989) A multidisciplinary approach to the evaluation and treatment of temporomandibular joint and cervical spine dysfunction. Cranio 7(3):205–213
105. Manfredini D, Cantini E, Romagnoli M, Bosco M (2003) Prevalence of bruxism in patients with different research diagnostic criteria for temporomandibular disorders (RDC/TMD) diagnoses. Cranio 21(4):279–285
106. Marbach JJ, Varoscak JR, Cloidt JC (1986) The diagnosis and treatment of three chronic facial pain disorders: deafferentation neuralgia, degenerative joint disease of the temporomandibular joint, and myofascial syndrome. J Mass Dent Soc 35(4):169–202
107. Marklund S, Wänman A (2008) Incidence and prevalence of myofascial pain in the jaw-face region. A one-year prospective study on dental students. Acta Odontol Scand 66(2):113–121
108. Martins-Junior RL, Palma AJ, Marquardt EJ et al (2010) Temporomandibular disorders: a report of 124 patients. J Contemp Dent Pract 11(5):71–78
109. Mc Ginty D, Epstein AN, Teitelbaum P (1965) The contribution of oropharyngeal sensations to hypothalamic hyperphagia. Anim Behav 13:413–418
110. Melis M, Lobo SL, Ceneviz C et al (2010) Effect of cigarette smoking on pain intensity of TMD patients: a pilot study. Cranio 28(3):187–192
111. Mense SS (1993) Nociception from skeletal muscle in relation to clinical muscle pain. Pain 54:241–289
112. Mitrirattanakul S, Merrill RL (2006) Headache impact in patients with orofacial pain. J Am Dent Assoc 137(9):1267–1274
113. Mohn C, Vassend O, Knardahl S (2008) Experimental pain sensitivity in women with temporomandibular disorders and pain-free controls: the relationship to orofacial muscular contraction and cardiovascular responses. Clin J Pain 24(4):343–352
114. Molina OF, Dos Santos J, Nelson SJ, Nowlin T (2000) Profile of TMD and bruxer compared to TMD and nonbruxer patients regarding chief complaint, previous consultations, modes of therapy, and chronicity. Cranio 18(3):205–218
115. Morgan DH, Hall WP, Vanwas SJ (1977) Diseases of the temporo-mandibular apparatus. A multidisciplinary approach. CV Mosby Co (ed), St Louis, 481p
116. Nassif NJ, Talic YF (2001) Classic symptoms in temporomandibular disorder patients: a comparative study. Cranio 19(1):33–41
117. Nicholson RA, Lakatos CA, Gramling SE (1999) EMG reactivity and oral habits among facial pain patients in a scheduled-waiting competitive task. Appl Psychophysiol Biofeedback 24(4):235–247
118. Niemi PM, Le Bell Y, Kylmala M et al (2006) Psychological factors and responses to artificial interferences in subjects with and without a history of temporomandibular disorders. Acta Odontol Scand 64(5):300–305
119. Nifosi F, Violato E, Pavan C et al (2007) Psychopathology and clinical features in an Italian sample of patients with myofascial and temporomandibular joint pain: preliminary data. Int J Psychiatry Med 37(3):283–300
120. Okeson JP (1995) Bell's orofacial pain, 5th edn. Quintes (ed), Chicago
121. Okesson SJP, Philips BA, Berry DTR et al (1991) Nocturnal bruxing events in subjects with sleep-disordered breathing and control subjects. J Craniomandib Disord Facial Oral Pain 5:258–264

122. Ottersen OP (2004) Afferent connections to the amygdaloid complex of the rat with some observations in the cat. III. Afferents from the lower brain stem. J Comp Neurol 202(3):335–356
123. Palesy PD (1997) Tendon and ligament insertions – a possible source of musculoskeletal pain. Cranio 15(3):194–202
124. Papy JJ, Hartmann F, Rey M, Cucchi G (1989) Temporal muscle EMG and somatosensory investigation of trigeminal pathways. In: EMG of jaw reflexes in man. Leuven Univ Press, Leuven, p 409
125. Park W, Nam W, Park HS, Kim HJ (2008) Intraosseous lesion in mandibular condyle mimicking temporomandibular disorders: report of 3 cases. J Orofac Pain 22(1):65–70
126. Parker MW, Chole JK (1995) Tinnitus, vertigo and temporomandibular disorders. Am J Orthod Dentofacial Orthop 107(2):153–158
127. Phillips JM, Gatchel RJ, Wesley AL, Ellis E 3rd (2001) Clinical implications of sex in acute temporomandibular disorders. J Am Dent Assoc 132(1):49–57
128. Plesh O, Sinisi SE, Crawford PB, Gansky SA (2005) Diagnoses based on the research diagnostic criteria for temporomandibular disorders in a biracial population of young women. J Orofac Pain 19(1):65–75
129. Poignonec S, Klamas G, Goudot P, Soudant J (1991) Articulation temporo-mandibulaire: anatomie, physiologie, rappel clinique. Sem Hôp Paris 67(22):1019–1027
130. Pullinger AG, Seligman DA (1987) TMJ osteoarthrosis: a differentiation of diagnostic sub groups by symptom historic and demographics. J Craniomandib Disord Facial Oral Pain 1:251–256
131. Quarti C, Renaud J (1972) Neuropsychologie de la douleur. Hermann (éd), Paris, 199p
132. Quemar JC, Lazar BD (1992) Multivariate analysis of craniomandibular disorders. Cranio 10(2):89–95
133. Rauhala K, Oikarinen KS, Raustia AM (1999) Role of temporomandibular disorders (TMD) on facial pain? Occlusion, muscle and TMJ pain. Cranio 17:254–261
134. Ren YF, Isberg A (1995) Tinnitus in patients with temporomandibular joint internal derangement. Cranio 13(2):75–80
135. Rigolet D (1976) Signes et diagnostic des troubles de l'occlusion. Act Odont Stomatol 114:253–273
136. Rollman GB, Gillespie JM (2000) The role of psychosocial factors in temporomandibular disorders. Curr Rev Pain 4(1):71–81
137. Rubinstein B, Axelsson A, Carlsson GE (1990) Prevalence of signs and symptoms of craniomandibular disorders in tinnitus patients. J Craniomandib Disord Facial Oral Pain 4:186–192
138. Rusiecki RS (1998) Chest pain as result of temporomandibular disorder (TMD). Gen Dent 46(4):352–355
139. Salonen L, Hellden L (1990) Prevalence of signs and symptoms of dysfunction in the masticatory system: an epidemiologic study in an adult Swedish population. J Craniomandib Disord Facial Oral Pain 4:241–250
140. Sarlani E, Grace EG, Reynolds MA, Greenspan JD (2004) Evidence for up-regulated central nociceptive processing in patients with masticatory myofascial pain. J Orofac Pain 18(1):41–55
141. Schokker RP, Hanson TL, Ansink BJJ (1990) Craniomandibular disorders in patients with different types of headache. J Craniomandib Disord Facial Oral Pain 4:47–51
142. Schwartz HC, Kendrick RW (1984) Internal derangements of the temporomandibular joint: description of clinical syndromes. Oral Surg Oral Med Oral Pathol 58(1):24–29
143. Selaimen CM, Jeronymo JC, Brilhante DP, Grossi ML (2006) Sleep and depression as risk indicators for temporomandibular disorders in a cross-cultural perspective: a case–control study. Int J Prosthodont 19(2):154–161
144. Sherman JJ, LeResche L, Huggins KH et al (2004) The relationship of somatization and depression to experimental pain response in women with temporomandibular disorders. Psychosom Med 66(6):852–860

145. Shimshak DG, De Furia MC (1998) Health care utilization by patients with temporomandibular joint disorders. Cranio 16(3):185–193
146. Silveira AM, Feltrin PP, Zanetti RV, Mautoni MC (2007) Prevalence of patients harboring temporomandibular disorders in an otorhinolaryngology department. Rev Bras Otorinolaringol (Engl Ed) 73(4):528–532
147. Sipilä K, Veijola J, Jokelainen J et al (2001) Association between symptoms of temporomandibular disorders and depression: an epidemiological study of the Northern Finland 1966 birth cohort. Cranio 19(3):183–187
148. Sjoholm TT, Piha SJ, Lehtinen I (1995) Cardiovascular autonomic control is disturbed in nocturnal teethgrinders. Clin Physiol 15(4):349–354
149. Slade GD, Diatchenko L, Bhalang K et al (2007) Influence of psychological factors on risk of temporomandibular disorders. J Dent Res 86(11):1120–1125
150. Steed PA, Wexler GB (2001) Temporomandibular disorders-traumatic etiology vs. nontraumatic etiology: a clinical and methodological inquiry into symptomatology and treatment outcomes. Cranio 19(3):188–194
151. Suvinen TI, Reade PC (1995) Temporomandibular disorders: a critical review of the nature of pain and its assessment. J Orofac Pain 9:317–339
152. Tanaka TT (1984) Recognition of the pain formula for head, neck and TMJ disorders: the general physical examination. CDA J 12(5):43–49
153. Travell JG, Simons DG (1983) Myofascial pain and dysfunction. The trigger-point manual. Williams & Wilkins (ed), Baltimore, 713p
154. Vallerand WP, Hall MB (1991) Improvement in myofascial pain and headaches following TMJ surgery. J Craniomandib Disord Facial Oral Pain 5:197–204
155. Velly-Miguel AM, Monplaisir J, Rompre PH et al (1992) Bruxism and other orofacial movements during sleep. J Craniomandib Discord Facial Oral Pain 6:71–81
156. Vimpari SS, Knuttila ML, Sakki TK, Kivela SL (1995) Depressive symptoms associated with symptoms of the temporomandibular joint pain and dysfunction syndrome. Psychosom Med 57:439–444
157. Wänman A, Agerberg G (1986) Mandibular dysfunction in adolescents. II: prevalence of signs. Act Odontol Scand 44(6):55–62
158. Wänman A, Agerberg G (1991) Etiology of craniomandibular disorders: evaluation of some occlusal and psychological factors in 19-years olds. J Craniomandib Disord Facial Oral Pain 5:35–44
159. Ware JC, Rugh JD (1988) Destructive bruxism: sleep stage relationship. Sleep 11:172–181
160. Watanabe Y, Ishikawa T, Kino K et al (2005) Relationship between oral sensory thresholds and depressive moods. J Med Dent Sci 52(1):73–80
161. Weideman CL, Bush DL, Yan-Go FL et al (1996) The incidence of parasomnias in child bruxers versus non-bruxers. Pediatr Dent 18(7):456–460
162. Weinberg S, Lapointe H (1987) Cervical extension-flexion injury (whiplash) and internal derangement of the temporomandibular joint. J Oral Maxillofac Surg 45(8):653–656
163. Wiesinger B, Malker H, Englund E, Wänman A (2007) Back pain in relation to musculoskeletal disorders in the jaw-face: a matched case–control study. Pain 131(3):311–319
164. Wright EF (2000) Referred craniofacial pain patterns in patients with temporomandibular disorder. J Am Dent Assoc 131(9):1307–1315
165. Wright EF, Bifano SL (1998) ENT clinic patients receive otologic symptom improvement from TMD therapy. J Orofac Pain 12(2):abstract no 34
166. Wright AR, Gatchel RJ, Wildenstein L et al (2004) Biopsychosocial differences between high-risk and low-risk patients with acute TMD-related pain. J Am Dent Assoc 135(4):474–483
167. Wruble MK, Lumley MA, Dudley MC, Mc Glynn FD (1989) Sleep-related bruxism and sleep variables: a critical review. J Craniomandib Disord Facial Oral Pain 3:152–158
168. Yap AU, Tan KB, Chua EK, Tan HH (2002) Depression and somatization in patients with temporomandibular disorders. J Prosthet Dent 88(5):479–484
169. Yap AU, Chua EK, Tan KB, Chan YH (2004) Relationships between depression/somatization and self-reports of pain and disability. J Orofac Pain 18(3):220–225

170. Yardin M (1995) Odontologie globale. Masson (éd), Paris
171. Yatani H, Studts J, Cordova M et al (2002) Comparison of sleep quality and clinical and psychologic characteristics in patients with temporomandibular disorders. J Orofac Pain 16(3):221–228
172. Young S, Jordan JC (1982) EMG activity of the sternomastoid muscles in relation to mouth movement. J Dent Res Abstract 61, 4:158
173. Yussuf H, Rothwell PS (1986) Temporomandibular joint pain-dysfunction in patients suffering from atypical facial pain. Br Dent J 161:208–212
174. Areso MP, Giralt MT, Sainz B et al (1999) Occlusal disharmonies modulate central catecholaminergic activity in the rat. J Dent Res 78(6):1204–1213

Objective Signs

Classically clinical investigation consists of *examination, palpation, and listening*. It can be addicted some tests. When confronted to orofacial complaints, clinicians must recall possible vascular or tumorous etiological reasons [77] or infections [82].

1 Examination

1.1 Extraoral Examination

The patient's posture should be carefully observed as it may reveal **postural dysfunction** [22, 26, 47, 103, 109]. A withdrawn facial expression may signal suffering or lassitude. In addition, it is advisable to measure the size of eyelid openings and compare the right and left sides [43]. Dental specialists can detect errors in the estimation of *vertical dimension of occlusion* (VDO) by evaluating the face proportions [114]. The examination of facial profiles helps evaluate certain types of maxillomandibular relations [75, 86] often associated with stomatognathic muscle pain felt on palpation [90].

1.2 Intraoral Examination

The following signs are usually checked by dentists, but some can be evaluated by any clinician who may then direct a patient suffering from pain or discomfort to a specialist. May an *occlusal rehabilitation* be necessary started, particularly if a deleterious parafunctional habit such as **severe clenching** is diagnosed? Occlusodontists have long observed that occlusion disorders may be accompanied by *grinding*. These troubles disturb the jaw lateral movements and may even result in blocking them. This explains why painful contractures affect the muscles

F. Hartmann, G. Cucchi, *Stress and Orality*,
DOI 10.1007/978-2-8178-0271-8_3, © Springer-Verlag France 2014

responsible for this movement (lateral and medial pterygoid muscles, temporalis). **Grinding** may be an individual response to occlusal prematurity [23]. But they may also be means to fight against malocclusion resulting from insufficient physiological wear or atypical wear [41]. Occlusal interference cannot be compensated by wear. Grinding has been widely evaluated by clinical experts and does not appear to be the most alarming factor [34, 48, 87, 103].

In contrast, **clenching** leaves no obvious trace upon clinical examination. The presence of keratosis or other traumatic mucosal lesion on the lateral edges of the tongue or on the inside of cheeks can signal parafunctional biting habits or simple occlusal disorders [93]. Maximum mouth opening can initially be measured with a pair of calipers or a ruler and be recorded. A minimum normal mouth opening for men is about 1.65 in. and about 1.5 in. for women (Fig. 1), but it obviously varies

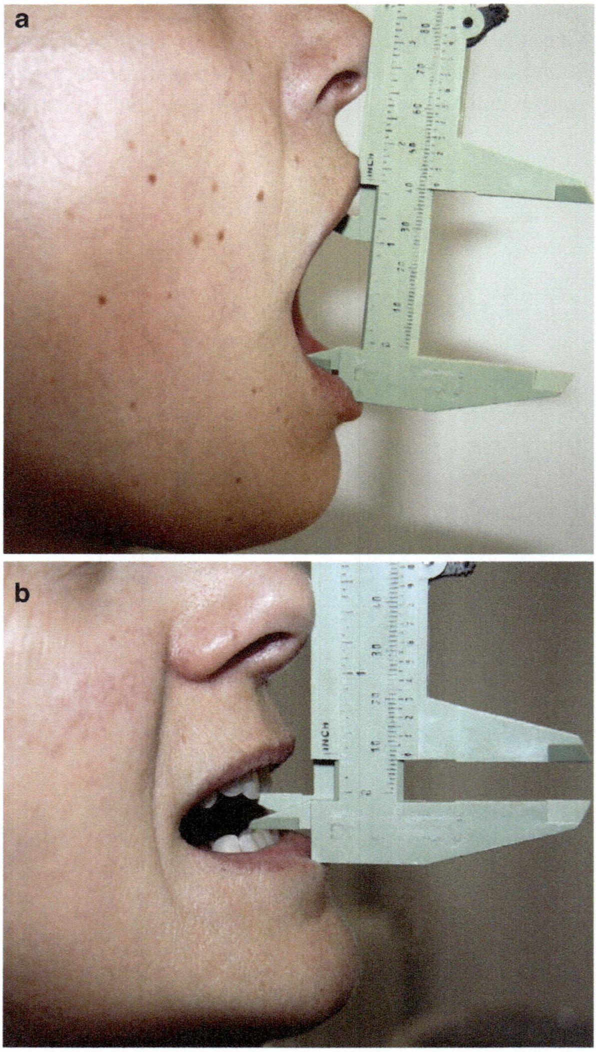

Fig. 1 (**a**, **b**) Measurement of the maximal mouth opening. (**a**) Normal; (**b**) limited

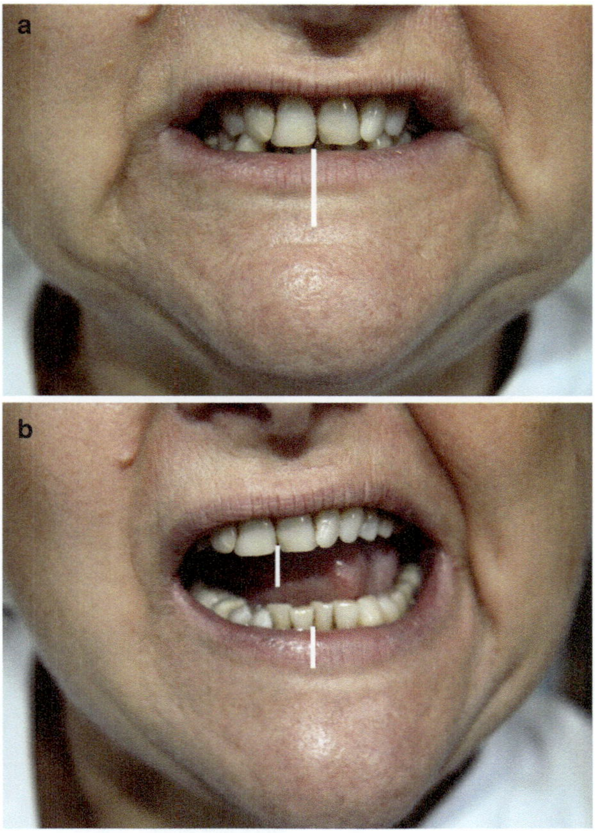

Fig. 2 (**a**, **b**) Jaw deviation during mouth opening. (**a**) Closed position; (**b**) opened position. During the mouth opening movement, the clinician must follow the inferior inter-incisal point in comparison to the medial vertical line

with the person's size. *Jaw deviation* can also be detected while the mouth is either opening or closing (Fig. 2). *Functional tongue malposition* [58, 103] during swallowing has been observed in studies particularly in subjects with an open jaw swallowing pattern (infantile deglutition) (Fig. 3) or with a lateral swallowing pattern, even sometimes lateral lingual interposition between the dental arches at rest. Close relations with anterior open bite (Fig. 4) have been noted [36]. The **tongue** is a complex muscular set; it is hard to control and requires minimal physiological space particularly in the posterior, that is, molar quadrant. With the exception of some cases of macroglossia, restricted space may be due to abnormally shaped dental arches resulting mainly from maxillomandibular dysmorphogenesis.[1] Functional lingual malposition (too low) often comes from a buccal breathing habit [88].

[1]There is still too little awareness of etiological factors that cause insufficient growth of the maxillary bones: for instance, new western world habits such as the decline in the practice of breastfeeding or overly soft food that reduces sensitive trigeminal stimulation (Fig. 5). Problems in the special relation between teeth and the maxillary volume are falsely considered as a normal tendency of human evolution. In fact, they result from etiological cultural factors that could be easily corrected.

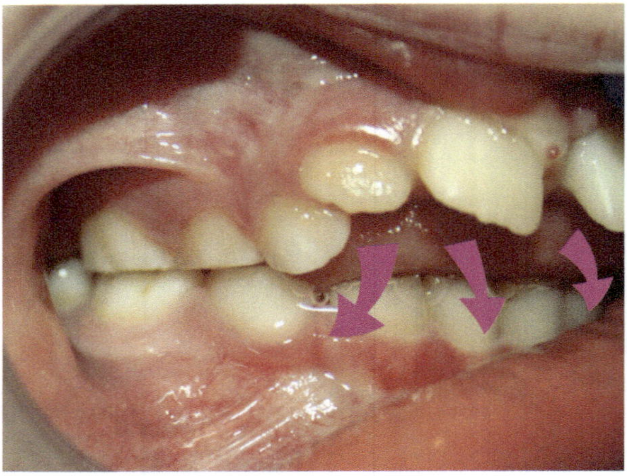

Fig. 3 Typical infantile deglutition (mixed denture). The *pink arrows* show the deleterious push from the tongue between anterior teeth

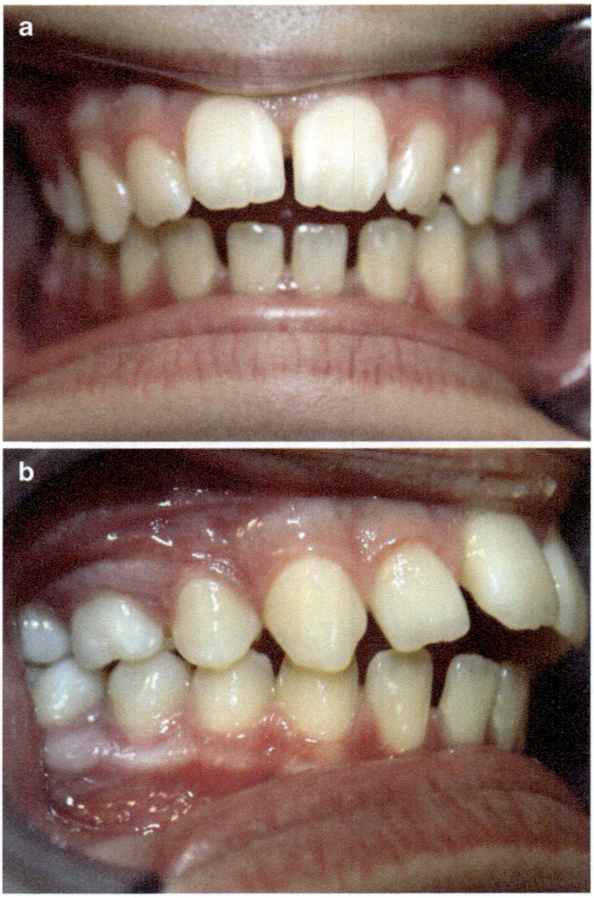

Fig. 4 (**a**, **b**) Anterior dental open bite in adult

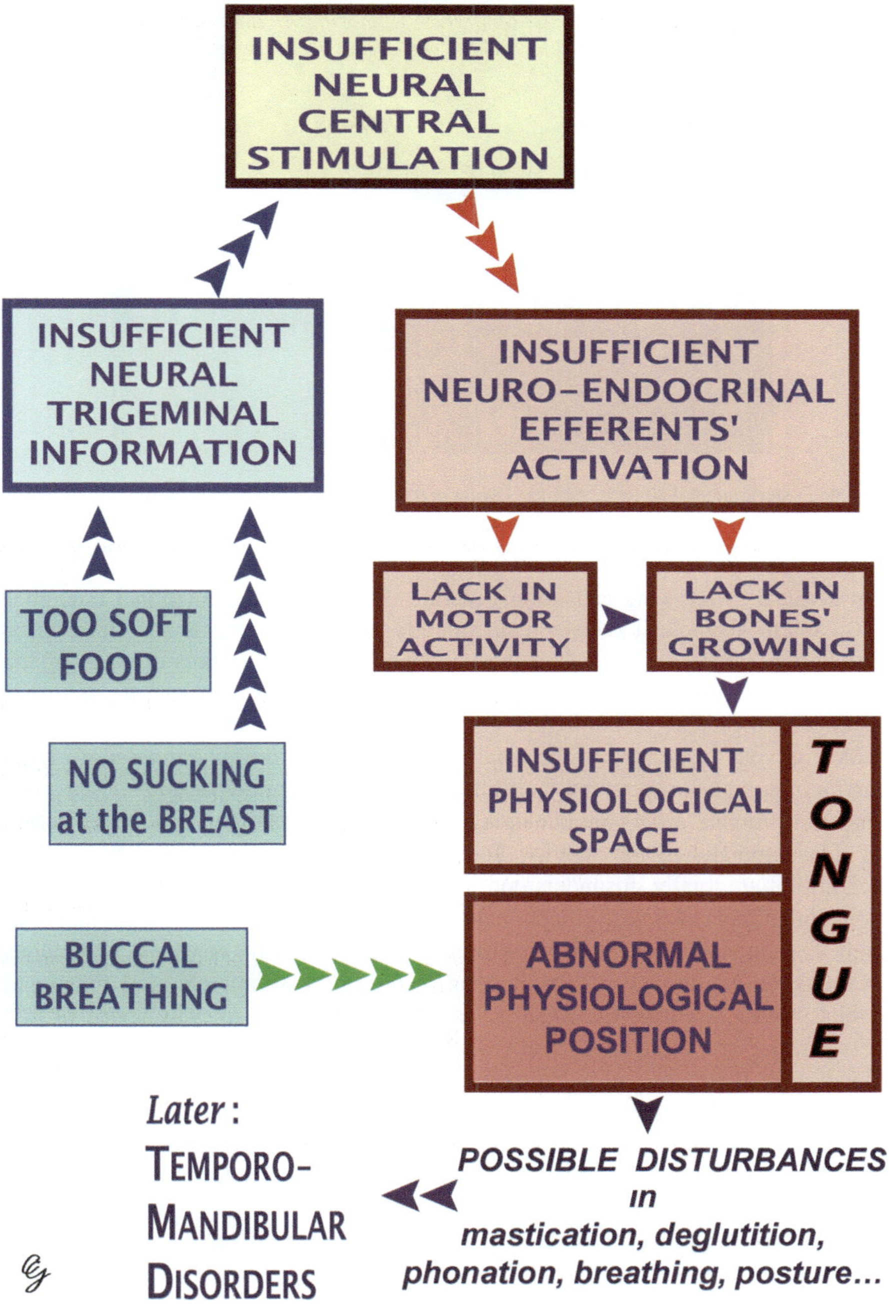

Fig. 5 Various cultural habits as potential factors of maxillar dysfunctional growing

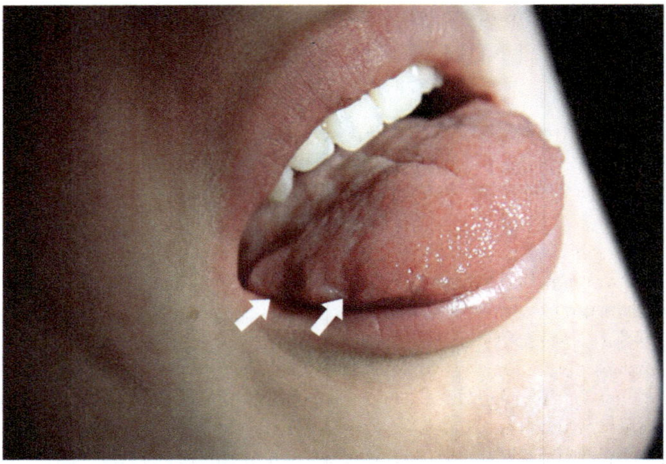

Fig. 6 Posterior dental contact printings (*white arrows*) on the lateral borders of the tongue

An atypical swallowing can often generate diverse oral dysfunctional outcomes [40], and to diagnose it keeps a main value for a favorable prognosis. The interval problem becomes evident when the clinician examines the lateral edges of the tongue: dental impressions may inform on the pressure coming from the posterior teeth (Fig. 6). Under physiological conditions, periodontal inputs[2] allow adequate motor nervous response to functional swallowing. *Missing or unbalanced dental tactile input volumes* between the right and left occlusal sides or *anomalous proprioceptive lingual inputs* are damaging conditions that can facilitate dysregulation of this automatic motor activity. Too many pathological outcomes of atypical deglutition are totally misunderstood: posture and locomotion disorders, dysfunctional breathing rhythm, dysfunctional cardiac rhythm, problems with phonation as well as human relation, and behavioral disturbances. This is why a meticulous examination of the patient's swallowing record and dynamic occlusal functional habits proves essential – as well as an evaluation of the freeway space (FWS) between the upper and lower teeth when the jaw is at rest and the head upright. Under normal circumstances, the space between the upper and lower dental arches should measure about 0.12 in. A reduced or insufficient FWS nearly always signals a lack of FWS due to dental prosthetic errors or excessive wear. It may result from stomatognathic muscle hyperactivity in jaw-closing muscles (clenching). Jaw depressor muscles (antagonist) react to the abnormal stretch by contracting themselves. This can trigger pain in some zones of the throat region. Some authors

[2]See chapter "Characteristics of Periodontal Proprioception."

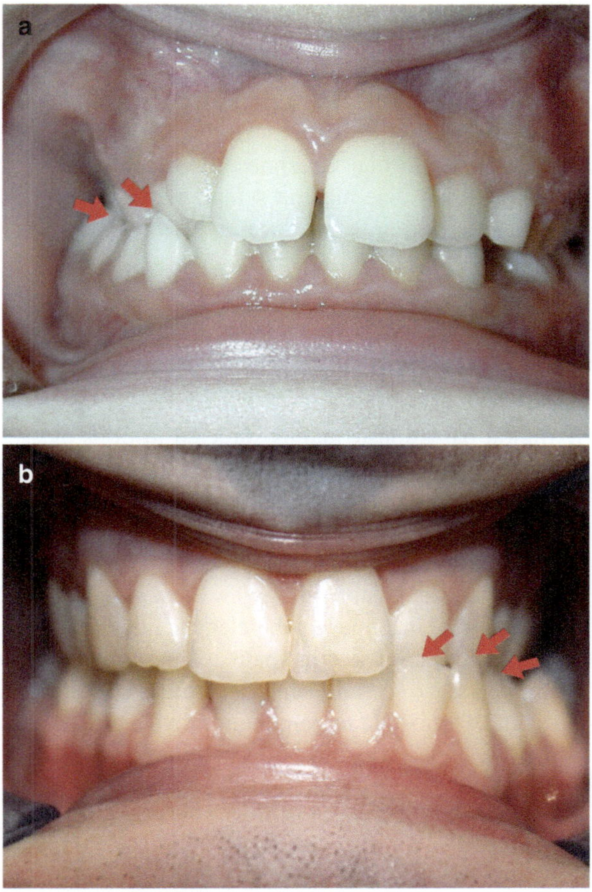

Fig. 7 (**a**, **b**) Dental crossbites (*red arrows*): lateral jaw movements may be disrupted

consider it essential to check the well-being of dental arches together with possible mucosal teeth indentation [27, 38, 110] while others believe that edentation has no significant relation with TMD [45, 72, 102]. A completely toothless patient may be at risk with TMD, as clinical observations may tell [96]. Epidemiologic studies revealed that toothless old patients with complete prosthetic restoration (particularly women) experienced a high percentage of TMJ clicking noises and tension neck-like symptoms [62]. Abnormalities in tooth position (eruption, rotation, etc.) should be taken into account [60]. According to studies on the subject, crossbites in children (Fig. 7a) or in adults (Fig. 7b) seem to be an important occlusal factor in the activity of posterior fibers in the ipsilateral temporalis muscle [78] and tend to encourage lateral displacement of the jaw at rest. More generally, occlusal disorders should be evaluated with a neuromuscular approach enlightened by scientific data. A sensitive method called the "shoulders method" [54] for detecting subtle occlusal disequilibration disorders is rather helpful.

2 Palpation

Even though this still can be subjective, *palpation of stomatognathic muscles* is one of the best ways of assessing severity of TMD [8, 9, 15, 20, 48, 51, 60, 91, 107, 111, 116, 117] with a major response in *females* [24]. Otherwise, the clinicians must remind that any sine materia symptom could worry the patient whereas the symptom materialization helps to reassure him or her [32].

2.1 Extraoral Palpation

Extraoral palpation is mainly directed towards *masseteris, temporalis,* and *supra-* and *infrahyoid muscles* (Figs. 8, 9, 10, 11, and 12) and towards muscles responsible for head posture such as the *trapezius, occipitalis,* and *sternocleidomastoidian muscle* (Figs. 13, 14, and 15). The SCM has been known to trigger certain persistent (noninfective) ear aches and dizziness [80, 112]. Some studies showed that the muscle experienced tension during jaw *clenching* [84, 123]. What's more, descriptions of frontal pain in subjects who clenched their teeth came as no surprise [115]. The region includes a projecting pain zone as previously described [80, 112] (Fig. 16). Many years ago, certain superficial areas including SCM proved to be frequently particularly sensitive to palpation: provoked pain by palpation in these three areas

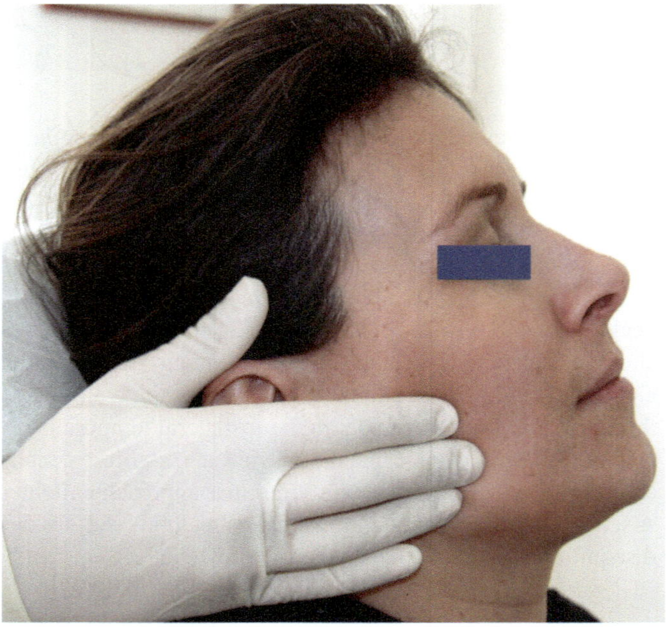

Fig. 8 Palpation of the m. masseteris

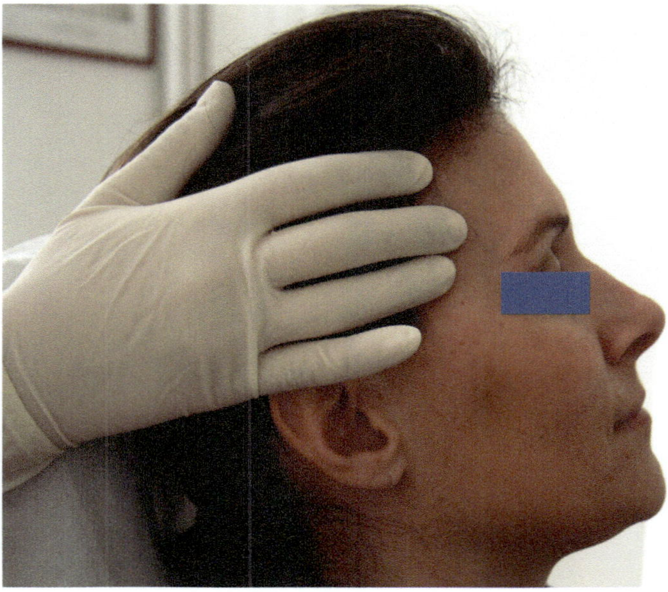

Fig. 9 Palpation of the m. temporalis (anterior fibers)

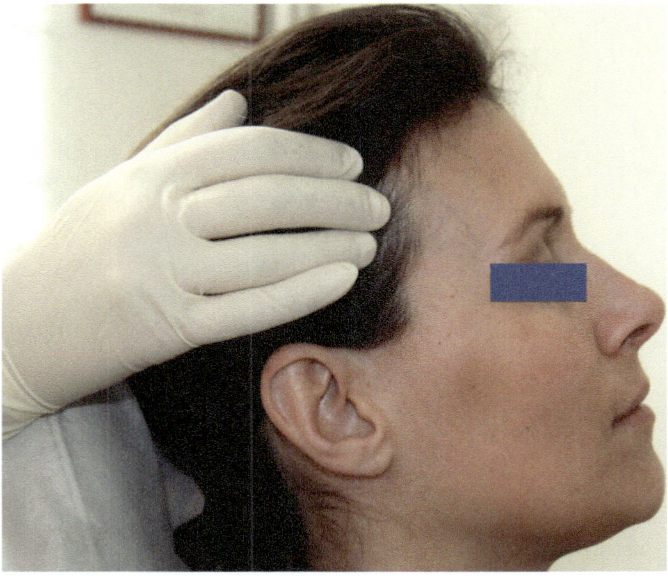

Fig. 10 Palpation of the m. temporalis (mild fibers)

generated a particular sign called the "*dental triad*" (Figs. 17 and 18) and revealed an occlusion disorder [50]. A close relation was found on palpation between stomatognathic muscles tenderness and cervical muscles tenderness [106]. The

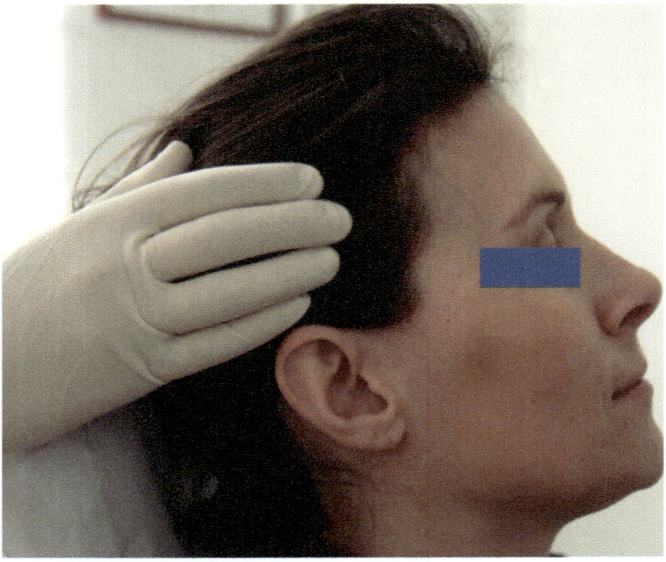

Fig. 11 Palpation of the m. temporalis (posterior fibers)

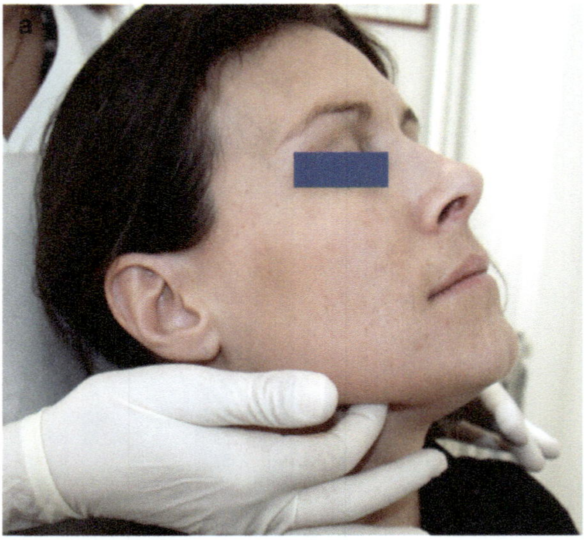

Fig. 12 (**a**, **b**) Palpation of the suprahyoid muscles

Fig. 12 (continued)

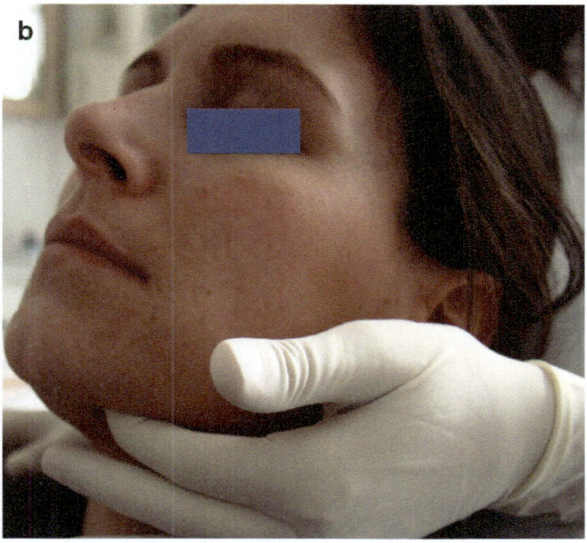

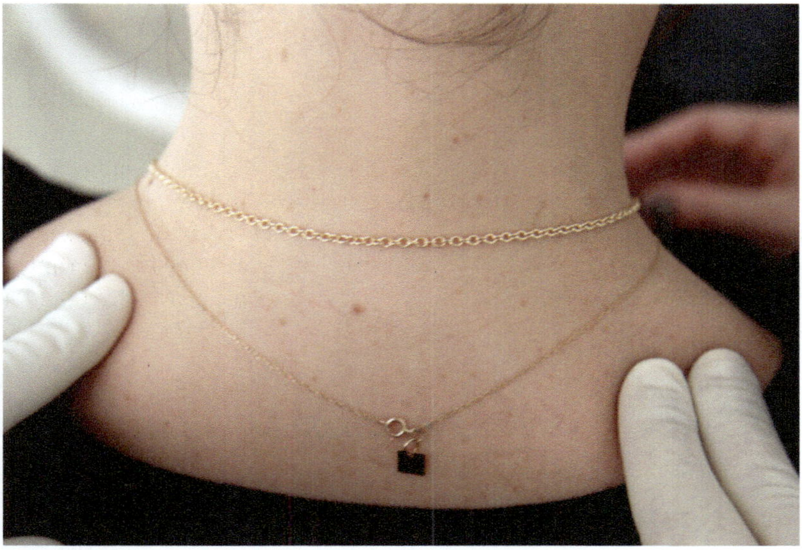

Fig. 13 Palpation of the m. trapezius

investigation of muscle sensibility to palpation should be extended to the arm, hand, and calf muscles.

TMJ palpation should be subdivided into the lateral aspect and the posterior aspect of the capsule (Figs. 19 and 20). Pain in the condylar process on palpation is a revealing symptom of TMJ disorders [61, 105].

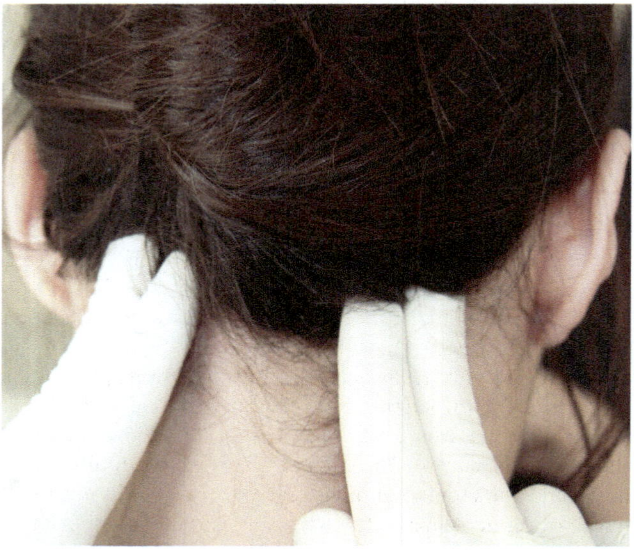

Fig. 14 Palpation of the m. occipitalis

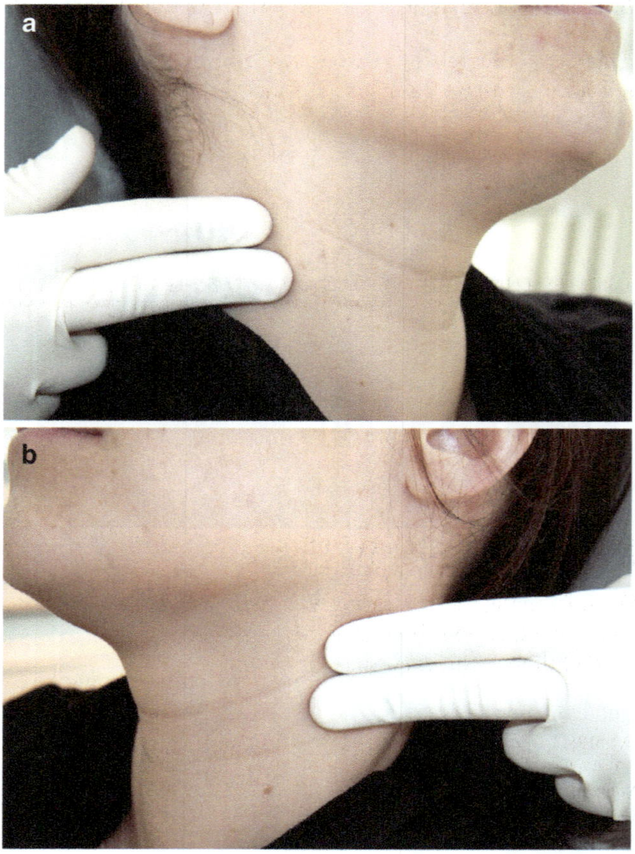

Fig. 15 (**a**, **b**) Palpation of the sternocleidomastoidian muscles

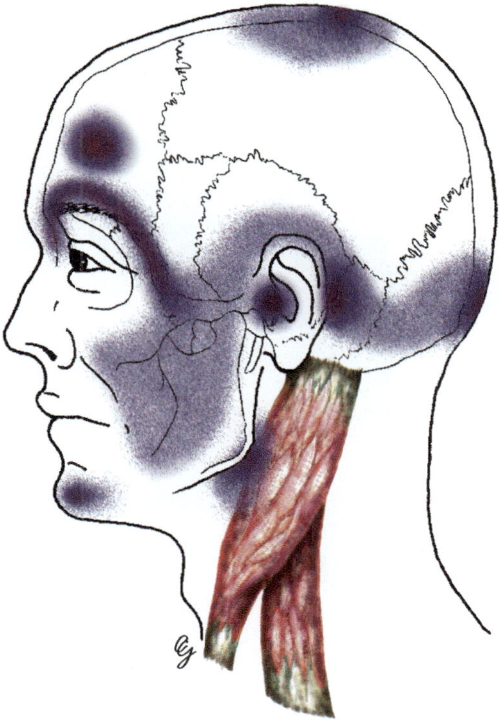

Fig. 16 Referred pain from the musculus sternocleidomastoideus (also involved in clenching) (Modified from Travell et al. [112])

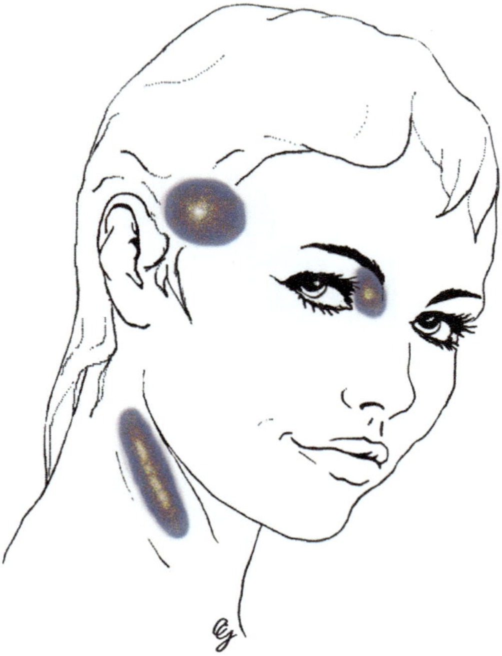

Fig. 17 The "dental triad". The three zones to be palpated: supra-medial aspect of orbit (near the point where nervus infratrochlearis emerges), temporal zone, and posterior border of SCM muscle. This sign was only considered positive when all three areas were painful when palpated

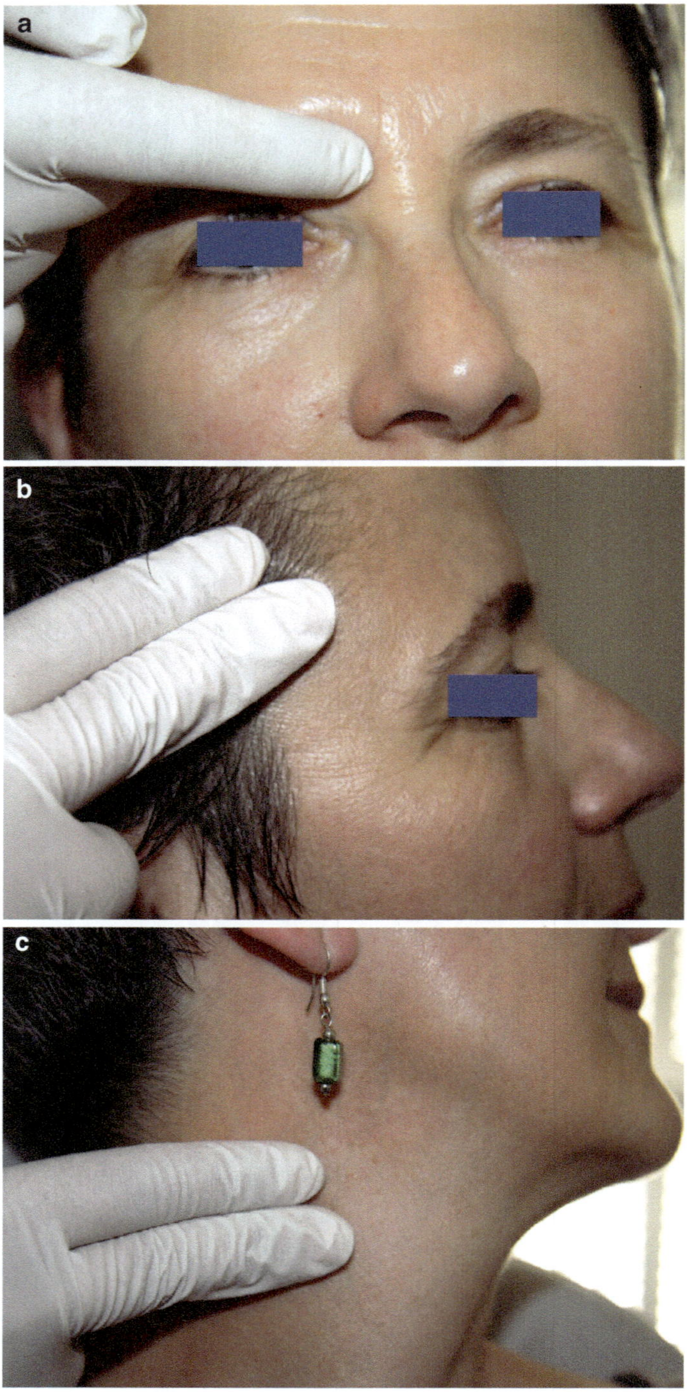

Fig. 18 (**a**–**c**) The "dental triad." (**a**) Supra-medial aspect of orbit (near the point where nervus infratrochlearis emerges), (**b**) temporal zone, and (**c**) posterior border of SCM muscle

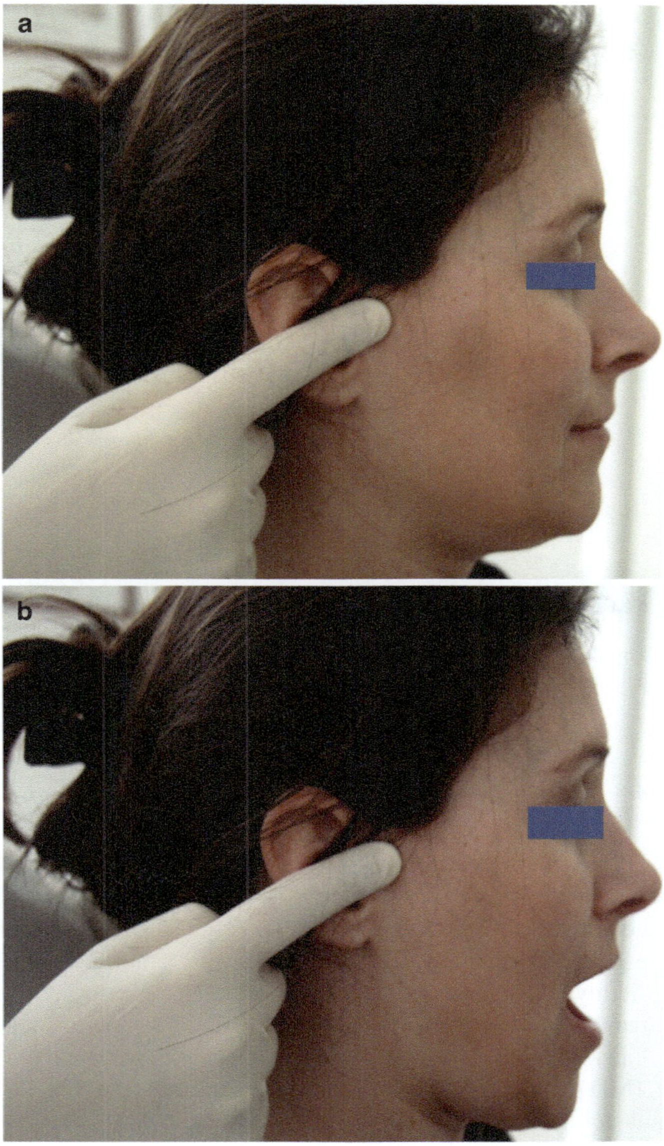

Fig. 19 (**a**, **b**) Palpating the jaw condyles: with two forefingers just before tragus, the clinician locates the jaw condyles as the patient makes light mandibular movements. Bilateral palpation performs while the mouth is closed (**a**), with and without pressure, then while the jaw is moved (**b**) with and without pressure

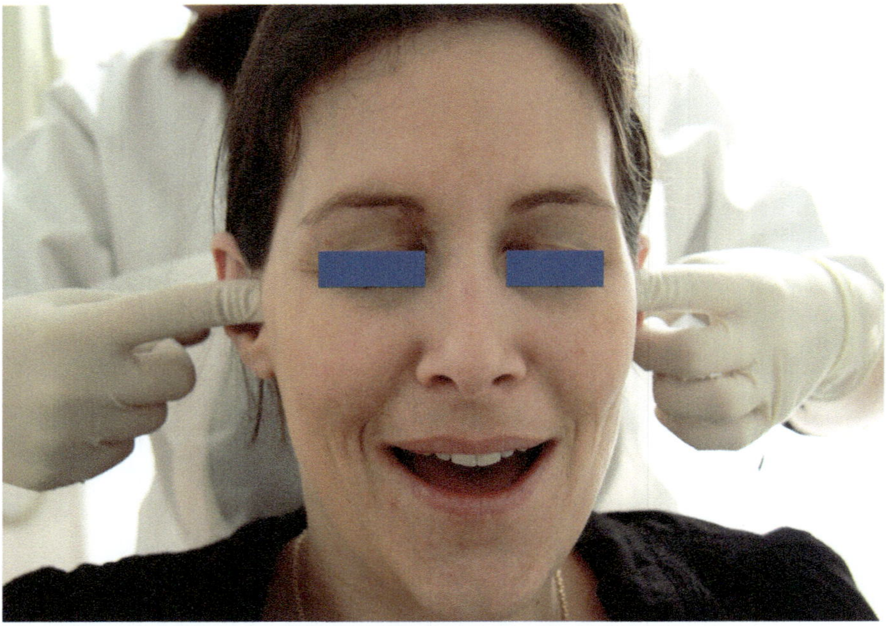

Fig. 20 Palpating the retro-articular space of the (TMJ): as the mouth is opened, the clinician palpates the retro-articular space with two forefingers

2.2 *Intraoral Palpation*

Intraoral palpation involves the *medial pterygoid muscles* (MPMs) (Figs. 21 and 22) and *muscles of the oral floor* (Fig. 23). Direct palpation (Fig. 24) of the lateral pterygoid muscles (LPMs) was the subject of debate based on different studies [3, 17], particularly anatomical studies on cadaveric subjects [108, 113]. However, the feasibility of such direct palpation has been recently evidenced by an anatomo-radiologic study on living subjects [6]. In our previous manual, we related a personal long-term statistical investigation about painful palpation of LPMs in a pathological TMD population: 464 women (Fig. 25) and 136 men (Fig. 26). Please note the prevalent bilateral sign both in women and men.

Fig. 21 Intraoral palpation of the m. pterygoideus medialis (MPMs). Please note that it is easier for the practitioner to use his right finger to palpate the patient's right side and his left finger for the patient's left side

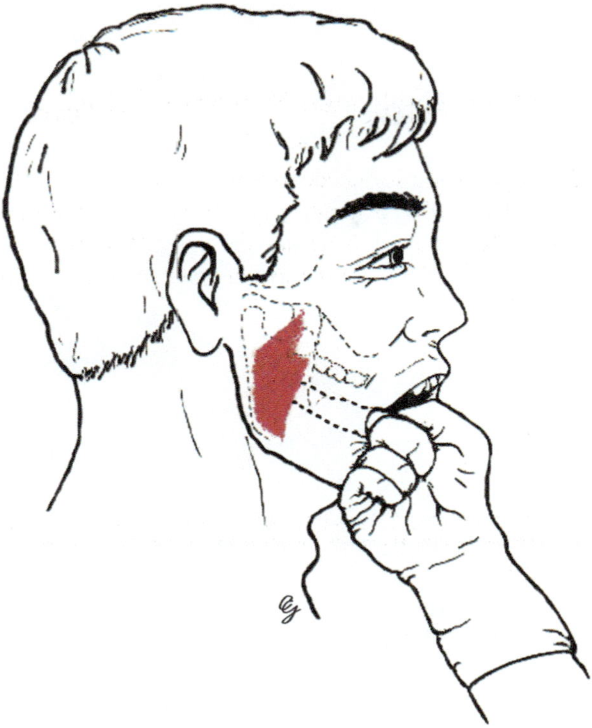

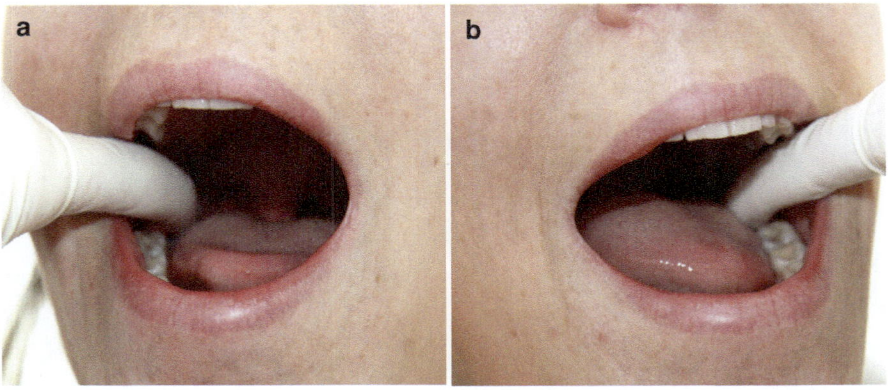

Fig. 22 (**a**, **b**) Intraoral palpation of m. pterygoideus medialis

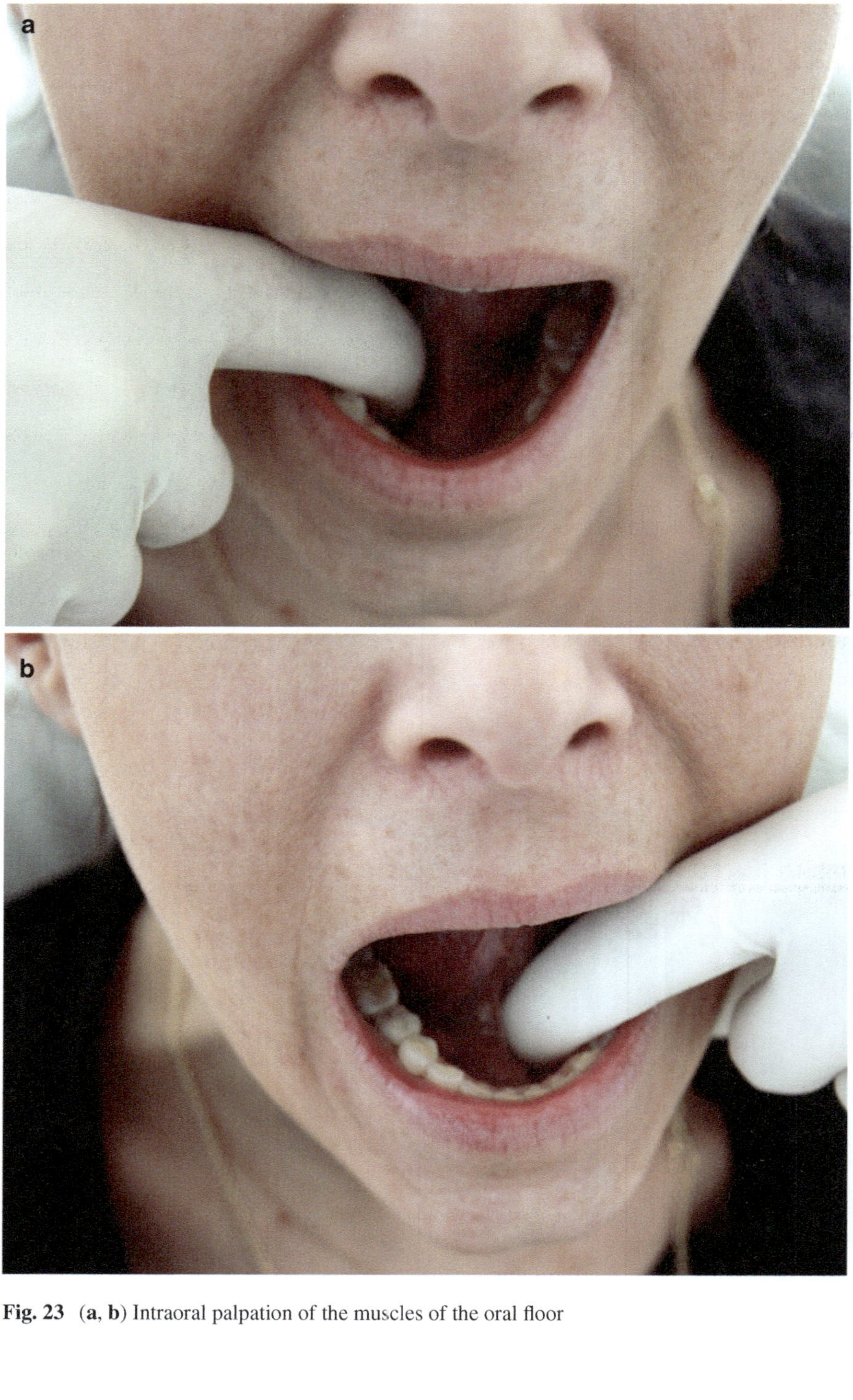

Fig. 23 (**a**, **b**) Intraoral palpation of the muscles of the oral floor

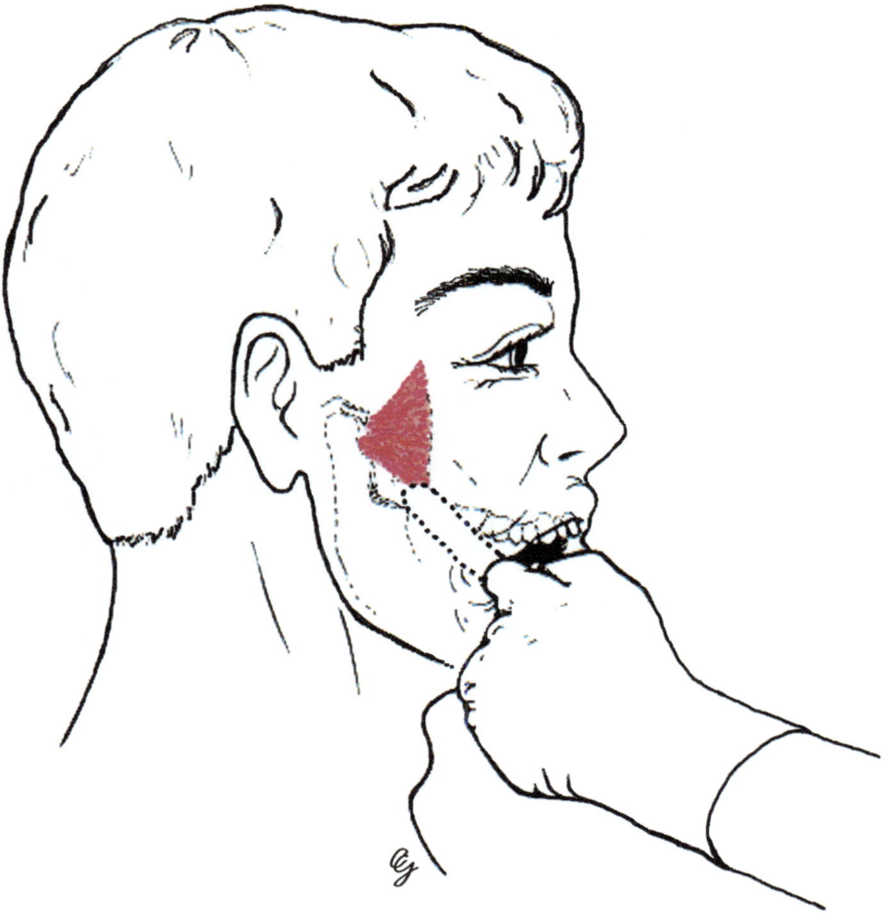

Fig. 24 Intraoral palpation of the m. pterygoideus lateralis (LPMs). Palpation is carried out with the index finger just laterally and behind the upper wisdom tooth, moving backwards and upwards. To help movement of the examining finger on inner aspect of temporal tendon, it is best to ask the patient to open his or her mouth about half way and to slightly lower the jaw to palpated side. Please note that it is easier for the practitioner to use his left finger to palpate the patient's right side and his right finger for the patient's left side. Painful palpation is part of what Travell [112] called, in a more general sense, "jump sign" or "twitch response." For some authors, this sensitivity to painful palpation was of the upmost importance in diagnosing TMD [12, 33, 48, 51, 92, 101, 118] above all when it is associated with uncompensated loss of posterior teeth. It might give objective evidence for spontaneous pain experienced in the area of TMJ [92]. Two tests can identify dysfunction of each head of the LPMs: pain on biting a tongue spatula in relation to its upper head and pain when pushing jaw forwards against resistance applied with hand on chin with regard to its lower head

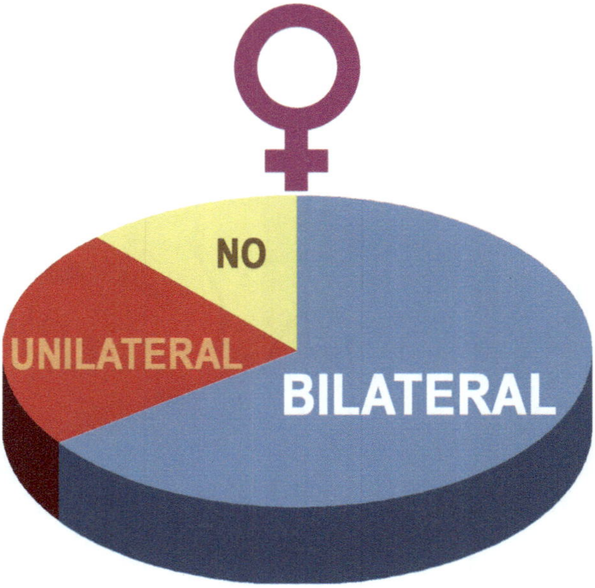

Fig. 25 Statistical percentage of pain on palpation of the LPMs in women [52]

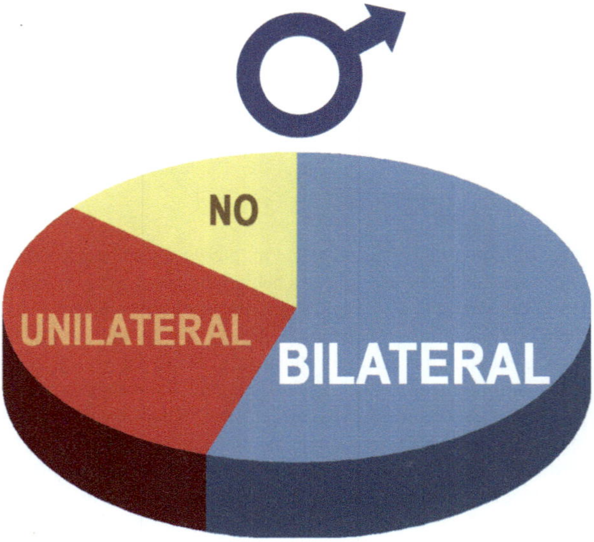

Fig. 26 Statistical percentage of pain on palpation of the LPMs in men [52]

3 Listening

Generally silent during normal mouth opening, TMJ may produce noises even in normal subjects whose jaw movements are extreme. However, the duration of the noise heard with a stethoscope should be much shorter in pathological cases such as subjects suffering from disc displacement than in normal subjects [42]. Classically, it is possible to distinguish between two kinds of noises. *Clicking sounds* are often premature [16, 83, 93]. *Screeching* or *crackling sounds* may indicate a degenerative change in patients with advanced TMJ dysfunctions [83], which can be confirmed by radiological investigations. To experts, signs such as clicking related to TMJ pain are frequently considered to have limited significance, depending on their own treatment strategy [104]. The following clinical classification of TMJ internal disorders has been defined [28]:

- type 1, jaw deviation with articular noises but normal mouth opening;
- type 2, same as type 1 with some occasional blockage;
- type 3, periarticular pain and limited mouth opening.

On the other hand, attentive listening of articular noises helps establish a more accurate diagnosis of articular dysfunction [28, 83]. Therefore, precocious clicking may reveal a recent but non-reducible lesion. Inversely crunching frequently signals tissular lesions [83, 97], but its treatment may trigger the existence of *non-reducible luxation*. TMJ internal derangement is clinically evidenced by dysfunctional signs in mouth opening movements [30, 79]. A precise classification is helpful to clinicians as it follows physiological neuromuscular principles [100].

For a long time, TMD were only considered as TMJ condylo-discal disorders, often related to dental occlusion disorders. They are now clearly recognized as originating from neuromuscular disorders involving stomatognathic muscles, even muscles responsible for head posture. Several arguments exist and must be considered for a more functional and neurophysiological approach of the problem [29, 30]. In physiological conditions, TMJ discs act as shock absorbers between the articular tubercle (tubercula articulares) and condylar process (processa condylaris) (Fig. 27). Ligaments protect soft structures (muscles) and hard structured TMJ in extreme positions that are physiologically unusual. Spastic conditions in muscles that mobilize TMJ may be facilitated by several acute or chronic physical factors. The incidence of TMJ internal derangement (disc displacement) has been found to be much more significant among male and female teenagers [57] though the cause remains unexplained. Different factors in the patient's medical history may be investigated by clinicians in order to refer the case to specialists.

3.1 Acute Factors *[2, 4, 5, 10, 30, 31, 44, 49, 63, 67, 71, 73, 95, 99, 100, 119, 120]*

Events such as direct shocks to TMJ or shocks to the chin [60, 104] or *whiplash injury* or sudden stretch could generate posterior attachment lesions and pain in the

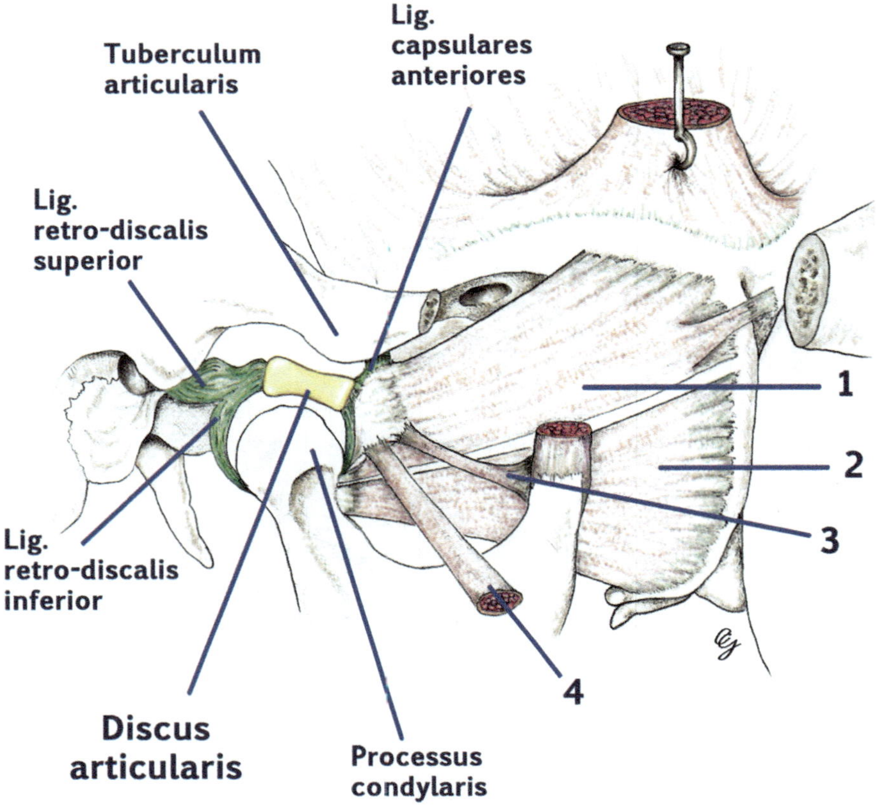

Fig. 27 The discomuscular functional apparatus of temporomandibular joints. *1* upper belly of the musculus pterygoideus lateralis, *2* lower belly of the m. pterygoideus lateralis, *3* discal belly of the m. temporalis, *4* discal belly of the m. masseteris

TMJ [13, 18, 98, 120] (Fig. 28). Physicians generally agree that acute injury with arthro-ligamentar lesion can cause articular pain and reflex contractures. Cranio-cervical trauma is one of the most frequent and disregarded isolated factors in the development of TMD [69]. Routine examination of the TMJ and stomatognathic muscles in each injured patient is recommended to clinicians [35, 68]. Many of the symptoms commonly attributed to cervical traumas (headache, facial pain, auricular pain, tinnitus, a feeling of ear fullness, swallowing problems, etc.) actually come from jaw traumas that occur simultaneously [39, 53]. A study of patients with cervical injury [11] showed an obvious link between painful sensibility of the nuchal muscles, accompanied by a restriction in the flexion-extension-rotation of these muscles, and painful palpation of the stomatognathic muscles. In TMD patients, the link between a motor vehicle accident (MVA) and TMD necessitates more complex and longer therapeutic procedures because the event makes the prognosis more difficult. Even low-speed shocks can generate important forces responsible for significant physical damage [74]. Yet, some authors still believe that TMJ internal

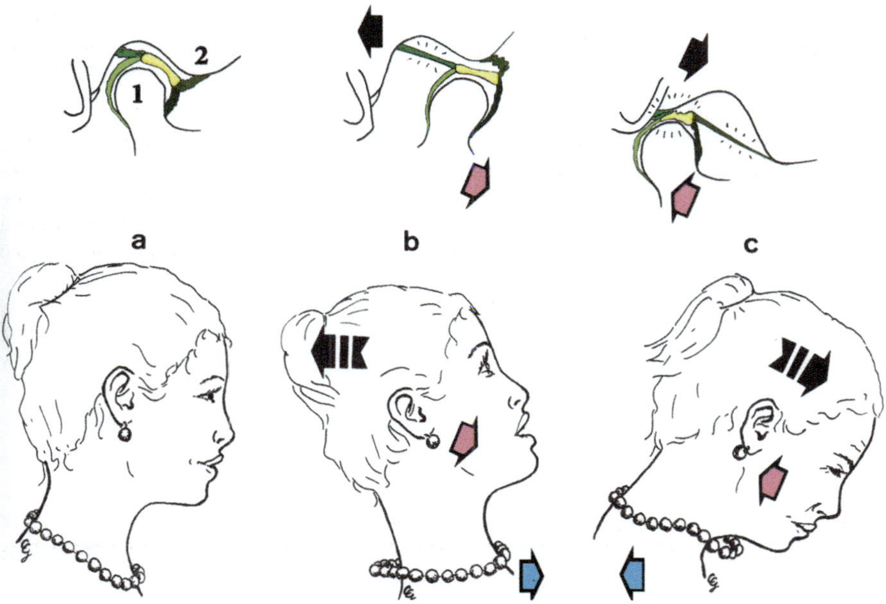

Fig. 28 Schematic lateral view of a TMJ whiplash trauma. *1* processus condylaris, *2* tuberculum articularis. (**a**) resting position, (**b**) hyperextension of the head/neck set, (**c**) hyperflexion of the head/neck set. Disc in *yellow*. TMJ ligaments in *green*. *Black arrows* movements of the skull. *Blue arrows* movements of the body. *Pink arrows* movements of the mandible

derangement should not be regarded as a primary cause of symptoms in whiplash patients [13, 14, 31, 46, 55, 56, 64, 65, 89]. Other circumstances may contribute to TMJ internal derangement:

- head hyperextension (cervical hyperlordosis) necessary before intubation prior to general anesthesia;
- forced fitting of a mouth-opener prior to stomatologic surgery without preliminary estimation of the patient maximal mouth opening when awake;
- prolonged dental sessions with the mouth wide open and no pause to relax stomatognathic muscles [30, 100, 120] as in long and difficult extractions of posterior teeth [4, 30].

3.2 *Chronic Factors*

When they persist, some factors create a functional overload on TMJ structures [83]. This happens in cases of:

- **Loss of VDO** [35, 66]
- **Dental occlusion disorder**, particularly posterior loss of adjustment [38]
- **Unilateral mastication** usually resulting from non compensated teeth loss [120] that can also be an alarming sign of functional asymmetry in stomatognathic muscles when searching for an analgesic position (premature)

During growth, it represents a major disturbing element in the craniofacial morphogenesis and a chronic factor in the onset of TMD [88]; *stomatognathic parafunctions, hyper-excitability of the stomatognathic muscles*, particularly LPMs [59, 100], may contribute through their articular attachments to a functional pathology of the disco-capsulo-muscular set [1, 21, 76]. Articular pain, frequently projected from spasmed LPMs [7, 43, 112], should increase if the patient tends to clench his teeth [121]. Furthermore, sustained contraction of the two LPMs in a stressed patient can contribute to the so-called acquired ligamentous laxity [17, 30]. Sustained compression of the condylar process on the posterior part of the disc will damage the posterior attachment and create anterior displacement of the disc [7, 70, 94]. Therefore, the increase in tension endured at this level can be facilitated by a loss in molar adjustment [30] following non-restored extractions and resorption of the bone base.

Sometimes painful and dysfunctional symptoms signal a classical rheumatismal pathology [122]. To make a differential diagnosis easier and exclude TMD, the patient should be asked a number of questions such as *"do you experience morning stiffness other than in the jaw?" "Over the past year, have you had recurrent swelling of joints other than in your TMJ?" "Do you feel muscle tenderness other than in your head or neck for more than 50 % of the time?"* This last question does not necessarily determine the absence of TMD.

In effect, TMD painful symptoms can largely extend to the anatomical fields of the head and neck. More rarely, TMJ internal derangement may result from infection or tumorous phenomena [73]. Unilateral condyle arthrosis accompanied by osteolysis can signal contralateral TMJ internal derangement [30]. Finally, psoriatic arthritis can affect TMJ and cause muscular tenderness, TMJ sounds, and jaw fatigue [25].

4 Other Tests

For a holistic approach to TMD, postural tests [19, 37, 47, 85] and kinesiologic tests [81] are very helpful for the clinician.

References

1. Abe S, Ouchi Y, Ide Y, Yonesu H (1997) Perspectives on the role of the lateral pterygoid muscle and the sphenomandibular ligament in temporomandibular joint function. Cranio 15(3):203–207
2. Afari N, Wen Y, Buchwald D et al (2008) Are post-traumatic stress disorder symptoms and temporomandibular pain associated? Findings from a community-based twin registry. J Orofac Pain 22(1):41–49
3. Ash MM (1986) Current concepts in the aetiology, diagnosis and treatment of TMJ and muscle dysfunction. J Oral Rehabil 13:1–20

4. Bakland LK, Christiansen EL, Strutz JM (1988) Frequency of dental in traumatic events in the etiology of temporo-mandibular disorders. Endod Dent Traumatol 4(4):182–185
5. Balla J (1989) The late whiplash syndrome. Aust NZ J Surg 50:610–614
6. Barriere P, Zink S, Riehm S et al (2009) Massage du muscle ptérygoïdien latéral dans le SADAM aigu. Rev Stomatol Chir Maxillofac 110:77–80
7. Bell WH (1989) Orofacial pains: classification, diagnosis, management, 3rd edn. Year Book Medical Pub Inc (ed), Chicago, 420p
8. Bernhardt O, Gesch D, Schwahn C et al (2005) Risk factors for headache, including TMD signs and symptoms, and their impact on quality of life. Results of the Study of Health in Pomerania (SHIP). Quintessence Int 36(1):55–64
9. Bernhardt O, Schiffman EL, Look JO (2007) Reliability and validity of a new fingertip-shaped pressure algometer for assessing pressure pain thresholds in the temporomandibular joint and masticatory muscles. J Orofac Pain 21(1):29–38
10. Bocchi L, Orso C (1983) Whiplash injury of the cervical spine. Ital J Orthop Traumatol 9:171–181
11. Braun B, Shifman EL (1991) The validity and predictive value of four assessment instruments for evaluation of the cervical and stomatognathic systems. J Craniomandib Disord Oral Facial Pain 5:239–244
12. Budtz-Jorgensen E, Luan W, Holm-Pedersen P, Fejerskov O (1985) Mandibular dysfunction related to dental, occlusal and prosthetic conditions in a selected elderly population. Gerodontics 1:28–33
13. Burgess J (1991) Symptom characteristics in TMD patients reporting blunt trauma and/or whiplash injury. J Craniomandib Disord Facial Oral Pain 5:251–257
14. Burgess J, Kolbinson DA, Lee PT, Epstein JB (1996) Motor vehicle accidents and TMDs: assessing the relationship. J Am Dent Assoc 127:1767–1772
15. Cacchiotti DA, Plesh O, Bianchi P, Mc Neill C (1991) Signs and symptoms in samples with and without temporomandibular disorders. J Craniomandib Disord Facial Oral Pain 5:167–172
16. Cardonnet TM, Clauzade M (1987) Diagnostic différentiel des dysfonctions de l'ATM. Cah Proth 58:125–169
17. Carpentier P, Yung JP, Marguelles R et al (1986) Microscopical study of the superior lateral pterygoid muscle's attachment. J Dent Res Abstract 65:1033
18. Carroll LJ, Ferrari R, Cassidy JD (2007) Reduced or painful jaw movement after collision-related injuries. A population-based study. J Am Dent Assoc 138(1):86–93
19. Clauzade M, Marty J-P (1998) Orthoposturodontie. SEOO (éd), Perpignan, p 214
20. Cooper BC, Kleinberg I (2007) Examination of a large population for presence of symptoms and signs of temporomandibular disorders. Cranio 25(2):114–126
21. Couly G, Guilbertes F, Cernea P, Bertrand JC (1976) A propos de l'articulation temporomandibulaire du nouveau-né. Les relations oto-méniscales. Rev Stomatol 77:673
22. D'Attilio M, Epifania E, Ciuffolo F et al (2004) Cervical lordosis angle measured on lateral cephalograms; findings in skeletal class II female subjects with and without TMD: a cross sectional study. Cranio 22(1):27–44
23. Dawson PE (1977) Les problèmes de l'occlusion. In: Traduction de Perelmuter S, Liger F (eds) Evaluation diagnostique et traitement. J Prélat (éd), Paris, 352p
24. Demir A, Uysal T, Basciftci FA, Guray E (2005) The association of occlusal factors with masticatory muscle tenderness in 10- to 19-year old Turkish subjects. Angle Orthod 75(1):40–46
25. Dervis E, Dervis E (2005) The prevalence of temporomandibular disorders in patients with psoriasis with or without psoriatic arthritis. J Oral Rehabil 32(11):786–793
26. De Wijer A, Steenks MH, De Leeuw J et al (1996) Symptoms of the cervical spine in temporomandibular and cervical spine disorders. J Oral Rehabil 23:742–750
27. Egermark-Eriksson I, Ingerval B, Carlsson GE (1983) The dependence of mandibular dysfunction in children on functional and morphologic malocclusion. Am J Orthod 83:187
28. Eversole L, Stone CE, Matheson D, Kaplan H (1985) Psychometric profiles and facial pain. Oral Surg 60(3):269–274

29. Farrar WB (1978) Characteristics of condylar path in internal derangement of TMJ. J Prosthet Dent 39:319
30. Farrar WB, Mc Carthy W (1982) A clinical outline of TMJ: diagnosis and treatment. Normandy Study Group for TMJ Dysfunction, 7th edn. Walker Co (ed), Montgomery
31. Fischer DJ, Mueller BA, Critchlow CW, LeResche L (2006) The association of temporomandibular disorder pain with history of head and neck injury in adolescents. J Orofac Pain 20(3):191–198
32. Fondras J-C (2005) La douleur, entre objet et sujet. Douleurs 6(1):23–27
33. Forssell H, Kangasniemi P (1984) Correlation of the frequency and intensity of headache to mandibular dysfunction in headache patients. Proc Finn Dent Soc 80:223–226
34. Forssell H, Kangasniemi P (1984) Mandibular dysfunction in patients with muscle contraction headache. Proc Finn Dent Soc 80:211–216
35. Friedman MH, Weisberg J (2000) The craniocervical connection: a retrospective analysis of 300 whiplash patients with cervical and temporomandibular disorders. Cranio 18(3): 163–167
36. Fujiki T, Inoue M, Miyawaki S et al (2004) Relationship between maxillofacial morphology and deglutitive tongue movement in patients with anterior open bite. Am J Orthod Dentofacial Orthop 125(2):160–167
37. Gagey PM, Toupet M, Heuschen S (1992) From ankle to hip strategy: aging as shown by the parameter VSY. In: Woollacott M, Horak F (eds) Posture and gait. Control mechanisms, vol II., pp 251–253
38. Gambade S, Marteau JM, Caix P (2006) Rôle du muscle ptérygoïdien médial dans les dysfonctions cranio-mandibulaires. Méd Bucc Chir Bucc 12(2):73–82
39. Garcia R Jr, Arrington JA (1996) The relationship between cervical whiplash and temporomandibular joint injuries. An MRI study. Cranio 14(3):233–239
40. Garliner D (1974) Myofunction therapy in dental practice: abnormal swallowing habits. Diagnosis, treatment: a course of study for the dental practitioner and speech pathologist, 2nd edn. Bartel Dental Book Co (ed), Brooklyn, 281p
41. Gaspard M (1979) L'appareil manducateur et la manducation (2 t). J Prélat (éd), Paris
42. Gay T, Bertolami CN, Donoff RB et al (1987) The acoustical characteristics of the normal and abnormal temporomandibular joint. J Oral Maxillo Fac Surg 45(5):397–407
43. Gelb H (1985) Clinical management of head, neck and TMJ pain and dysfunction: a multidisciplinary approach to diagnosis and treatment. WB Saunders Co (ed), Philadelphia/London/Toronto
44. Gelb H, Gelb M (1989) Taking the mystique out of the diagnosis and treatment of craniomandibular (TMJ) disorders. Int Dent J 39(2):129–139
45. Godoy F, Rosenblatt A, Godoy-Bezerra J (2007) Temporomandibular disorders and associated factors in Brazilian teenagers: a cross-sectional study. Int J Prosthod 20(6):599–605
46. Goldberg MB (1999) Posttraumatic temporomandibular disorders. J Orofac Pain 13(4):291–294
47. Guillaume P (1993) Remarques sur l'examen clinique postural. Crit Postur 58:10
48. Hall E, Terezhalmy GT, Pelleu GB, Bethesda PD (1986) A set of descriptors for the diagnosis of dental pain syndrome. Oral Surg Oral Medic Oral Pathol 61:153–157
49. Harkins S, Marteney J (1985) Extrinsic trauma: a significant precipitation factor in temporomandibular dysfunction. J Prosthet Dent 54:271–272
50. Hartmann F (1979) Les douleurs cranio-faciales d'origine dentaire. Medit Medic 3:7–15
51. Hartmann F, Cucchi G (1987) Muscle ptérygoïdien et SADAM: diagnostic précoce et traitement. Rev Odont Stomatol 16(3):209–218
52. Hartmann F, Cucchi G (1993) Les dysfonctions cranio-mandibulaires (SADAM). Nouvelles perspectives médicales. Springer-Verlag (éd), Paris, 176p
53. Hartmann F, Sauget Y, Orofino J (1990) Incidences des chocs sur la posture et le mouvement de l'articulation temporo-maxillaire. Arch Inter Physiol Bioch 98(4):C16–C17
54. Hartmann F, Cucchi G, Antrassian J et al (1985) Neurophysiologie et équilibration en prothèse adjointe totale. Cah Proth 51:79–90

55. Heise AP, Laskin DM, Gervin AS (1992) Incidence of temporo-mandibular joint symptoms following whiplash injury. J Oral Maxillofac Surg 50:825–828
56. Howard RP, Benedict JV, Raddin JH, Smith HL (1991) Assessing neck extension-flexion as a basis for temporo-mandibular joint dysfunction. J Oral Maxillofac Surg 49:1210–1213
57. Isberg AM, Isacsson G, Williams WN, Loughner BA (1987) Lingual numbness and speech articulation deviation associated with temporomandibular joint disk displacement. Oral Surg Oral Med Oral Pathol 64:9–14
58. Jeanmonod A (1988) Occlusodontie. Applications cliniques. Cah Proth (éd), Paris
59. Juniper RP (1984) Temporomandibular joint dysfunction: a theory based upon electromyographic studies of the lateral pterygoid muscle. Br J Oral Maxillofac Surg 22:1–8
60. Kampe T, Hannerz H, Strom P (1991) Five-year follow-up of mandibular dysfunction in adolescents with intact and restored dentitions: a comparative anamnestic and clinical study. J Craniomandib Disord Facial Oral Pain 5:121–128
61. Keersmaekers K, De Boever JA, Van Den Berghe L (1996) Otalgia in patients with temporomandibular joint disorders. J Prosthet Dent 75(1):72–76
62. Klemetti E (1996) Signs of temporomandibular dysfunction related to edentulousness and complete dentures: an anamnestic study. Cranio 14(2):154–157
63. Klobas L, Tegelberg A, Axelsson S (2004) Symptoms and signs of temporomandibular disorders in individuals with chronic whiplash-associated disorders. Swed Dent J 28(1):29–36
64. Kolbinson DA, Epstein JB, Burgess JA, Senthilselvan A (1997) Temporomandibular disorders, headaches, and neck pain after motor vehicle accidents: a pilot investigation of persistence and litigation effects. J Prosthet Dent 77:46–53
65. Kolbinson DA, Epstein JB, Senthilselvan A, Burgess JA (1997) A comparison of TMD patients with or without prior motor vehicle accident involvement: treatment and outcomes. J Orofac Pain 11(4):337–345
66. Kreisberg MK (1986) Headache as a symptom of craniomandibular disorders I: pathophysiology. Cranio 4(2):135–142
67. Krogstad BS, Jokstad A, Dahl BL, Soboleva U (1998) Somatic complaints, psychologic distress and treatment outcome in two groups of TMD patients, one previously subjected to whiplash injury. J Orofac Pain 12(2):136–143.
68. Kronn E (1993) The incidence of TMJ dysfunction in patients who have suffered a cervical whiplash injury following a traffic accident. J Orofac Pain 7(2):209–213
69. Levandosky J (1993) Mandibular whiplash. Part II: an extension flexion injury of the temporomandibular joints. Funct Orthod 10(2):45–51
70. Mahan PE, Thomas PD, Wilkinson M et al (1983) Superior and inferior bellies of the lateral pterygoid muscle EMG activity at basic jaw positions. Res Educ 50(5):170–178
71. Mannheimer J, Attanasio R, Cinotti WR, Pertes R (1989) Cervical strain and mandibular whiplash effects upon the craniomandibular apparatus. Clin Prev Dent 11(1):29–32
72. Mc Namara JA, Seligman DA, Okeson JP (1994) Occlusion, orthodontic treatment and temporomandibular disorders: a review. J Orofac Pain 9:73–89
73. Mc Neill C (1990) Craniomandibular disorders: guidelines for evaluation, diagnosis and management. American Academy of Craniomandibular Disorders, Quintesc Pub (ed), Chicago, pp 13–53
74. Miller DB (1998) Low velocity impact, vehicle damage and passenger injury. Cranio 16(4):226–229
75. Miller JR, Mancl L, Critchlow C (2005) Severe retrognathia as a risk factor for recent onset painful TMJ disorders among adult females. J Orthodont 32(4):249–256
76. Minagi S, Watanabe H, Takashi S, Hiromichi T (1990) The relationship between balancing side occlusal contact patterns and TMJ sounds in humans: proposition of the concept of balancing-side protection. J Craniomandib Disord Facial Oral Pain 4:251–256
77. Mock D (1999) The differential diagnosis of temporomandibular disorders. J Orofac Pain 13(4):246–250
78. Moller E, Troelstrup B (1975) Functional and morphological asymmetry in children with unilateral cross-bite. J Dent Res Abstract 54:L45

79. Mongini F (1984) The stomatognathic system. Quintes Pub Co Inc (ed), Chicago/Berlin/London/Rio de Janeiro/Tokyo
80. Morgan DH, Hall WP, Vanwas SJ (1977) Diseases of the temporo-mandibular apparatus. A multidisciplinary approach. CV Mosby Co (ed), St Louis, 481p
81. Nahmani L, Zarrinpour A, Lumbroso C (1995) La mise en articulateur selon le concept posturo-kinésiologique. Orthod Franç 66:605–626
82. Ogi N, Nagao T, Toyama M, Ariji E (2002) Chronic dental infections mimicking temporomandibular disorders. Aust Dent J 47(1):63–65
83. Ogus HD, Toller PA (1981) Common disorders of temporomandibular joint. J Wright & Sons (ed), Bristol
84. Palazzi C, Miralles R, Soto MA, Santander H, Zuñiga C, Moya H (1996) Body position effect on EMG activity of sternocleidomastoid and masseter muscles in patients with myogenic cranio-cervical-mandibular dysfunction. Cranio 14(3):200–209
85. Perez P, Pradier P, Daures JP, Bouges S (1997) Dépistage des précontraintes posturales sur les ATM: axiogrammes posturaux. In: Lacour M, Gagey PM, Weber B (eds) Posture et environnement. Sauramps Méd (éd), Montpellier, 87p
86. Perry HT (1969) Myofascial pain dysfunction syndrome: the orthodontic view point. J Am Dent Assoc 79:137
87. Pinto OF (1966) Temporomandibular joint problems in underwater activities. J Prosthet Dent 16:772–781
88. Planas P (1992) La réhabilitation occlusale. (Traduction: Chateau M, Kolf J) Masson (éd), Paris
89. Probert TCS, Wiesenfeld D, Reade PC (1994) Temporomandibular pain dysfunction disorder resulting from road traffic accidents – An Australian study. Int J Oral Maxillofac Surg 23:338–341
90. Pullinger AG, Seligman DA, Solberg WK (1988) Temporomandibular disorders. Part II: occlusal factors associated with TMJ tenderness and dysfunction. J Prosthet Dent 59:363–367
91. Rammelsberg P, LeResche L, Dworkin S, Mancl L (2003) Longitudinal outcome of temporomandibular disorders: a 5-year epidemiologic study of muscle disorders defined by research diagnostic criteria for temporomandibular disorders. J Orofac Pain 17(1):9–20
92. Reik L (1985) Unnecessary dental treatment in headache patients for temporomandibular joint disorders. Headache 25(5):246–248
93. Rigolet D (1983) Le syndrome de dysfonctionnement des ATM. Ann Oto Laryngol 98:527
94. Ronquillo HI, Guay J, Tallents RH et al (1988) Comparison of internal derangements with condyle fossa relationships, horizontal and vertical overlap, and Angle class. J Craniomandib Disord Facial Oral Pain 2:137–140
95. Roydhouse RH (1973) Whiplash and temporomandibular dysfunction. Lancet 1:1394–1395
96. Runyan DA, Shimoda LM, Mc Gowan MJ (1989) Treatment for acute craniomandibular dysfunction symptoms in edentulous patients with unserviceable or no existing complete dentures. J Prosthet Dent 62(5):542–545
97. Sadowsky C, Muhl ZF, Sakols EI, Sommerville JM (1985) Temporomandibular joint sound related to orthodontic therapy. J Dent Res 64(12):1392–1395
98. Sale H, Isberg A (2007) Delayed temporomandibular joint pain and dysfunction induced by whiplash trauma: a controlled prospective study. J Am Dent Assoc 138(8):1084–1091
99. Schneider K, Zernicke RF, Clark G (1989) Modeling of jaw-head-neck dynamics during whiplash. J Dent Res 68(9):1360–1365
100. Schwartz HC, Kendrick RW (1984) Internal derangements of the temporomandibular joint: description of clinical syndromes. Oral Surg Oral Med 58(1):24–29
101. Scott DS, Lundeen TF (1980) Myofascial pain involving the masticatory muscles: an experimental model. Pain 8:207–215
102. Seligman DA, Pullinger AG (1991) The role of functional occlusal relationships in temporomandibular disorders: a review. J Craniomandib Disord Facial Oral Pain 5:265–279
103. Serviere F (1988) Dysfonction linguale et SADAM. Inf Dent 15(14):1211–1217

104. Spruijt RJ, Hoogstraten J (1991) The research on temporomandibular joint clicking: a methodological review. J Craniomandib Disord Facial Oral Pain 5:45–50
105. Steigerwald D, Verne SV, Young D (1996) A retrospective evaluation of the impact of TMJ arthroscopy on the symptoms of headache, neck pain, shoulder pain, dizziness and tinnitus. Cranio 14(1):46–54
106. Stiesch-Scholz M, Fink M, Tschernitschek H (2003) Comorbidity of internal derangement of the temporomandibular joint and silent dysfunction of the cervical spine. J Oral Rehabil 30(4):386–391
107. Stockstill JW, Gross AJ, Mc Call WD Jr (1989) Interrater reliability in masticatory muscle palpation. J Craniomandib Disord 3(3):143–146
108. Stratmann U, Mokrys K, Meyer U et al (2000) Clinical anatomy and palpability of the inferior lateral pterygoid muscle. J Prosthet Dent 83(5):548–554
109. Tanaka TT (1984) Recognition of the pain formula for head, neck and TMJ disorders: the general physical examination. Calif Dent Assoc J 12(5):43–49
110. Tanne K, Tanaka E (1993) Association between malocclusion and temporomandibular disorders in orthodontic patients before treatment. J Orofac Pain 7:156–162
111. Travell JG (1981) Identification of myofascial trigger point syndrome: a case of atypical facial neuralgia. Arch Physio Med Rehabil 62:100–106
112. Travell JG, Simons DG (1983) Myofascial pain and dysfunction. The trigger-point manual. Williams & Wilkins (ed), Baltimore, 713p
113. Turp JC, Minagi S (2001) Palpation of the lateral pterygoid region in TMD-where is the evidence? J Dent 29(7):475–483
114. Urbanowicz M (1987) Alteration of vertical dimension and its effect on head and neck posture. Cranio 5:51–53.
115. Villarosa GA, Moss RA (1995) Oral behavior patterns as factors contributing to the development of head and facial pain. J Prosth Dent 54(3):427–430
116. Wänman A (1995) The relationship between muscle tenderness and craniomandibular disorders: a study of 35-years old from the general population. J Orofac Pain 9(3):235–243
117. Wänman A, Agerberg G (1986) Two-year longitudinal study of symptoms of mandibular dysfunction in adolescents. Act Odont Scand 44(6):321–331
118. Wänman A, Agerberg G (1986) Mandibular dysfunction in adolescents. II: prevalence of signs. Act Odont Scand 44(6):55–62
119. Webb C (1995) Whiplash: mechanisms and patterns of tissue injury. J Aust Chir Assoc 15(2):60–69
120. Weinberg S, Lapointe H (1987) Cervical extension-flexion injury (whiplash) and internal derangement of the temporomandibular joint. J Oral Maxillofac Surg 45(8):653–656
121. Westling L, Carlsson GE, Helkimo M (1990) Background factors in CMD with special references to general joint hypermobility, parafunctions and trauma. J Craniomandib Disord Facial Oral Pain 4:89–98
122. Wright EF, Des Rosier KF, Bifano SL (1997) The prevalence and prediction of rheumatic disorders among temporomandibular disorder patients. J Orofac Pain 11(2):abstract n°29
123. Young S, Jordan JC (1982) EMG activity of the sternomastoid muscles in relation to mouth movement. J Dent Res Abstract 61, 4:158

Stomatognathic Parafunctions

Oral parafunctions are defined as motor sequences that aim at satisfying oral needs but implicate compensating and substituting muscles or muscular sets when their onset is inadequate. Specialists recognize two major forms: **teeth grinding** and **teeth clenching**. *Grinding* is an isotonic muscular contraction. The jaw moves horizontally and affects dental tissues (enamel) or supporting tissues (periodontium). Obvious signs such as premature wearing on faces can be observed during clinical inspections. It can also be noticed by spouses at night (sounds). Inversely *clenching* may remain totally unnoticed. Clenching contraction is isometric without any lateral excursive movement [3]. Due to impossible structural compensation, this parafunctional form is particularly harmful to soft tissues (muscles) in the short term. This may explain the link observed between parafunction and muscle pain and discomfort [20]. When it continues for long periods of time, the parafunction can create more complex secondary local problems such as arthrosis in the TMJ. While links between oral parafunction and TMD symptoms are hard to establish [2], some authors have noted a significant connection between oral habits (grinding) and neck pain in children aged between 4 and 6 [32]. There is evidence of the involvement of stomatognathic muscle spasticity responding to *central factors* (psycho-emotional) and/or *peripheral factors* (dental occlusal disorders, lingual dysfunction, working or sleeping malposition, severe traumatism, etc.). A recent functional MRI study seemed to correlate occlusal disturbances and emotions as potentially convergent factors to magnify with clenching the neural processing into the brain [25]. Most patients are unaware of their involuntary clenching habit [19] and not willing to admit it, as the habit is deeply ingrained in their behavior. They gradually become conscious of it in the days following the first consultation. This is a very important point in the process of making a diagnosis. It is indeed necessary to give the patient sufficient time for his self-discovery of any parafunctional habit. The process is easier if done outside the consultation room, particularly during activities that require attention and concentration, such as driving a car, working on a computer, pealing vegetables, sewing, and performing mental calculation. In our previous manual [11], we showed the percentage of consciousness of parafunctional clenching in a personal group of patients (Fig. 1). Other resting or sleeping postures are

F. Hartmann, G. Cucchi, *Stress and Orality*,
DOI 10.1007/978-2-8178-0271-8_4, © Springer-Verlag France 2014

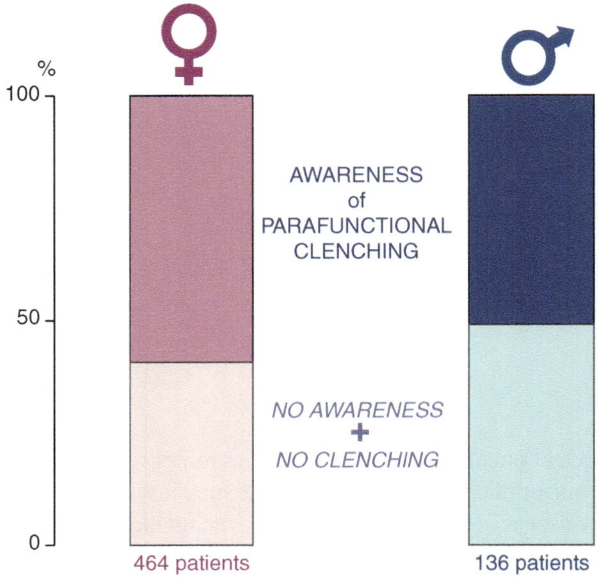

Fig. 1 Percentage of awareness of parafunctional clenching in pathological groups according to gender

stressful [31]: watching television, leaning head on hands, resting elbows on knees, or reading while stretched out or lying on one side. This is particularly obvious in professional occupations such as typists or dental surgeons. The overall picture is consistent with insidious repetitive factors such as chronic micro-traumas that help trigger certain muscular spasms. Several cases of TMD have been reported in *divers* [1] and *musicians* [4, 5, 12, 13, 26]. This predisposition to TMD is confirmed by studies [18]: *violinists* and *violists* frequently clench their teeth during concerts and as many as 40 % of them complain of either growing or aggravated neck pain [13]. It is clinically important to ask the patient *"do you occasionally or frequently clench your jaw muscles and hold your teeth together tightly?"* because clenching seems to initiate the **most deleterious forms of TMD** [6, 10, 14–16, 23, 24, 28, 30]. Parafunctional habits can cause trauma in the form of micro-trauma, and this can play an important role in initiating and maintaining reported signs and symptoms [19]. Links between muscular symptoms and psychosocial stressful factors in TMD patients are evidenced by the significant correlation between clenching and muscular pain [9]. Therefore, the role of sociocultural factors affecting the patient at a psycho-affective level and the psychosocial dimension of the patient's history must be taken into account [33]. This helps evaluate the different constraints exercised on the patient's psycho-affective life by professional stressors and more largely relational stressors. In any case, severity levels of parafunctional habits must be evaluated to facilitate etiological TMD therapy [22]. In children, however, causal links between oral parafunction and TMD signs or symptoms are less evident [2]. There are several oral parafunctions (Fig. 2). A good metaphor to make a distinction between grinding and clenching is to compare teeth grinding to the visible tip of the "*parafunctional iceberg*" while **clenching is its hidden part** (Fig. 3). Indeed

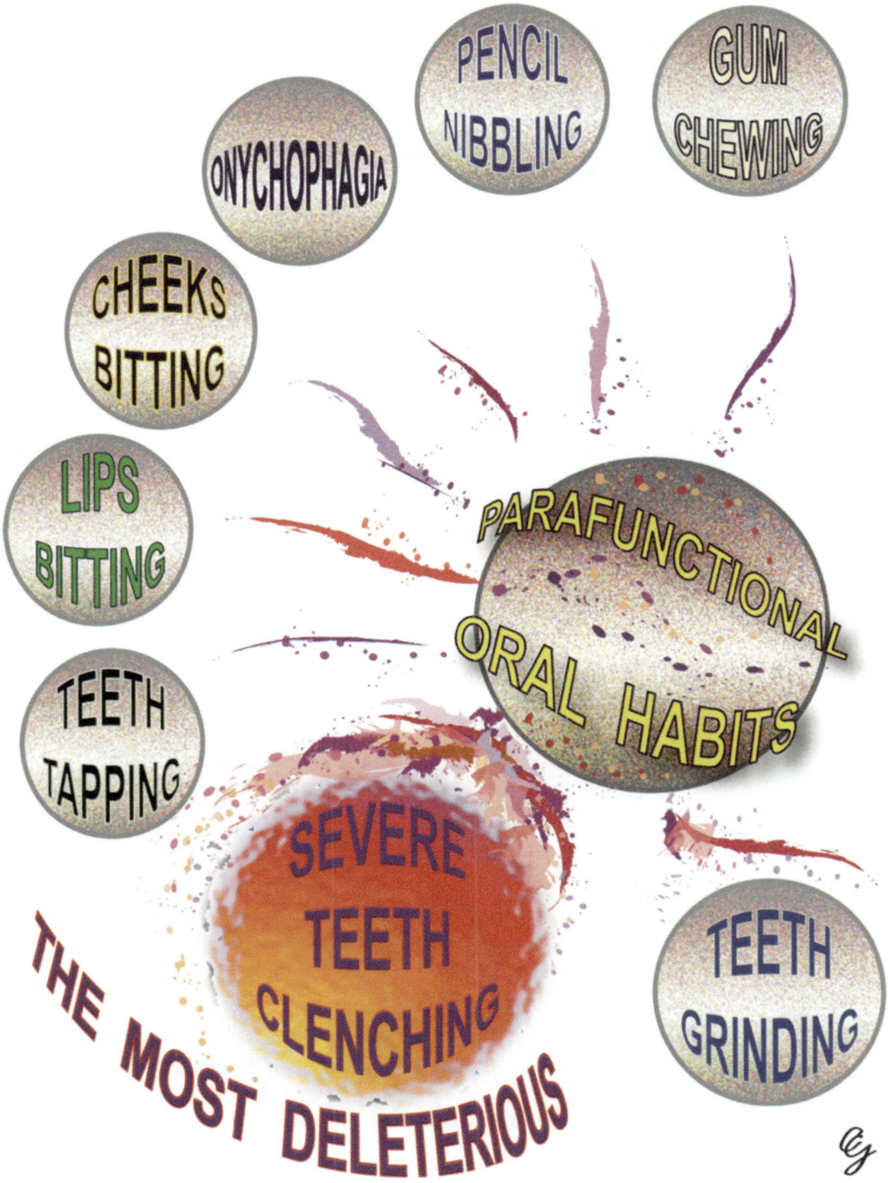

Fig. 2 Some oral parafunctional habits

grinding is easily observed during clinical examination. Clenching, clinically obscure (Fig. 4), on the other hand, has long been misunderstood. Today, given its detrimental and invalidating effect, this parafunction requires the clinician's undivided attention, whatever his specialty. Aside from bruxism, medical history will sometimes reveal a number of associated tics such as pencil nibbling, nail chewing,

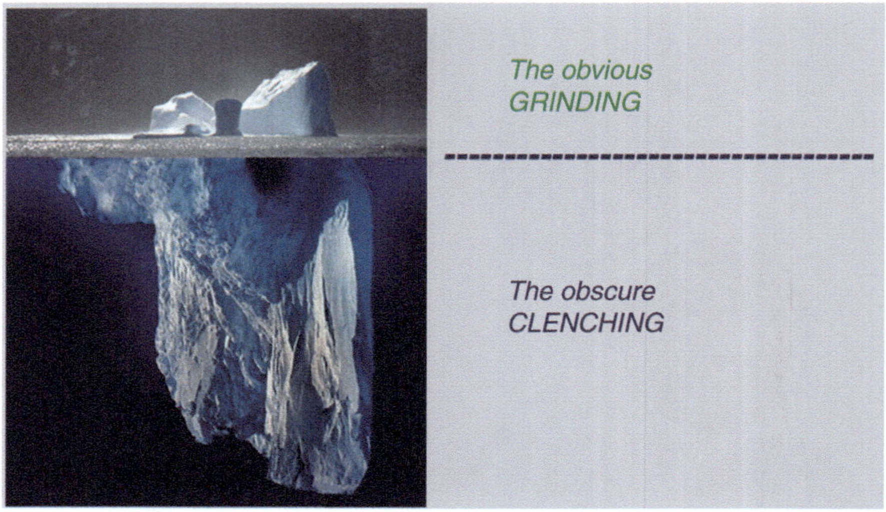

Fig. 3 The "parafunctional iceberg." As compared to clinically recognizable grinding, clenching may be considered as a tricky oral parafunction, that is, invisible during the clinical examination of dental arches

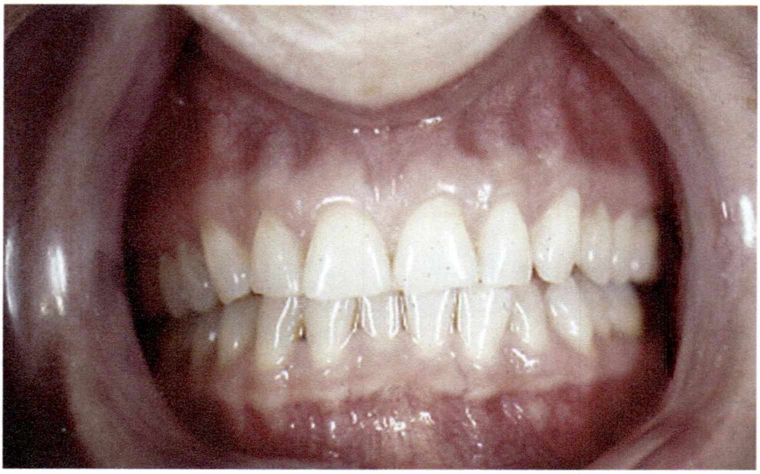

Fig. 4 Rather fine dental arches, aren't they? And yet she clenches!

lip or cheek biting particularly in female adolescents [7], teeth contacting habits [17], and gum chewing [16]. According to psychology experts, most of these habits are compensating phenomena due to psycho-emotional-blocked attitudes in *introverted subjects*. However, clinicians can be alerted of a patient's pencil biting habit when he obtains relief by positioning something between the upper and lower dental arches. The vertical dimension of occlusion is probably underestimated or inadequate (see chapter "Objective Signs"). The patient must then be referred to a dentist.

Information on the patient's eating habits can also prove useful, particularly when there is a tendency to chewing on one side only [8, 21, 29]. Some specialists [27] choose to observe the actual masticatory moods of their patients themselves by having them chew gum during their clinical examination.

References

1. Aldridge RD, Fenlon MR (2004) Prevalence of temporomandibular dysfunction in a group of scuba divers. Br J Sports Med 38:69–73
2. Barone A, Sbordone L, Ramaglia L (1997) Craniomandibular disorders and orthodontic treatment need in children. J Oral Rehabil 24(1):2–7
3. Boyd CH (1987) The effect of head position on EMG evaluations of representative mandibular positioning muscle groups. Cranio 5:51–53
4. Bryant GWT (1989) Myofacial pain dysfunction and viola playing. Br Dent J 166:335–336
5. Corcoran DF (1985) Dental problems in musicians. J Int Dent Assoc 31(1):4–7
6. Egermark-Eriksson I, Carlsson GE, Magnusson T (1987) A Long-Term Epidemiologic Study of the Relationship between occlusal Factors and Mandibular Dysfunction in Children and Adolescents. J Dent Res 66(1):67–71
7. Feteih RM (2006) Signs and symptoms of temporomandibular disorders and oral parafunctions in urban Saudi Arabian adolescents: a research report. Head Face Med 16(2):25
8. Fujita Y, Motegi E, Nomura M et al (2003) Oral habits of temporomandibular disorder patients with malocclusion. Bull Tokyo Dent Coll 44(4):201–207
9. Hagberg C, Hagberg M, Kopp S (1994) Musculoskeletal symptoms and psychosocial factors among patients with craniomandibular disorders. Acta Odontol Scand 52:170–177
10. Hartmann F, Sarrat P, Gaudy JF et al (1988) Muscle ptérygoïdien latéral, dissection anatomique et imagerie médicale. Perspectives dans le traitement du SADAM. Act Odont Stomatol 163:545–566
11. Hartmann F, Cucchi G (1993) Les dysfonctions cranio-mandibulaires (SADAM). Nouvelles perspectives médicales. Springer-Verlag (éd), Paris, 176p
12. Hirsch JA, Mc Call WD, Bishop B (1982) Jaw dysfunction in violin and viola players. J Am Dent Assoc 104:838–843
13. Howard JA, Lovrovich AT (1989) Wind instruments: their interplay with orofacial structures. Med Prob Perf Art 4(2):59–72
14. Kampe T, Hannerz H, Strom P (1996) Ten-year follow-up study of signs and symptoms of craniomandibular disorders in adults with intact and restored dentitions. J Oral Rehabil 23(6):416–423
15. Kampe T, Tagdae T, Tagdae G, Edman G, Karlsson S (1997) Reported symptoms and clinical findings in a group of subjects with long-standing bruxism. J Oral Rehabil 15:314–325
16. Kernbaum S (1990) Eléments de pathologie infectieuse 5ème éd. Simep/Specia, Paris
17. Kino K, Sugisaki M, Haketa T et al (2006) Teeth contacting habit as a contributing factor to chronic pain in patients with temporomandibular disorders. J Med Dent Sci 53(2):103–109
18. Kovero O, Kokonen M (1996) Signs and symptoms of temporo-mandibular disorders in adolescent violin players. Acta Odontol Scand 54(4):271–274
19. Lobbezoo-Scholte AM, De Leeuw JRJ, Steenks MH et al (1995) Diagnostic subgroups of craniomandibular disorders. J Orofac Pain 9(1):24–43
20. Manfredini D, Cantini E, Romagnoli M, Bosco M (2003) Prevalence of bruxism in patients with different research diagnostic criteria for temporomandibular disorders (RDC/TMD) diagnoses. Cranio 21(4):279–285
21. Miyake R, Ohkubo R, Takehara J, Morita M (2004) Oral parafunctions and association with symptoms of temporomandibular disorders in Japanese university students. J Oral Rehabil 31(6):518–523

22. Molina OF, Dos Santos J, Nelson SJ, Nowlin T (2000) Profile of TMD and bruxer compared to TMD and nonbruxer patients regarding chief complaint, previous consultations, modes of therapy, and chronicity. Cranio 18(3):205–218
23. Molina OF, Dos Santos J, Mazzetto M (2001) Oral jaw behaviors in TMD and bruxism: a comparison study by severity of bruxism. Cranio 19(2):114–122
24. Moss RA, Lombardo TW, Villarosa GA et al (1995) Oral habits and TMJ dysfunction in facial pain and non-pain subjects. J Oral Rehabil 22(1):79–81
25. Otsuka T, Watanabe K, Hirano Y et al (2009) Effects of mandibular deviation on brain activation during clenching: an fMRI preliminary study. Cranio 27(2):88–93
26. Pinto OF (1966) Temporomandibular joint problems in underwater activities. J Prosthet Dent 16:772–781
27. Planas P (1992) La Réhabilitation Neuro-Occlusale. (Traduction: Chateau M, Kolf J) Masson (éd), Paris
28. Quemar JC, Lazar BD (1992) Multivariate analysis of craniomandibular disorders. Cranio 10(2):89–95
29. Reinhardt R, Tremel T, Wehrbein H, Reinhardt W (2006) The unilateral chewing phenomenon, occlusion, and TMD. Cranio 24(3):166–170
30. Serviere F (1988) Dysfonction linguale et SADAM. Inf Dent 15(14):1211–1217
31. Travell JG, Simons DG (1983) Myofascial pain and dysfunction. The trigger-point manual. Williams & Wilkins (ed), Baltimore, 713p
32. Widmalm SE, Gunn SM, Christiansen RL, Hawley LM (1995) Association between CMD signs and symptoms, oral parafunction, race and sexe, in 4–6 years old African-American and Caucasian children. J Oral Rehabil 22(2):95–100
33. Yardin M (1995) Odontologie globale. Masson (éd), Paris

Part I
In Conclusion

There is evidence of pain and discomfort in constellation, caused by TMD particularly when the structures largely project out of the anatomico-physiological eating territory. When clinical examination yields no results, and previous antalgic, anti-inflammatory, or neuroleptic drug treatments fail, practitioners should consider TMD as a potential source of headaches and even pain affecting areas topographically distant from the oral sphere. Patients may be diagnosed as suffering from migraine or fibromyalgia or chronic fatigue. These are frequent diagnoses among introverted and highly stressed females. Yet, more comprehensive investigations may reveal the existence of a particular harmful oral parafunctional tendency of **clenching** teeth firmly together through a durable tight contraction of the jaw-closing muscles. Experience shows that, unlike grinding, *this motionless type of parafunctional habit repeatedly goes unnoticed.* Practitioners should look for objective evidence in establishing a diagnosis: of particular value is the feeling of pain revealed on palpation of the stomatognathic muscles. In addition, the patient's medical history is helpful in assessing peripheral factors, either postural, occlusal, lingual, traumatic, psycho-emotional, biosocial, or other general factors which sometimes combine to generate or aggravate an illness that is still disconcerting to most.

Part II
Pathophysiology

Introduction

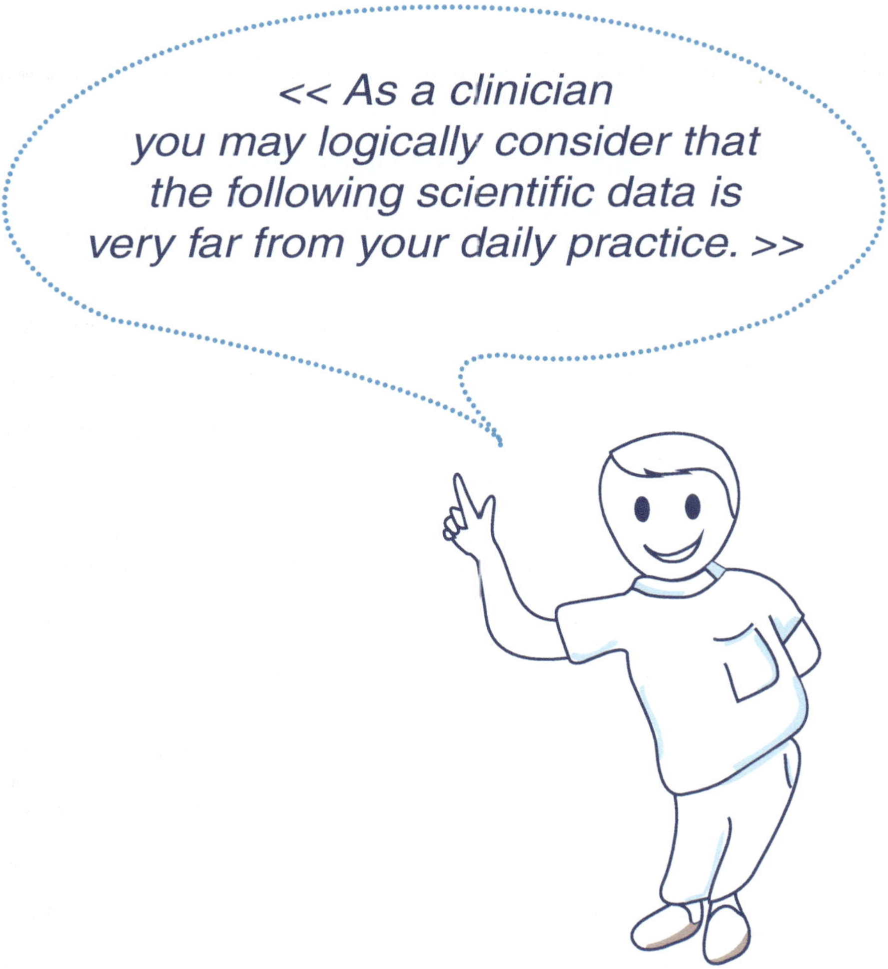

F. Hartmann, G. Cucchi, *Stress and Orality*,
DOI 10.1007/978-2-8178-0271-8_5, © Springer-Verlag France 2014

In fact, pathophysiological data are highly simplified and selected in order to explain the mechanisms of TMD. Based on their personal experience, clinicians should ask themselves the following question: besides TMD, do other little known parafunctional oral habits also play a part in the mechanisms of atypical forms of migraine, fibromyalgia, chronic fatigue, etc.? The question should be carefully validated by further clinical evaluations.[1] However, when faced with unresolved clinical forms, such data can help clinicians identify and eliminate oral habits – particularly the complex deleterious oral parafunction referred to as **severe teeth clenching**. In any case, significant therapeutic results can be expected. TMD classically affect the stomatognathic musculature, the two temporomandibular joints (TMJ), and some associated structures.

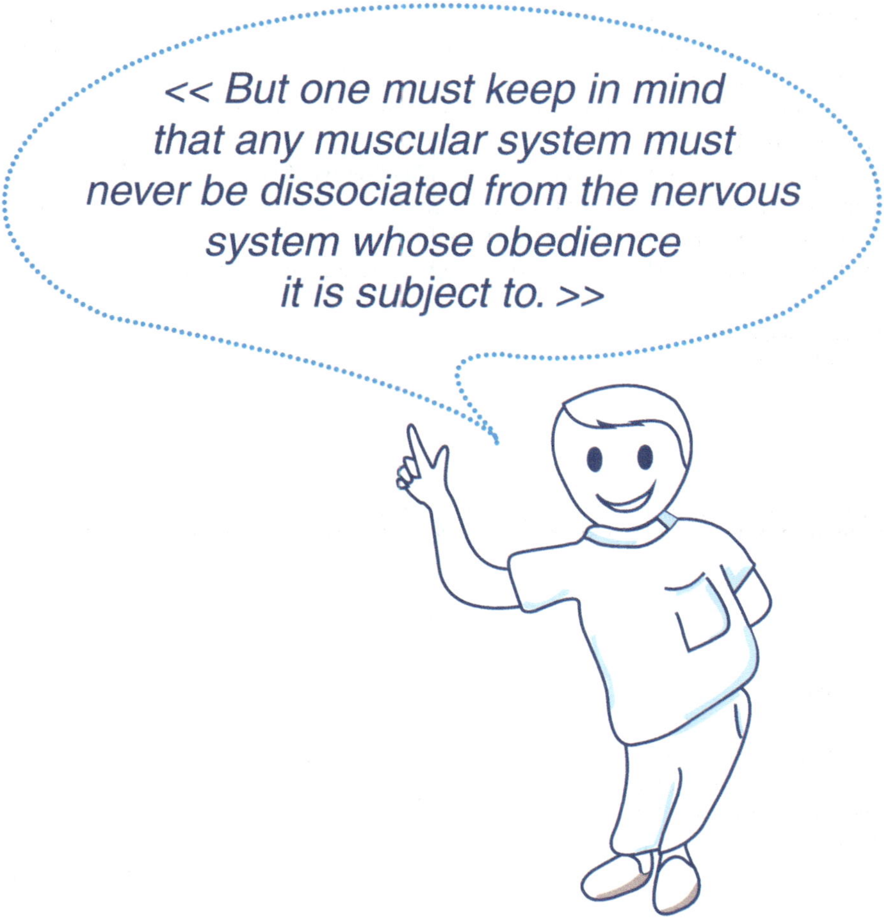
<< But one must keep in mind that any muscular system must never be dissociated from the nervous system whose obedience it is subject to. >>

[1] In fact, most of the data originate from recordings on cats, rats, or monkeys; to extend the data to human physiological conditions, it needs to be substantiated.

There, the condition extends to the brain and its functional roles. Today neurophysiologists agree that the more they recognize the importance of a system, the more highly differentiated its sensory component appears to be. Furthermore, physiologists currently admit that spastic conditions generate maximized inputs. The famous β–γ buckles create intense and/or frequent sensory afferents (proprioceptive as well as nociceptive). When this happens in the *oral sphere*, the most affected nerves are the **paired trigeminal nerves** (V). The paired (V), right and left, are mixed nerves – both sensory and motor (Fig. 1). They greatly innervate the stomatognathic system and send various inputs from the orofacial sphere's tissues (Fig. 2). Furthermore, **the (V) have the most important anatomical representation at the level of the brain stem** (Figs. 3 and 4).

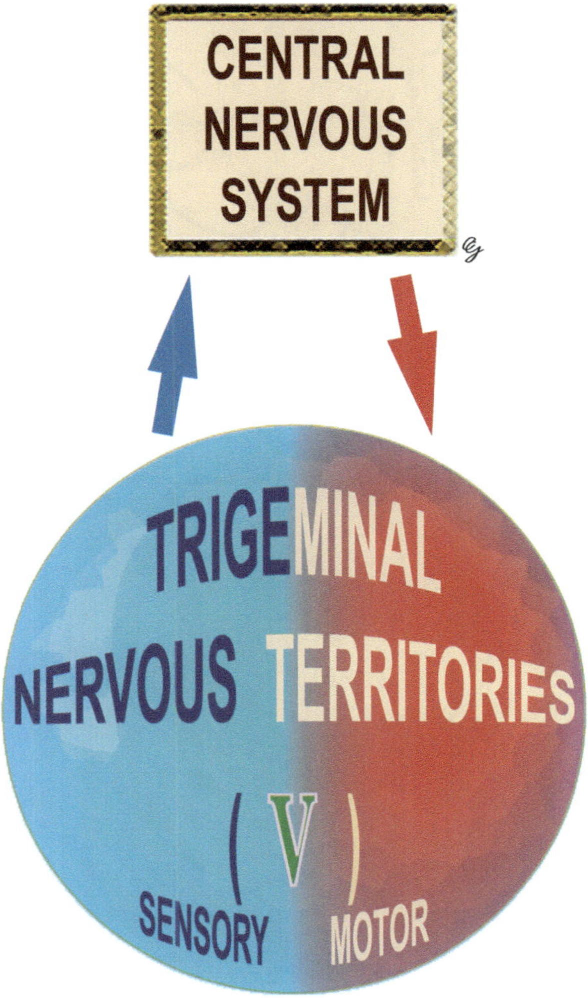

Fig. 1 Trigeminal sensory-motor and mixed complex related to the central nervous system

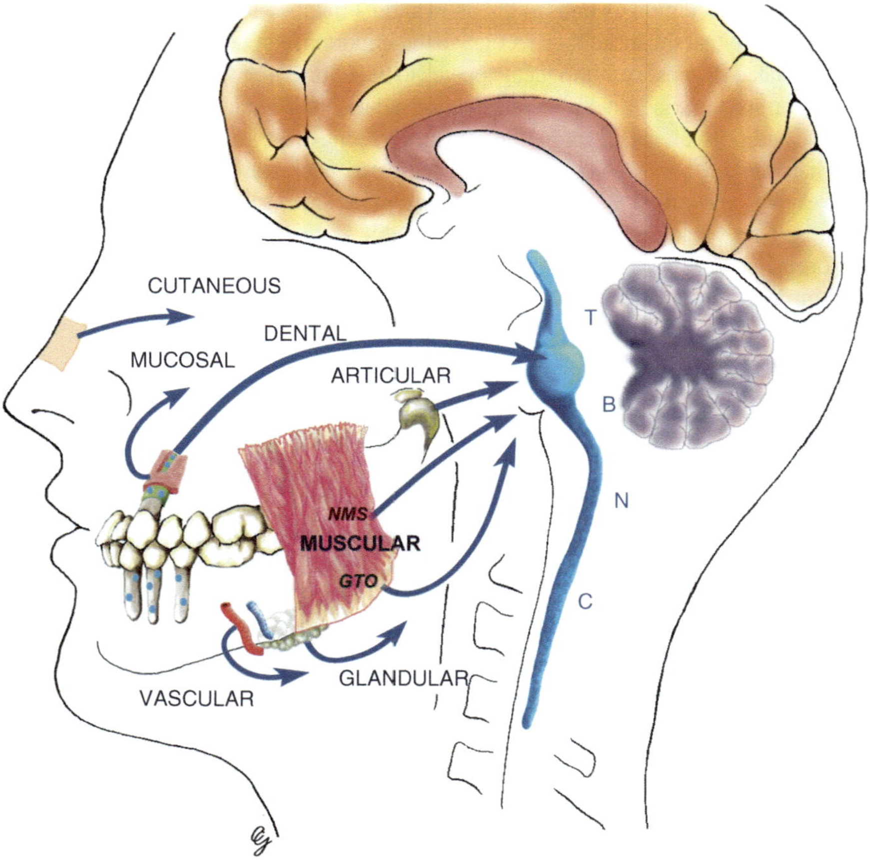

Fig. 2 Trigeminal afferents to the trigeminal brainstem nuclear complex (TBNC)

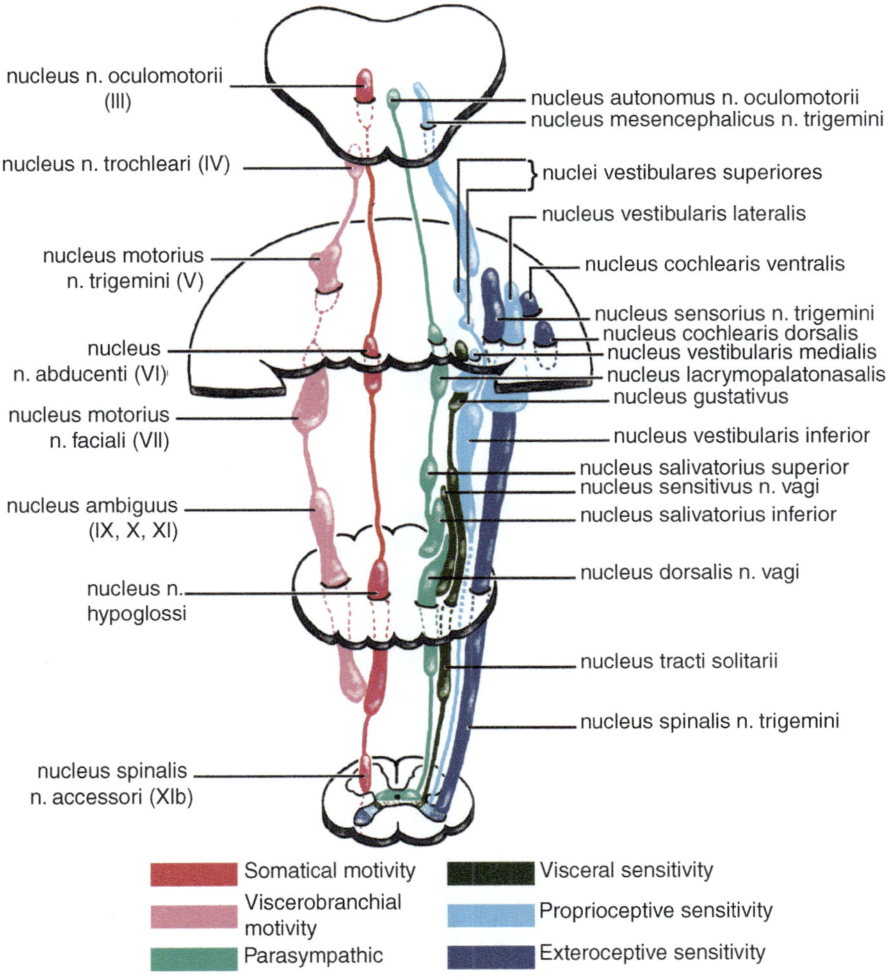

Fig. 3 Nuclei of the cranial nerves (Modified from Bossy [3])

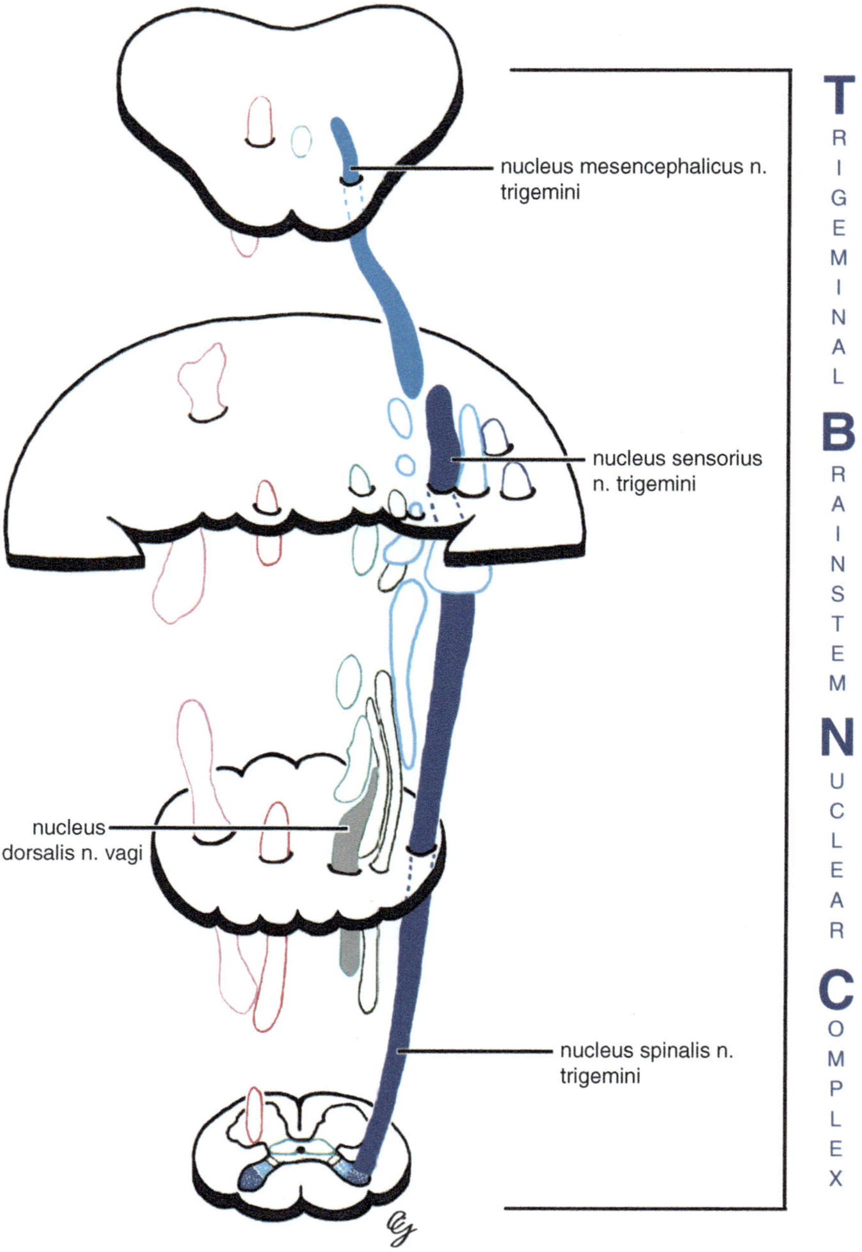

Fig. 4 Trigeminal brainstem nuclear complex (*TBNC*). The sensory nuclei of the (TBNC) are shown in full color. Compare with the nucleus dorsalis nervi vagi (X) shown in gray; both lead to breathing, cardiac contraction, and digestion. No comment

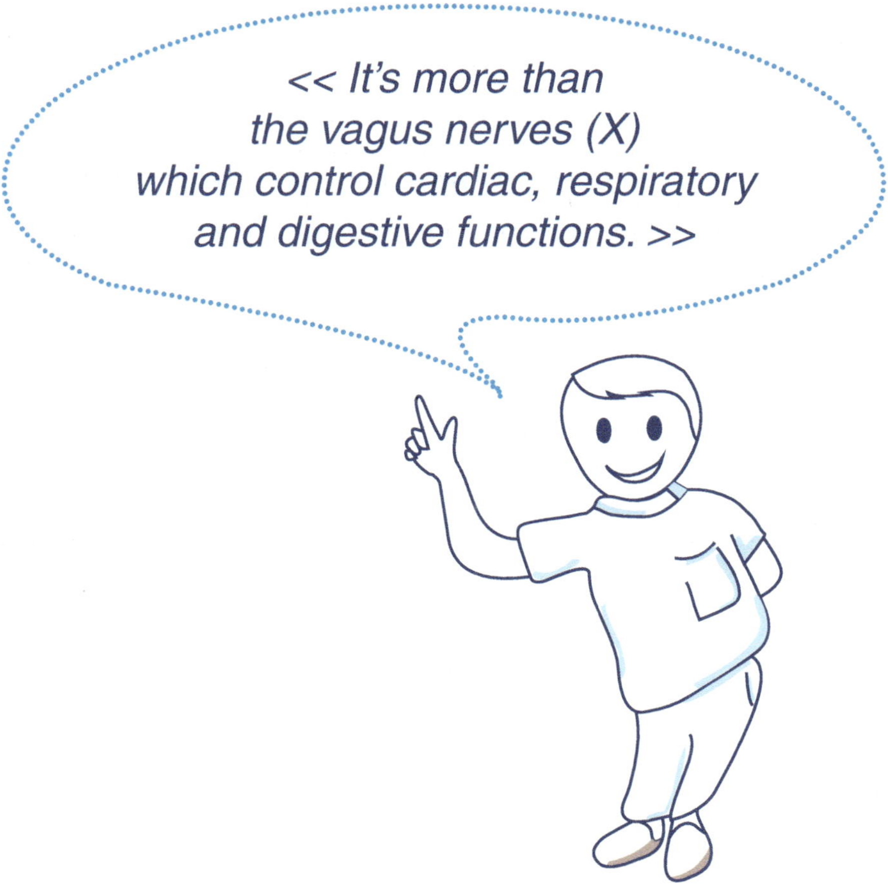
<< It's more than
the vagus nerves (X)
which control cardiac, respiratory
and digestive functions. >>

Yet some neuroscientific data are strangely underestimated. They relate to *rich* and *various nervous connections* between *trigeminal* and *non-trigeminal centers* and shed light on many implications of the paired (V) in various vital physiological functions such as eating, breathing, speaking, hearing, and standing. The fact that a harmonious regulation of the system needs correct inputs coming from the periphery can be easily understood. In spastic oral disorders, abnormal trigeminal afferents are potentially able to *overflow trigeminal centers and disturb non-trigeminal ways*. This kind of "overflowing" phenomenon, generally referred to as "sensitization" by specialists, depends on two factors. The first one is the intensity, durability, and/or frequency of peripheral inputs. The second is the set of conditions of receptivity in the central nervous system.[2]

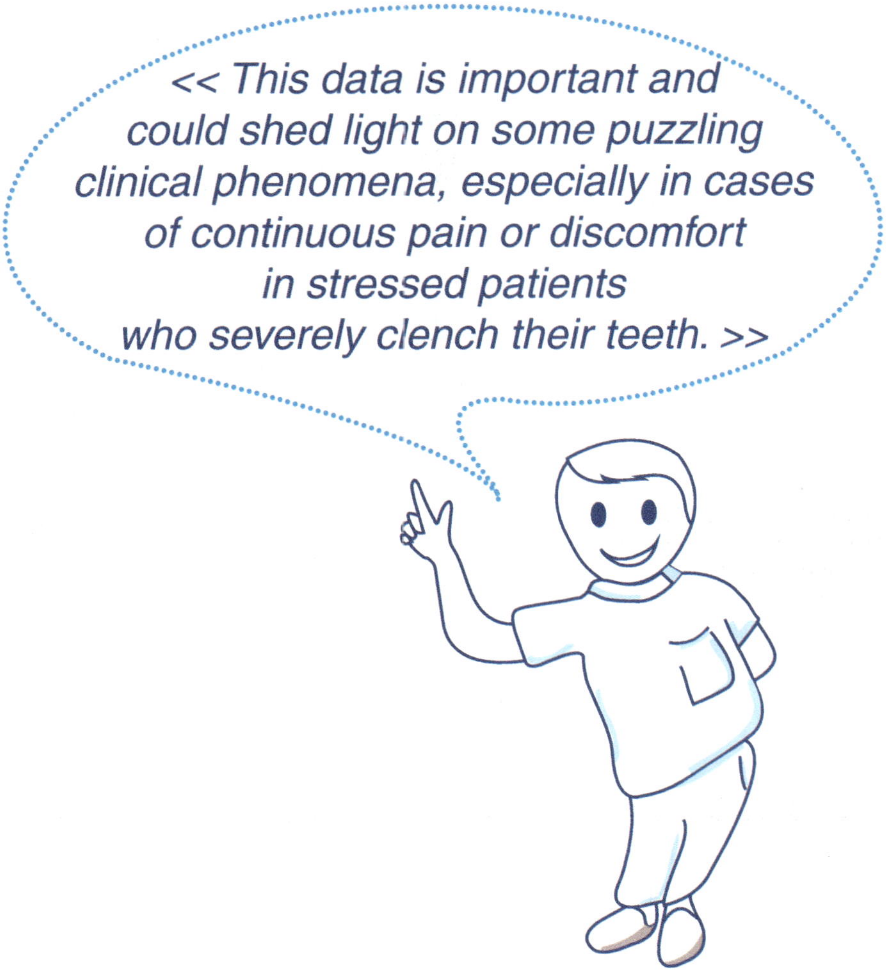

With this in mind, any clinician can reflect on the reasons why uncommon forms of clinical disorders (migraine, fibromyalgia, chronic fatigue, etc.) have failed to respond to classical therapeutic procedures.

---

[2]As a reminder, there is no partition within the nervous system; the only obstacle that nervous inputs must clear are the synapses, that is, the junctions between neurons. Therefore, intense and/or durable inputs run through more easily than low and/or short ones. This phenomenon is facilitated when the central nervous tissues become more sensitive as a result of negative psycho-emotional and peripheral factors. Specialists usually refer to this phenomenon as "sensitization" [1, 2]. We suggest the possible role of trigeminal parafunctional overstimulation (severe clenching) in perpetuating and even increasing sensitization.

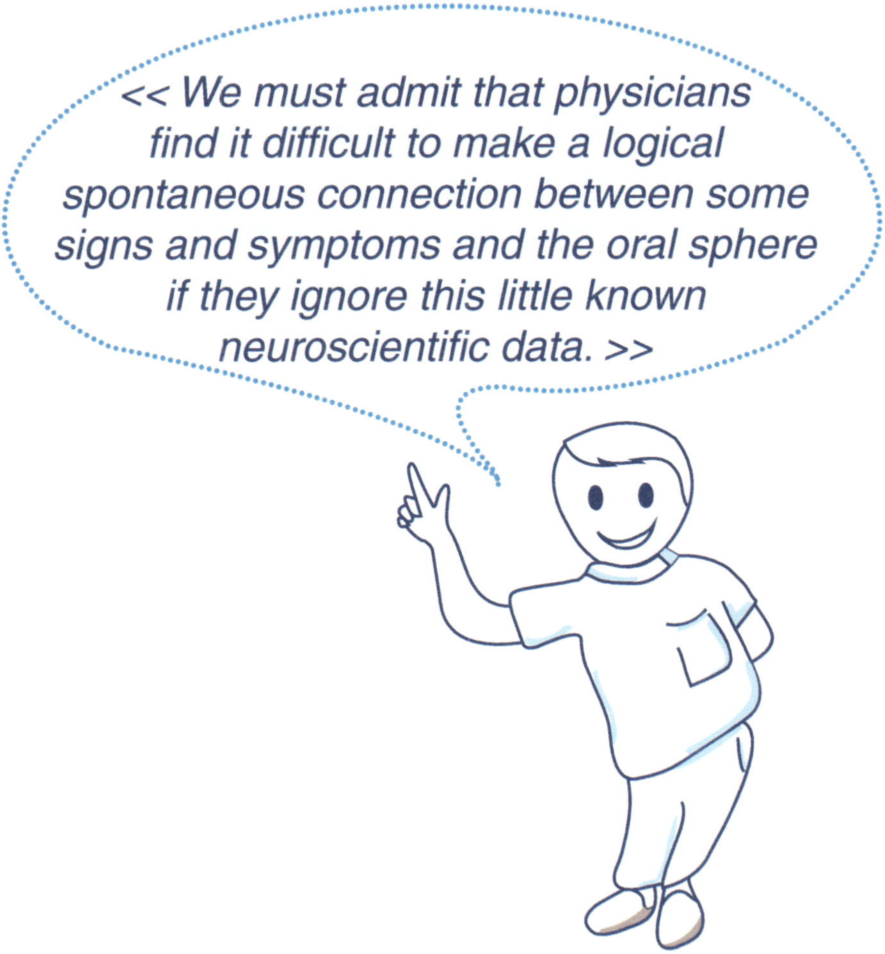

Key questions are have the paired (V) played a special role in emphasizing the pathophysiological phenomena that triggered the neuroendocrine response to stress? How could it relate to the onset of the previously mentioned disorders (migraine, fibromyalgia, chronic fatigue, etc.)?

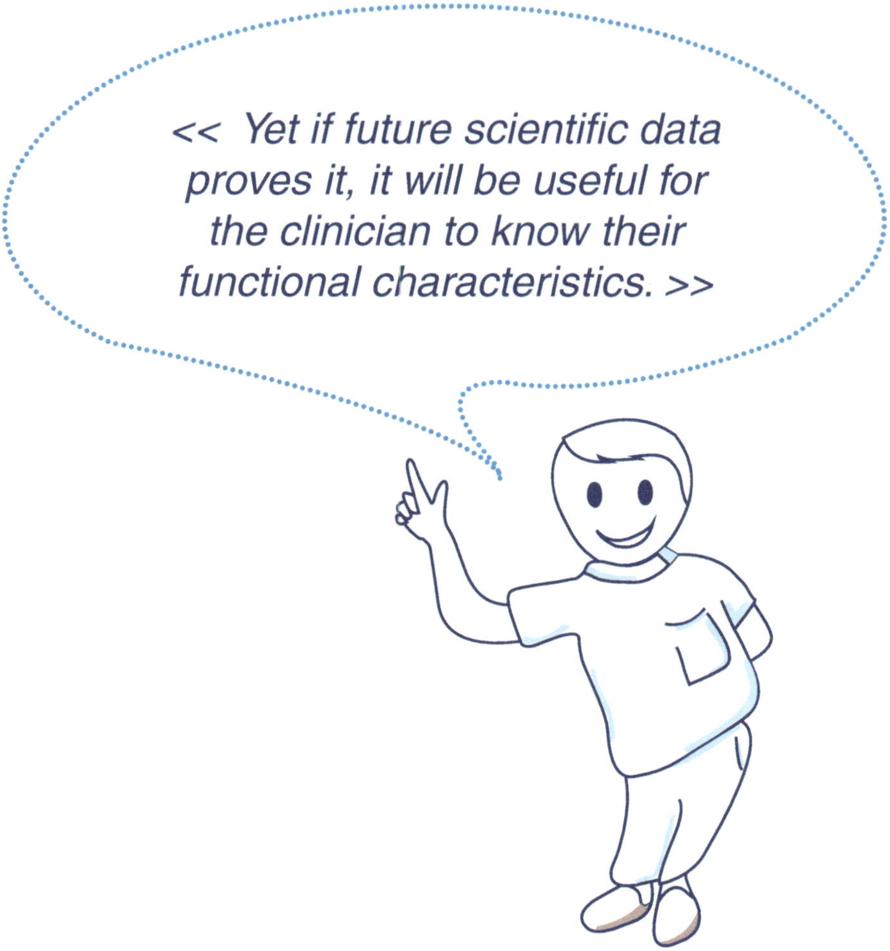

<< Yet if future scientific data proves it, it will be useful for the clinician to know their functional characteristics. >>

Chapter "The Trigeminal Nerve Pathways and Their Central Projections" recalls important fundamental data about the hodology of trigeminal ways and connections which remain too often unexploited by clinicians. Indeed, two important steps must be taken. Dentists evaluating TMD must also pay close attention to the patient's complaint about areas distant from the trigeminal area. As for physicians, they must consider the *oral sphere as a potential source of dysfunction of unexpectedly remote areas*.

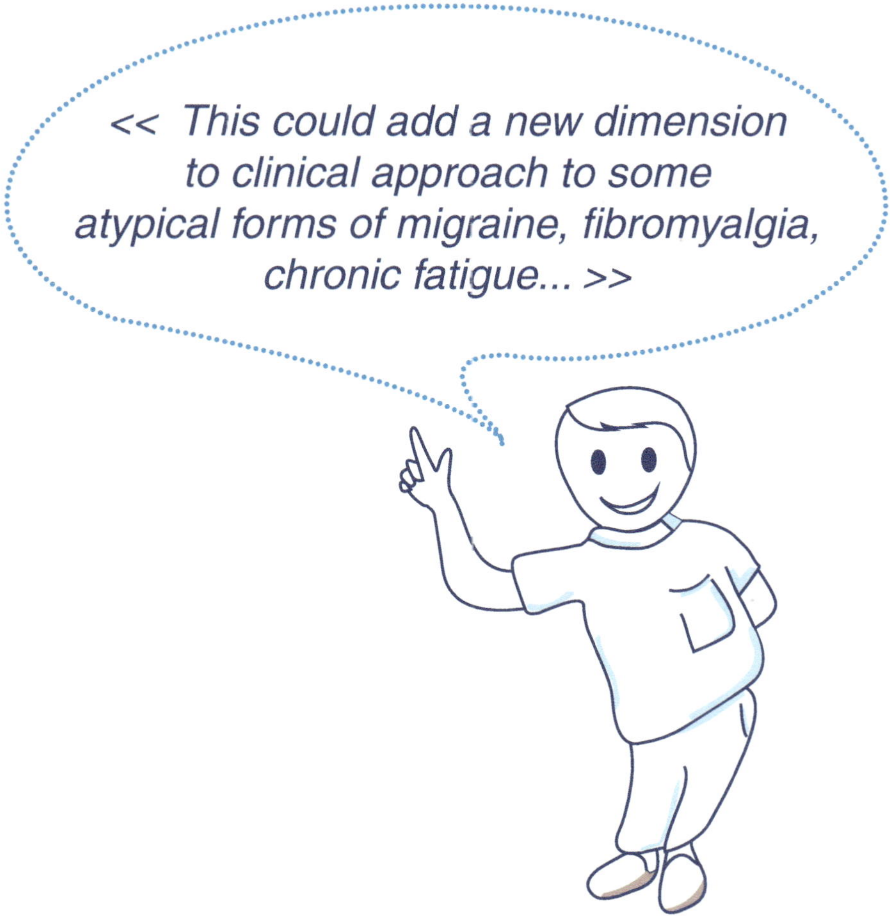

Chapter "Useful Physiological Reminders" contains some useful physiological reminders that may help understand the pathophysiological theory suggested by chapter "Pathophysiological Conditions" about possible TMD mechanisms and their clinical manifestation.

References

1. Arendt-Nielsen L, Mense S, Graven-Nielsen T (2003) Assessment of muscle pain and hyperalgesia. Experimental and clinical findings. Germ Schmerz 17(6):445–449
2. Arendt-Nielsen L, Graven-Neilsen T (2003) Central sensitization in fibromyalgia and other musculoskeletal disorders. Curr Pain Headache Rep 7(5):355–361
3. Bossy J (1990) Anatomie clinique: Neuro-anatomie. Springer Verlag (éd), Paris

Characteristics of Periodontal Proprioception

The dental organ is a privileged functional zone because it is a rich sensory innervated element, the first one involved in the digestive process. Histological and electrophysiological modern techniques have clearly shown the tooth periodontal sensory innervation.[1] Most ordinary people consider teeth as a potential source of acute pain and nothing more than *a piece of bone set in a bone* useful to crush food and give a pretty smile.

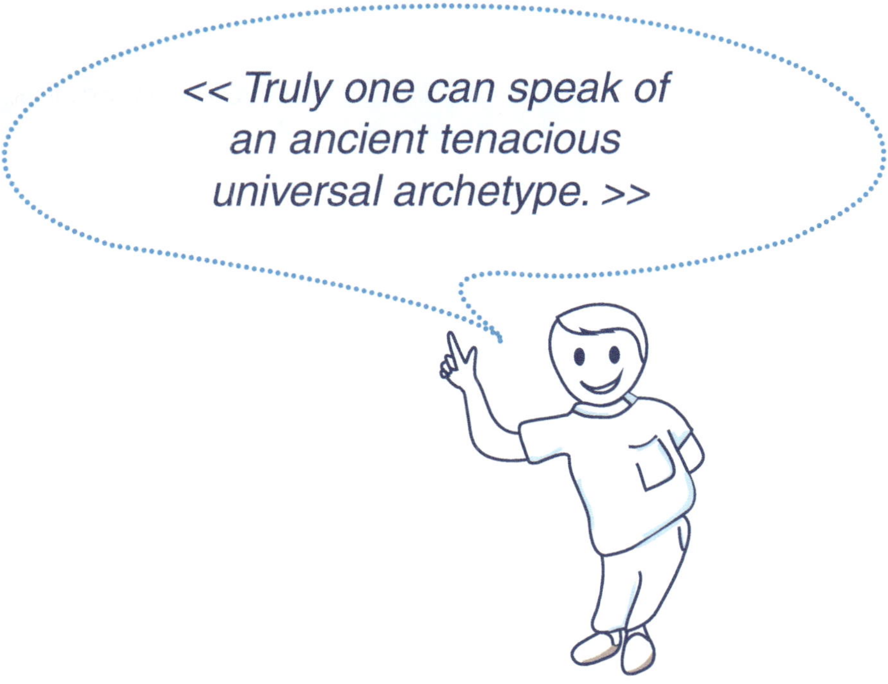

[1]Periodontium = ligament which links the tooth to the maxillary bone.

F. Hartmann, G. Cucchi, *Stress and Orality*,
DOI 10.1007/978-2-8178-0271-8_6, © Springer-Verlag France 2014

Fig. 1 Lioness holding cub

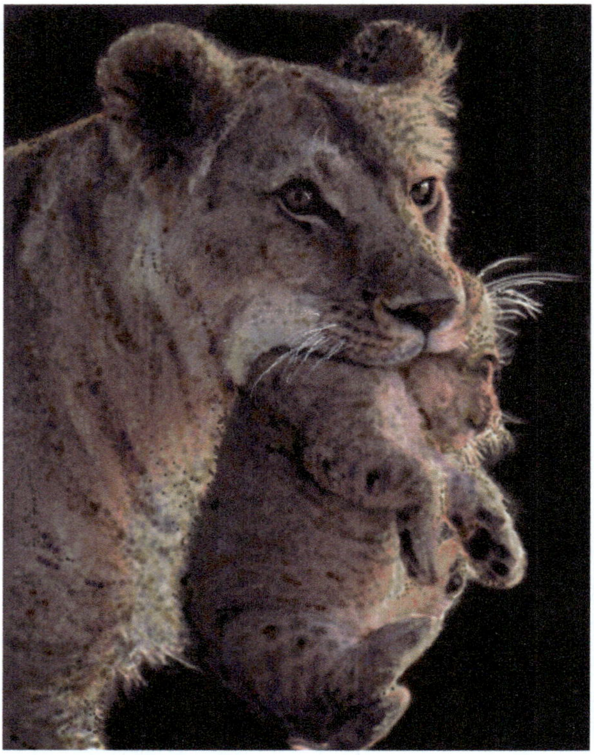

Indeed few are aware of the *very subtle tactile sensitivity* – the role of the periodontal apparatus in the painless capacity of teeth. Just think of a female tiger or a lioness whose jaws could tear and mangle her prey (Fig. 1). Have you ever wondered how she is able to hold her cubs gently and safely between those same jaws? Humans have inherited that same sensitivity which makes it possible for oriental merchants to calibrate pearls by placing them between their incisors.[2] Periodontal inputs seem mostly helpful for the brain's coordination of vital functions such as eating.[3] According to their response to different types of stimuli, two main types of **periodontal receptors** (PR) have been found (Fig. 2): **physiological PR** and **nociceptive PR**.

[2]They are precise to the micron, that is, thousandths of millimeter. Some objects are so small that they are hardly perceptible between thumb and forefinger, but they are sensed between upper and lower teeth. In a personal study with blind children and young adults who had to feel a calibrated hair between their teeth, we found that the discriminative tactile rate was decreasing as we moved from the front teeth to the back teeth.

[3]This is explained by the particular role of teeth in the digestive system. They participate in regulating food mastication and play a significant stereognostic role in the identification of the forces used to hold and manipulate food between teeth [45]. They inform the nervous centers to modulate the

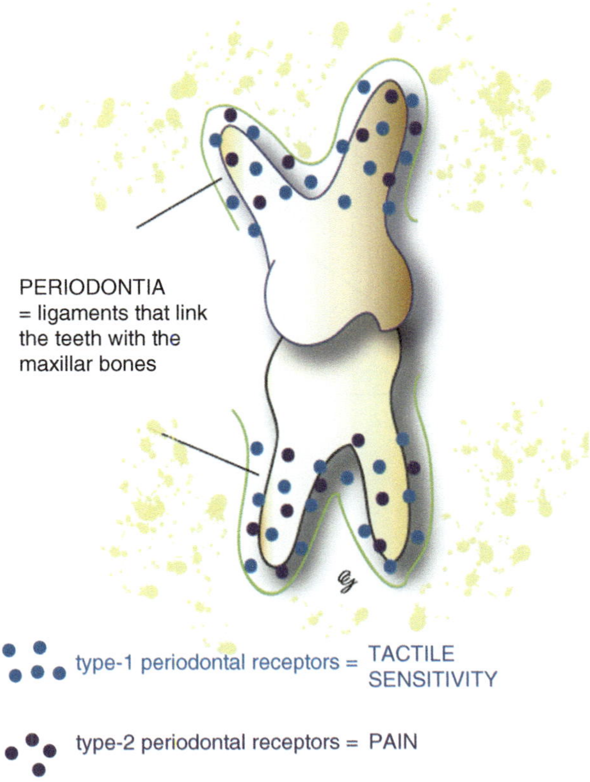

Fig. 2 Physiological and nociceptive periodontal receptors

1 Physiological Receptors

These mechanical receptors detect forces applied to the tooth [8, 11, 14, 33, 40]. They are called *type 1 receptors* [34] and have three characteristics. They are sensitive to the *intensity of forces applied to the dental corona* (Fig. 3). They are sensitive to the *direction of the stimulus* as previously pointed at [37]. They respond according to the *velocity of the forces* applied to the dental corona. Trigeminal ways send these inputs to the brain, especially to the primary and secondary somatosensory cortices SI[4] and SII [41] (Fig. 4), recently confirmed in the humans [36, 45]. In physiological conditions the volumes of sensory tactile periodontal inputs must

motor neurons of masticatory and swallowing muscles for maximal functional efficiency. Other functional roles include modifying the salivary flow, remodeling the alveolar bone, and participating in maxillary and mandibular bone growing. In the nociceptive field they produce alarm signals in case of threat to the dental tissues.

[4]The key role of incisors in the blind mole rat could explain the large representation in the S1 somatosensory cortex (31 %) [6].

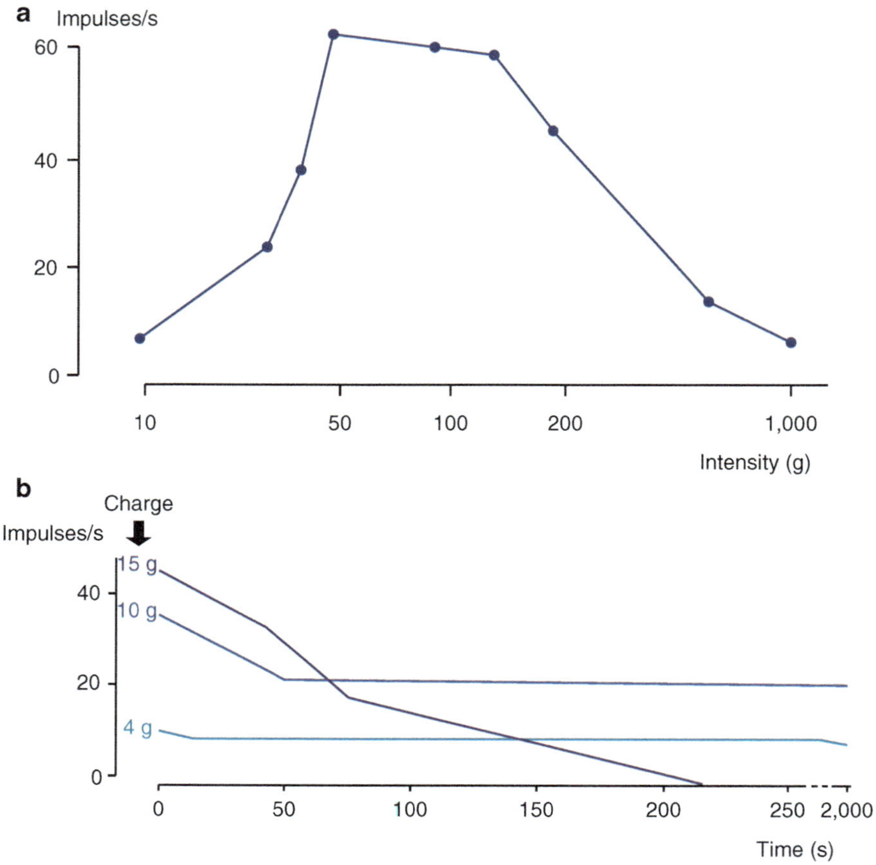

Fig. 3 Physiological response of the periodontal receptors (PR) to the stimulus intensity (**a**) and to timing (**b**). (**a**) Please note three characteristic parts in the graph. For this receptor, the plateau is reached when the intensity goes beyond a 50 g force. (**b**) When intensity stays at a low level (4 and 10 g), the discharge decreases and then stabilizes; for stronger stimulation (50 g), the discharge regularly decreases and disappears at 200 s. When the stimulating force is maintained for a rather long time, about 80 % of the receptors keep pulsing. The durations of their responses are inversely variable depending on the intensity of stimulation: they are known as *slow-adaptive receptors*. The lower the threshold of excitability, that is, less efficient stimulation (some grams), the slower the adaptation: therefore, when very light pressure is applied, the response lasts for a long time. These findings are useful when considering orthodontic procedures [29]. The other 20 % are *rapid-adaptive receptors* with a discharge duration below 4–5 s, specially for heavy pressures. They are mainly situated in the coronary region [5]. Thus, three subgroup receptors were described: (1) the spontaneously pulsing receptors, (2) the slow-adaptive receptors, and (3) the rapid-adaptive receptors which seem to be fewer than the others [30]. One admits that physiological (PR) are type similar but have a variable capacity to adaptation

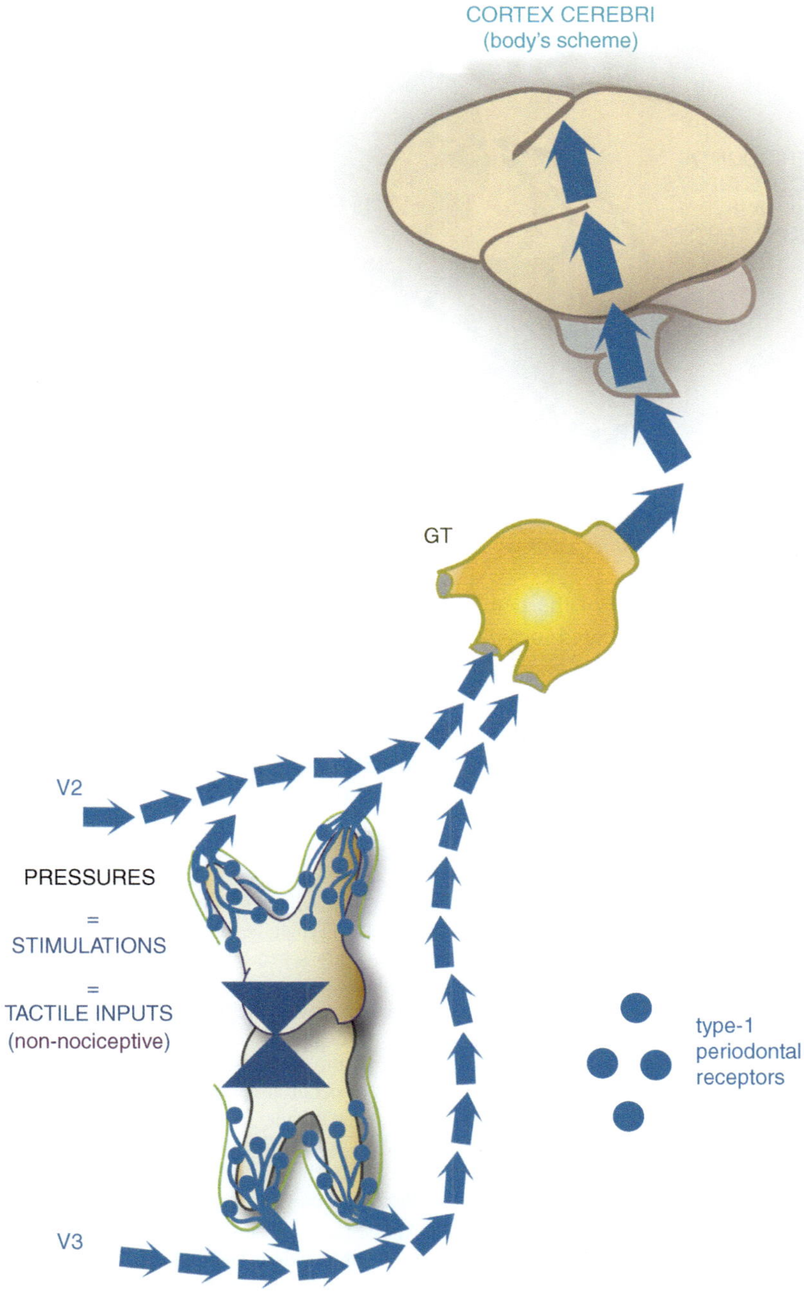

Fig. 4 Physiological response from PR sending tactile inputs to the brain

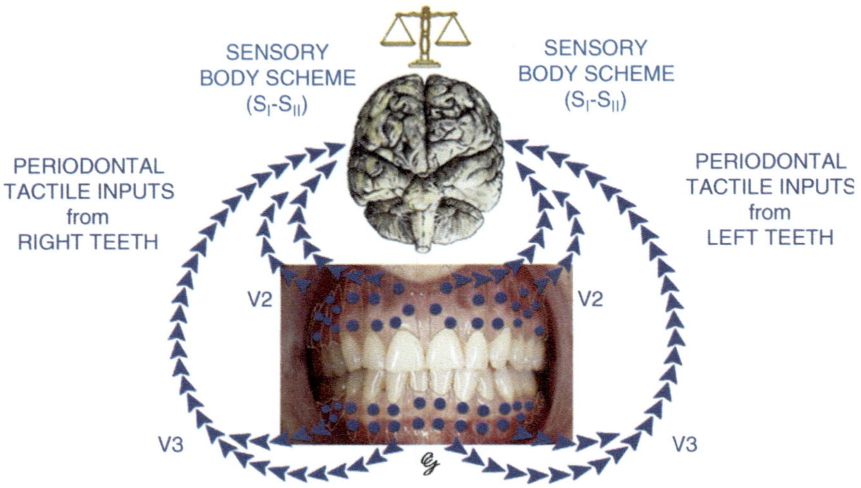

Fig. 5 Balanced periodontal inputs going to the brain in physiological conditions. SI-SII, cortical sensory receptive areas. *Blue points* type 1 periodontal receptors

come from both sides of the dental arches in a balanced mood.[5] Several sensory properties can be attributed to type 1 PR.[6] However, scientific data do not yet exist to know how they react to abnormally excessive mechanical forces. Some speak of human parafunctional stomatognathic spastic conditions (severe teeth clenching). An fMRI investigation should be highly useful to get a clear answer. Two entirely opposite theories are suggested: one based on a strong reaction and the other on no reaction. There may also be intermediate conditions.

[5]The cerebral sensory cortex expects to receive the same sensory volume on the right side and on the left side (Fig. 5). We speak of non-nociceptive – that is, tactile – inputs. Let's use a clinical example: your dentist has just fit a crown in your mouth. Typically, you must not be aware of this new component. In neurophysiological terms, your body scheme must accept it. People often believe – wrongfully so – "No pain: no problem." In fact the component should in no way *exist* when you lightly tap the upper and lower teeth together. Any tactile feeling of imbalance must be immediately pointed out by the patient and fixed by the dentist. If not, dysfunctional reflexes from the trigeminal territory may occur since adjustment by the nervous system is very difficult, even impossible in most cases. Indeed, leaving this kind of occlusal abnormality unchanged may be considered as a neurophysiological error and a professional fault. To help perform a very sophisticated equilibration, we previously described an easy method called the *shoulder method* [16, 18]. The patient's awareness of his neural tactile sensitivity directs the dentist to perform a more balanced occlusion as compared to low-tech methods (paper, varnish, scan, etc.).

[6]Tact, stereognosis (capacity in recognizing thickness, form, and texture of food), proprioception which permits to everyone to spatially situate one's teeth position. The first and the second moods are conscious; the third is unconscious. Type 1 PR keeps a major role in learning functions and movements. The proprioceptive control on the behavioral sets appears to be higher during new works learning and realizing [21, 22]. The PR could initiate a negative feedback [7, 12, 32, 46] due to very fine biting force discrimination when TMJ receptors failed [47]. Remember about the tiger female and its cub. Muscle receptors do not pulsate within the 1 mm band preceding the closing of the mouth [3]. But during mastication, the conditions change [15, 43, 44]: the PR sensibility decreases [28]. Their dental protecting role towards excessive biting forces, specially at the end of the masticatory cycle, is confirmed by some studies [13, 38]. Otherwise a periodontal and neuromuscular bundle co-activation of the masseteric has been shown [4, 9]. There is a closing mouth

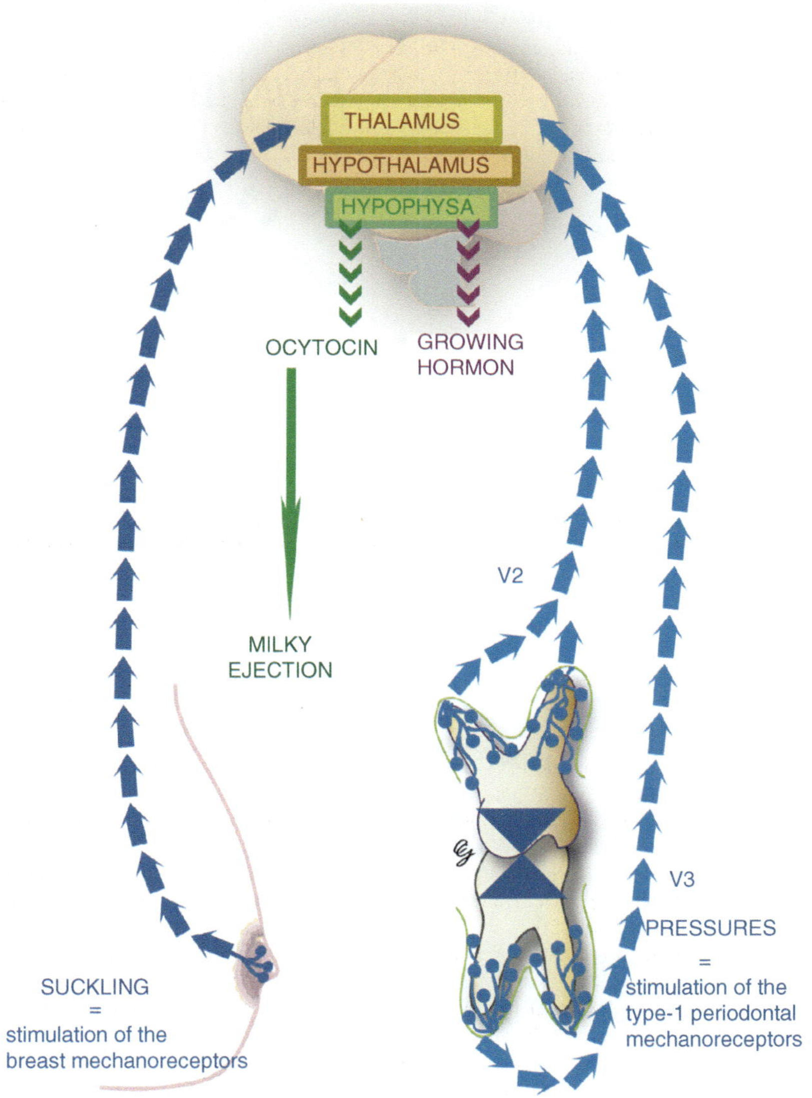

Fig. 6 Similar neuroendocrine mechanical responses between tooth and breast (Model)

---

masseteric reflex due to ipsilateral PR stimulation [48, 49]. The study in humans [25, 26, 45] confirmed the animal recorded results. A positive feedback of PR exists for chewing force control when a substantial influence of joint receptors on movement control does not [42]. It has been also evoked their role into maxillary growing mechanisms [10, 17] (Fig. 6). Finally the type 1 PR also intervene in human parotid secretion control [1, 19, 20]. According to some studies, mechanical receptors exist in intradental region, and both can provide a continuum of dynamic afferent inputs necessary for tactile sensitivity of teeth [8]. Intraoral touch receptors, spindles in jaw-closing muscles, and specialized PR have especially powerful effects on physiological movement parameters [31]. The periodontal tissue also receives a major sympathetic innervation as shown by histological, histochemical, and electrophysiological studies [24, 27]. Otherwise when teeth are lost, the tactile information is relayed by mucosal receptors [23, 39]. Neurophysiologists call that as a vicarious phenomenon.

2 Nociceptive Receptors[7]

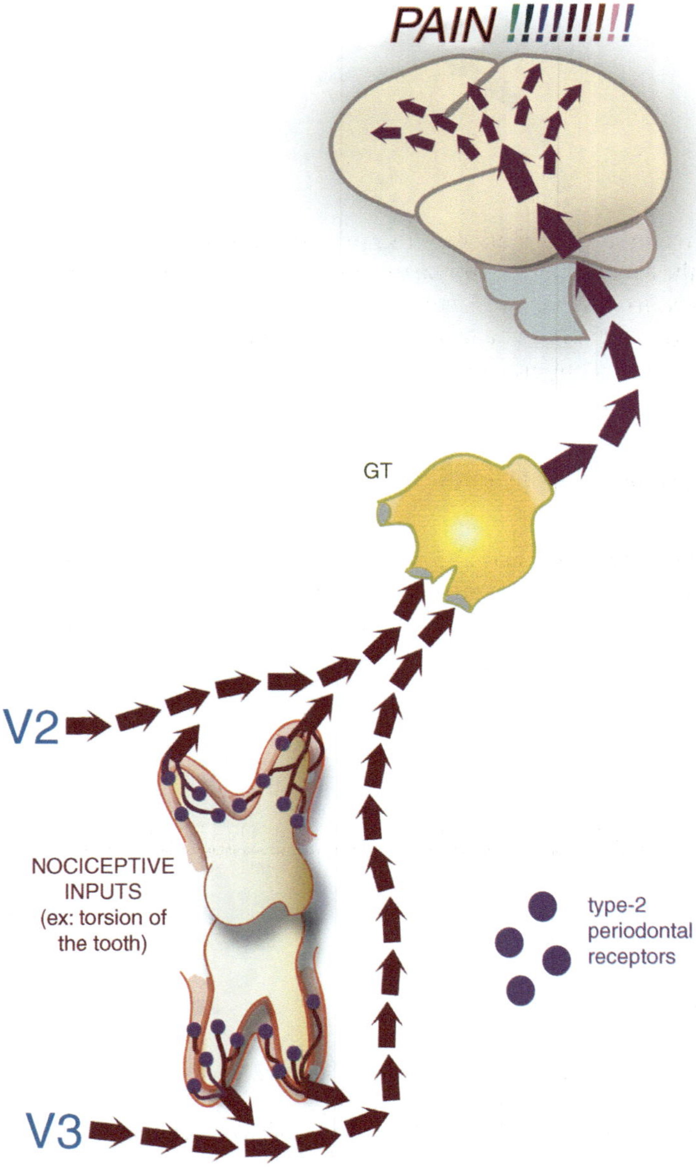

Fig. 7 Nociceptive PR sending pain inputs to the brain

[7]Some PR responding to experimental particularly nociceptive stimuli have been shown with the cat [35] and the monkey [2]. They are called as *type 2 receptors* (Fig. 7). These stimulations are tooth hard torsion, warming (40–50 °C), and intra-ligamentar injection of algogenic substances (bradykinin, potassium chlorure). In pathological conditions it depends of the tooth lesion. The nociceptive PR never react to any coronal pressure, even a strong one. They seem to be a different type of PR which are connected to small-size nervous fibers (myelinated and nonmyelinated), whereas physiological PR are connected to large-size myelinated fibers.

References

1. Anderson DJ, Hector MP (1987) Periodontal mechanoreceptors and parotid secretion in animals and man. J Dent Res 66:518–523
2. Aubert M, Hartmann F, Mei N, Salenc C (1978) La sensibilité dentaire chez le Chat. Rev Biol Ecol Médit 5(2):61–94
3. Bonfil JJ (1975) Sensibilité fusoriale des muscles masticateurs, intercuspidation canine et position mandibulaire de repos. Etude chez le chat aigu. J Biol Bucc 3:77–90
4. Brodin P, Turker KS, Miles TS (1993) Mechanoreceptors around the tooth evoke inhibitory and excitatory reflexes in the human masseter muscle. J Physiol 464:711–723
5. Cash M, Linden RWA (1982) The distribution of mechanoreceptors in the periodontal ligament of the mandibular canine tooth of the cat. J Physiol 330:439–447
6. Catania KC, Remple MS (2001) Somatosensory cortex dominated by the representation of teeth in the naked mole-rat brain. Proc Natl Acad Sci USA 99(8):5692–5697
7. Dessem D, Iyadurai OD, Taylor A (1988) The role of periodontal receptors in the jaw-opening reflex in the cat. J Physiol 406:315–330
8. Dong WK, Shiwaku T, Kawakami Y, Chudler EH (1993) Static and dynamic responses of periodontal ligament mechanoreceptors and intradental mechanoreceptors. J Neurophysiol 69(5):1567–1582
9. Funakoshi M, Nakashima N (1980) Excitation of masseter muscle spindle induced by periodontal stimulation. J Dent Res Abstract 422:992
10. Gasson N, Stutzmann J, Petrovic AG (1975) Les mécanismes régulateurs de l'ajustement occlusal interviennent-ils dans le contrôle de la croissance du cartilage condylien? Orthod Franç 46:77–101
11. Hannam AG (1976) Periodontal mechanoreceptors. In: Anderson DJ, Matthews B (eds) Mastication. Wright & Sons Limited, Bristol, pp 42–49
12. Hannam AG, Matthews B (1969) Reflex jaw opening in response to stimulation of periodontal mechanoreceptors in the cat. Arch Oral Biol 14:415–419
13. Hannam AG, Matthews B, Yemm R (1986) The unloading reflex in masticatory muscles of man. Arch Oral Biol 13:361–367
14. Hartmann F, Mei N, Vedel J-P (1979) Bases neurophysiologiques de l'occlusion. Encycl Med Chir Paris Stomatol 22008:C-10
15. Hartmann F, Vedel J-P, Mei N (1982) Physiologie et physiopathologie de la mastication. Encycl Med Chir Paris Stomatol 22008:A-15
16. Hartmann F, Cucchi G, Antrassian J et al (1985) Neurophysiologie et équilibration en prothèse adjointe totale. Cah Proth 51:79–90
17. Hartmann F, Mei N, Salenc C, Trub M (1985) Periodontal sensitivity and bone growth. Actual Odontostomatol 39(151):673–683
18. Hartmann F, Cucchi G (1993) Les dysfonctions cranio-mandibulaires (SADAM). Nouvelles perspectives médicales. Springer-Verlag (éd), Paris, 176p
19. Hector MP (1984) Evidence for the involvement of periodontal mechanoreceptors in the control of parotid secretion. J Dent Res 63(4):490
20. Hector MP, Linden RW (1987) The possible role of periodontal mechanoreceptors in the control of parotid secretion. Q J Exp Physiol 72:285–301
21. Hellsing G (1987) Human jaw muscle motor behavior. Part I: motor drive. Swed Dent J 11:251–261
22. Hellsing G (1987) Human jaw muscle motor behavior. Part II: reflex and receptor mechanism. Swed Dent J 12:47–56
23. Heraud J (1988) Etude des différences d'épaisseurs infimes perçues au niveau occlusal chez le sujet denté et édenté (1ère partie). Thèse 3ème cycle Sci Odont Marseille
24. Holland GR (1989) Sympathetic-sensory axon to axon contacts in the dental pulp. Proc Finn Dent Soc 85:375–378
25. Johansson RS, Olsson KA (1976) Microelectrode recording from human oral mechanoreceptors. Brain Res 118:307–311
26. Johnsen SE, Trulsson M (2003) Receptive field properties of human periodontal afferents responding to loading of premolar and molar teeth. J Neurophysiol 89:1478–1487
27. Karita K, Izumi H, Tabata T et al (1989) The blood flow in the periodontal ligament regulated by the sympathetic and sensory nerves in the cat. Proc Finn Dent Soc 85:289–294

28. Kiliardis S, Tzakis M, Carlsson S (1990) Short-term and long-term effects of chewing training on occlusal perception of thickness. Scand J Dent Res 98:159–166
29. Kohno T, Matsumoto Y, Kanno Z et al (2002) Experimental tooth movement under light orthodontic forces: rates of tooth movement and changes of the periodontium. J Orthod 29(2): 129–135
30. Loescher AR, Robinson PP (1989) Receptor characteristics of periodontal mechanosensitive units supplying the cat's lower canine. J Neurophysiol 62(4):971–978
31. Lund JP, Kolta A (2006) Generation of the central masticatory pattern and its modification by sensory feedback. Dysphagia 21(3):167–174
32. Matthews B, Yemm R (1971) Response of masseter and digastric muscle to mechanical stimulation of teeth in decerebrate cats. J Dent Res 50:697
33. Mei N, Hartmann F, Roubien R (1971) Functional characteristics of dental ligament mechanoreceptors in cats. J Physiol Paris 63(6):137
34. Mei N, Hartmann F, Roubien R (1975) Caractéristiques fonctionnelles des mécano-récepteurs des ligaments dentaires chez le chat. J Biol Buccale 3:29–39
35. Mei N, Hartmann F, Aubert M (1977) Periodontal mechanoreceptors involved in pain. In: Anderson DJ, Matthews B (eds) Pain in the trigeminal region. Elsevier, Amsterdam, p103
36. Miyamoto JJ, Honda M, Saito DN et al (2006) The representation of the human oral area in the somatosensory cortex: a functional MRI study. Cereb Cortex 16(5):669–675
37. Ness AR (1954) The mechanoreceptors of the rabbit mandibular incisor. J Physiol 126:475–493
38. Ochardson R, Sheena H, Mac Farmale H (1980) The effect of local periodontal anaesthesia on the maximum biting force achieved by human subjects. Arch Oral Biol 25:799–804
39. Orofino J (1990) Exteroception et dimension verticale chez l'édenté. Cah Proth 77:56–63
40. Pfaffmann C (1939) Afferent impulses from the tooth due to pressure and noxious stimulation. J Physiol 97:207–219
41. Salenc C (1979) Projection des nerfs maxillaires et des récepteurs dentaires sur le cortex cérébral du chat. Thèse 3rd cycle Sci Odont Marseille
42. Schindler HJ, Stengel E, Spiess WE (1998) Feedback control during mastication of solid food textures – a clinical-experimental study. J Prosthet Dent 8(3):330–336
43. Sekine H, Kishi M, Yamakura D et al (1995) Significance of periodontal pressoreceptive sensation for hardness discrimination of foods. In: Morimoto T, Matsuya T, Takada K (eds) Brain and oral functions. Elsevier Sciences, Amsterdam
44. Trulsson M (2007) Force encoding by human periodontal mechanoreceptors during mastication. Arch Oral Biol 52(4):357–360
45. Trulsson M, Francis ST, Bowtell R, McGlone F (2010) Brain activations in response to vibrotactile tooth stimulation: a psychophysical and fMRI study. J Neurophysiol 104:2257–2265
46. Turker KS, Jenkins M (2000) Reflex responses induced by tooth unloading. J Neurophysiol 84(2):1088–1092
47. Williams WN, Lapointe LL, Mahan PE, Cornell CE (1984) Discrimination des forces de morsure après modification ou diminution de la sensibilité des ATM et des incisives. J Dent Res Abstract 63:288
48. Yamada Y, Ash MM (1984) Reflex responses in jaw muscle to mechanical tooth stimulation. J Dent Res 63:323
49. Yamada Y, Stohler CS, Shimada K, Ash MM Jr (1985) Short and long latency jaw-opening reflex responses elicited by mechanical stimulation in man. Arch Oral Biol 30:197–200

The Trigeminal Nerve Pathways and Their Central Projections

The trigeminal system comprises the trigeminal nerves and their associated central nuclei. The nervous subdivision is devoted to the sensory innervation of the face and oral cavity and the motor control of the stomatognathic system. The V branches divide distally into three main nerves: the *ophthalmic* (V1), the *maxillary* (V2), and the *mandibular* (V3) *nerves*. The major part of the trigeminal sensory hodology systematically follows the three-stage nerve pattern (Fig. 1): periphery to brainstem, brainstem to diencephalon, diencephalon to telencephalon (cerebral cortex[1]). Information goes through the thalamocortical ways, most likely through the ways coming from the medulla. Thus, trigeminal ways carry both sensory and nociceptive inputs. A clear functional distinction between lemniscal and extralemniscal ways is now discarded. So that *abnormally intense and/or durable and/or frequent trigeminal non-nociceptive inputs* (sensitive overstimulation) *can be integrated as nociceptive one by the CNS*. By the way they both become potential factors of reticular overactivity when they across these main nervous filters[2]. This notion may be significant to understand clinical outcome of some parafunctional oral habits as **severe clenching**, producing **abnormal trigeminal inputs**. Most sensory trigeminal afferents (periphery) project to a collection of brainstem nuclei. Together with the mesencephalic (MeN) and motor (MoN) trigeminal nuclei, these form the *trigeminal brainstem nuclear complex* (TBNC). Its great anatomical extension underlines the fundamental physiological significance of the sensory information it deals with. Furthermore, ascending and descending internal connections between the TBNC interneurons were identified [72] (Fig. 2). The TBNC relays inputs to superior nervous centers (thalamus, cerebellum, cortex cerebri). It is at the source of motor reflexes. It provides ascending sensory activities prior to conduction to upper integrative structures. It is useful for more elaborate oral motor activities which participate in the accuracy and memorization of personal living situations. For a

[1] Cortex cerebri.

[2] Please see Fig. 4 in chapter "Useful Physiological Reminders" about the factors of reticular activity and Fig. 8 in chapter "The Behavioral Side of Clenching" about "on-off" reticular units under psycho-emotional influences.

F. Hartmann, G. Cucchi, *Stress and Orality*,

DOI 10.1007/978-2-8178-0271-8_7, © Springer-Verlag France 2014

long time the functional organization of the TBNC has been considered as a very schematic representation [14, 36, 37, 49, 71] depending on the different types of afferent fibers reaching separate subnuclei. But studies [8, 41] have revealed a rather complex nervous structure. Non-trigeminal inputs were previously known to project to the TBNC[3]. But several trigeminal projections from the TBNC have also been identified, to the telencephalon through various relays, to the cerebellum.

Neuroscientific studies have shown that trigeminal afferents could directly project to non-trigeminal nervous structures, that is, without being relayed by the TBNC. They are called *primary afferents* (Fig. 3).

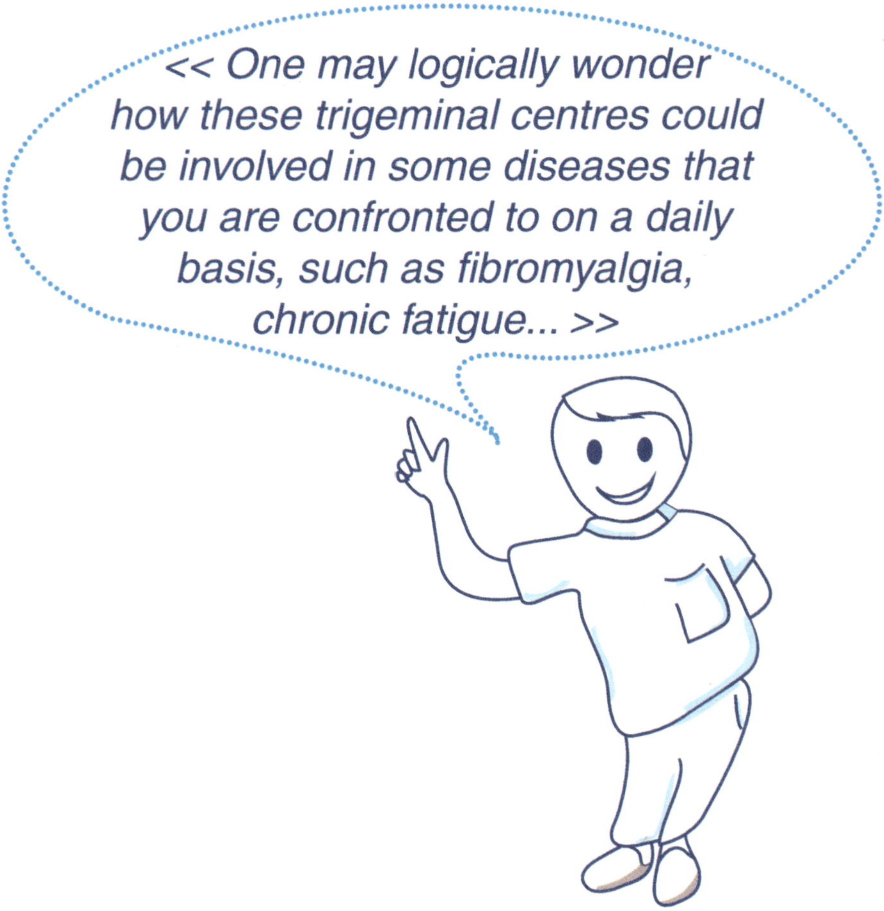

[3]Projections from the (VIIb), (IX), and (X) nerves and C1–C3 sensory roots to the (NS) [12, 24, 30, 50, 75, 79, 96, 101], the area postrema to the ipsilateral (MeN) [60]. Vagal and glossopharyngeal inputs project to the nucleus paratrigeminalis dorsalis; this nucleus and adjacent areas can be a convergence zone for intraoral, mandibular, and dental trigeminal afferents [21, 45, 46, 99] and vagal, glossopharyngeal, and oropharyngeal afferents [2, 100, 101]. This mixed projection zone can be largely involved in trigemino-spinal reflexes, in trigemino-visceral integrated phenomena, and in orofacial reflexes and oral motor behaviors such as swallowing. What's more

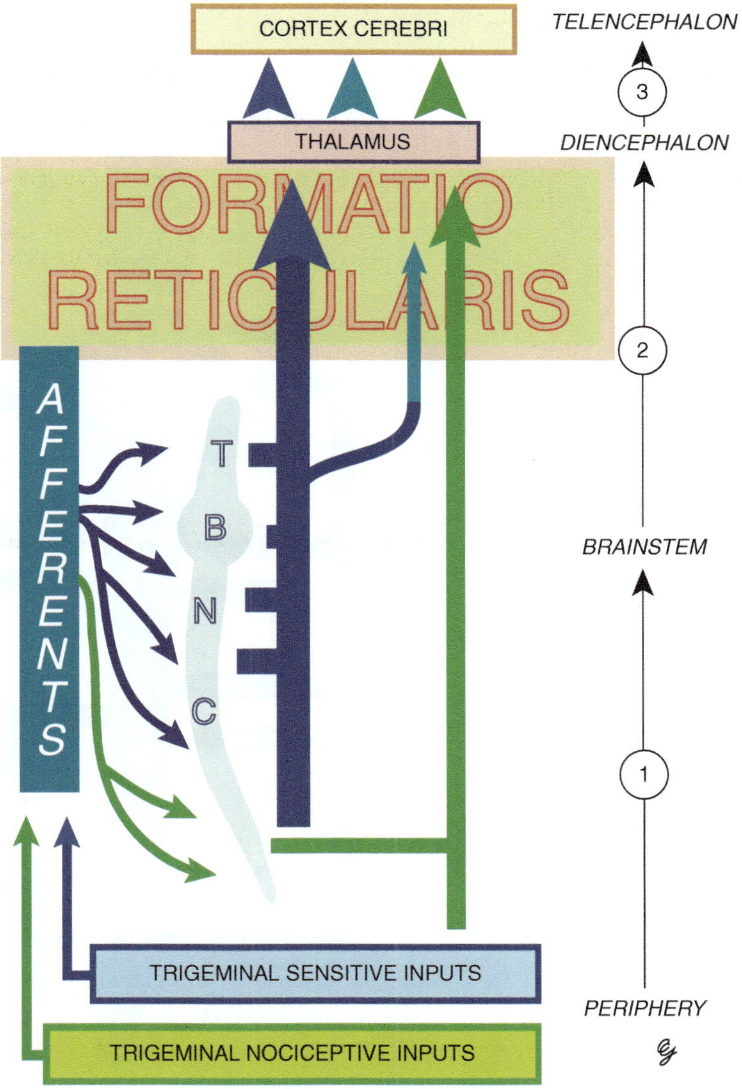

Fig. 1 Sensory and nociceptive trigeminal pathways. They follow the classical 3-stage sensory nervous system from periphery towards telencephalon

different integrative modalities for trigeminal nociceptive inputs between males and females [9, 10] have been noted at the level of SnC which can explain some clinical human gender discrepancies in TMD. The projections to the trigeminal motor nucleus (MoN) may connect oral receptors and stomatognathic muscles; they facilitate masticatory and swallowing reflexes [2, 3, 27, 30, 38, 46, 48, 53, 57, 58, 65, 69, 93, 112]. In this way, human periodontal receptors can initiate positive or negative feedback [2, 35, 45, 46, 48, 70].

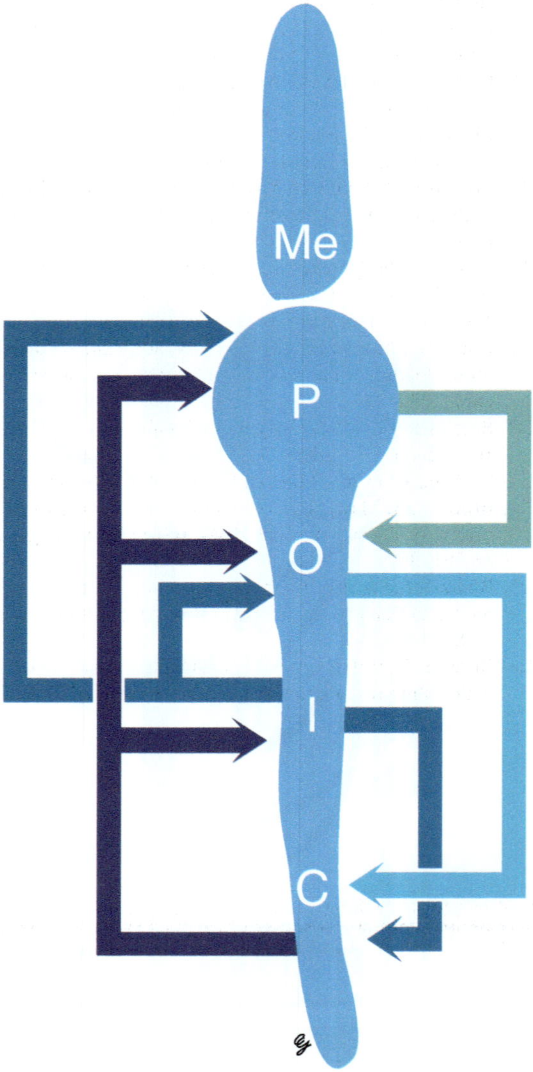

Fig. 2 Interconnections between the TBNC nuclei (Modified from Olsson et al. [72])

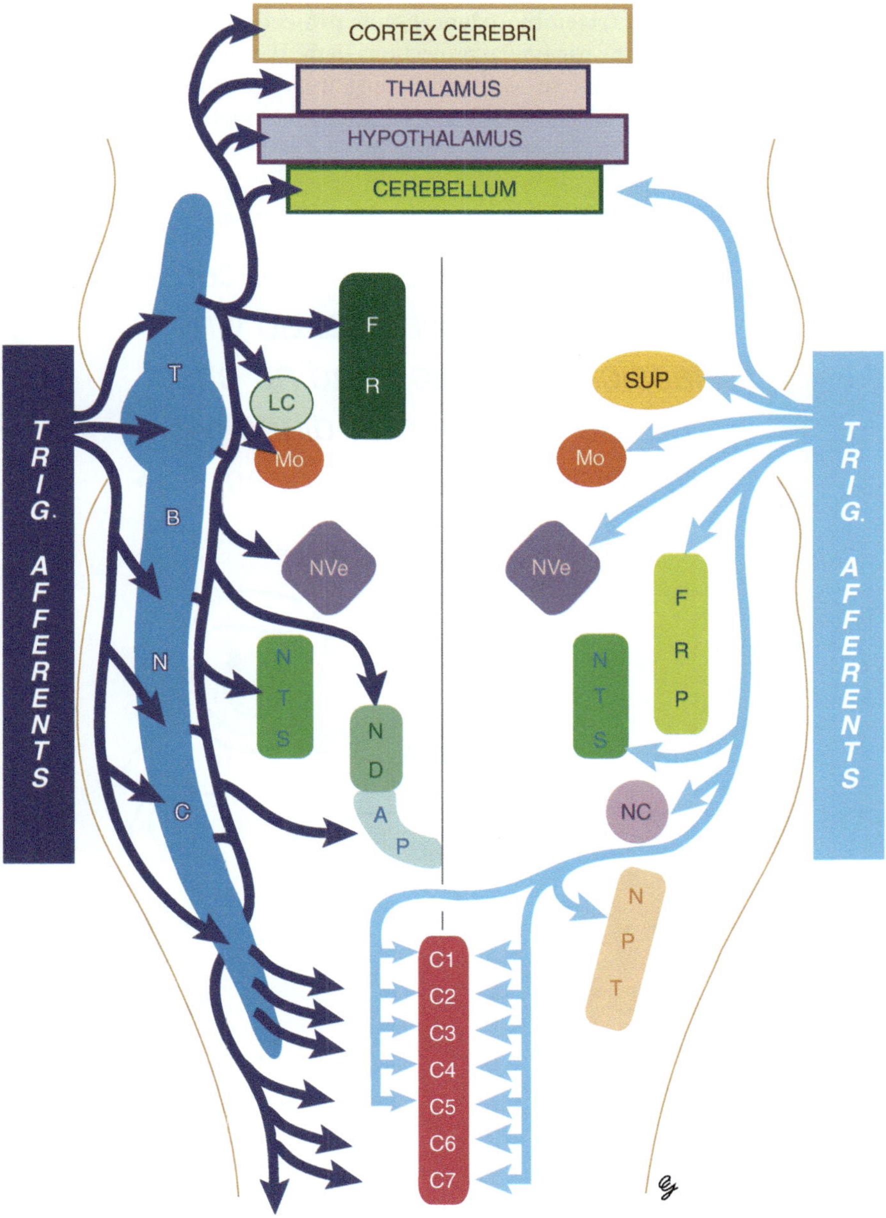

Fig. 3 Projections of trigeminal afferents to the brain according to fundamental data [5, 62, 63, 88, 109]. *Light blue arrows* primary afferents (without relay in the TBNC). *Deep blue* other afferents (with relay in the TBNC). *AP* area postrema, *FR* formatio reticularis, *FRP* formatio reticularis parvocellularis, *LC* locus coeruleus, *Mo* nucleus motorius nervi trigemini, *NC* nucleus cuneatus, *ND* nucleus dorsalis nervi vagi, *NPT* nucleus paratrigeminalis, *NTS* nucleus tracti solitarii, *NVe* nuclei vestibulares, *SUP* nucleus supratrigeminalis, *TBNC* trigeminal brainstem nuclear complex

The long ascending trigemino-telencephalic projection pathways.

A synthetic view of the trigeminal projections to the diencephalons was outlined [7]. In fact they are as diverse as those coming from the spinal cord. It can be classified as follows: the trigemino-solitary and trigemino-pontomesencephalic projections[4] [1, 33, 67, 68, 76, 77, 94].

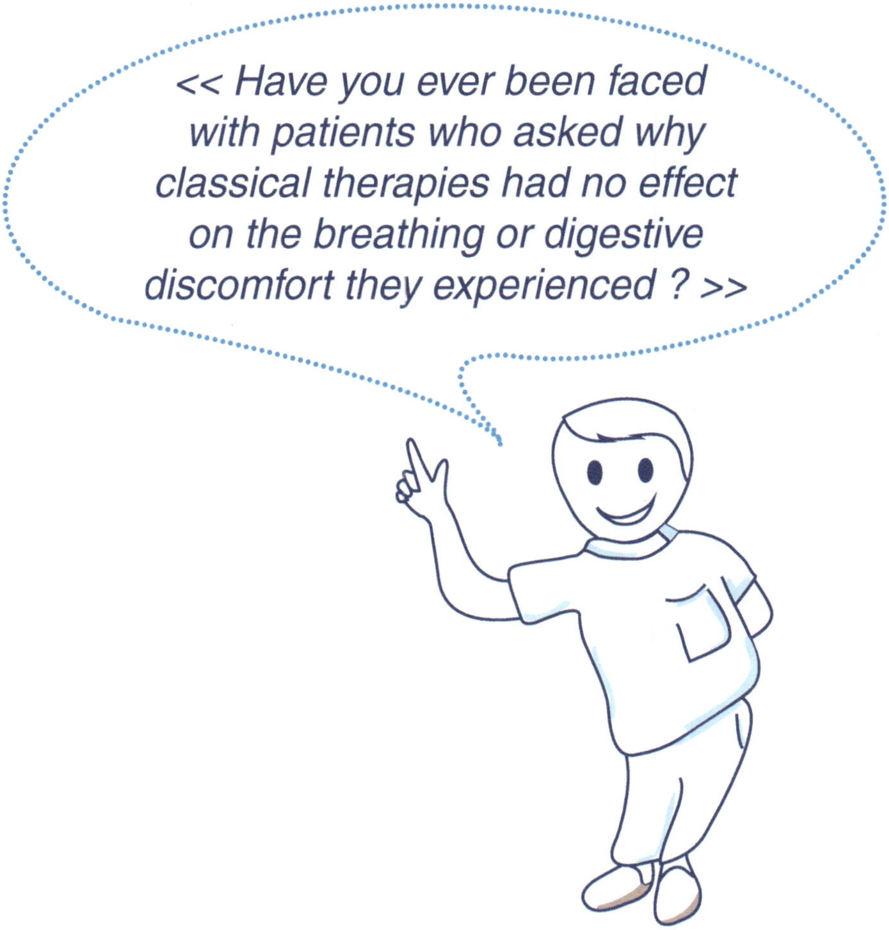
<< Have you ever been faced with patients who asked why classical therapies had no effect on the breathing or digestive discomfort they experienced ? >>

[4]They terminate at the central areas which direct visceral and vegetative inputs. These play a role in intensifying painful sensations and/or associated autonomic manifestations of cardiac and respiratory rhythmic variations.

The trigemino-reticular projections[5] [25, 39, 86, 114].

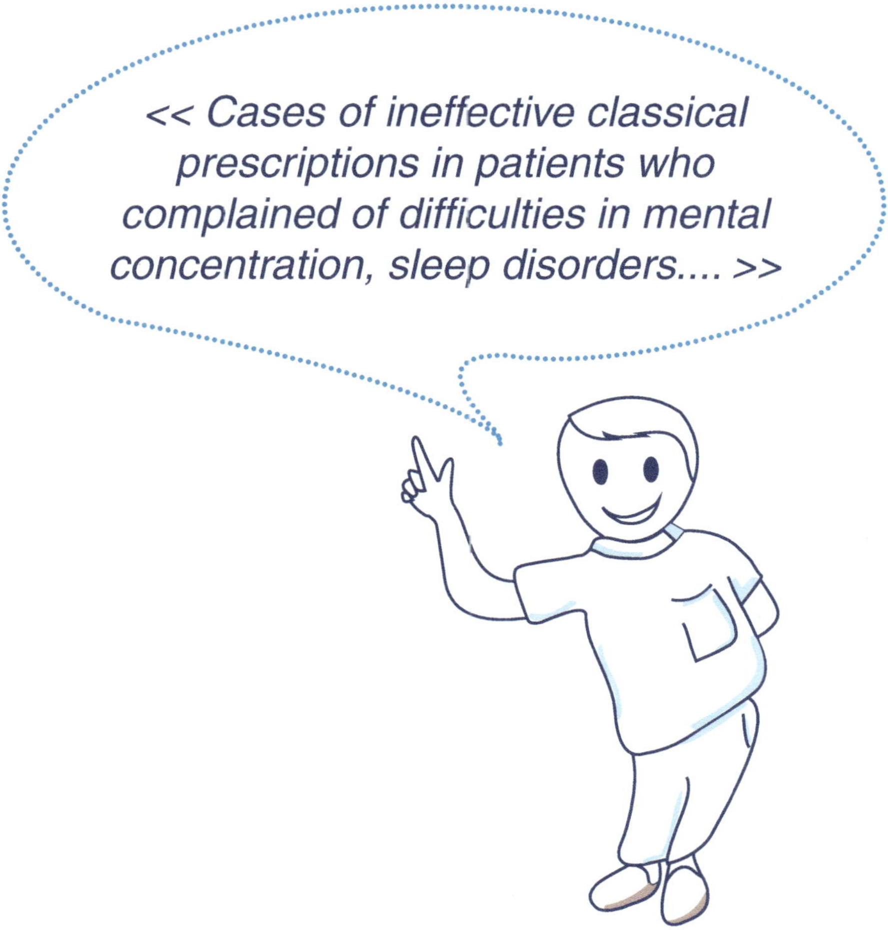

[5]They terminate at various levels of the bulbar and pontine reticular formation: they are involved in motor and vasomotor reactions and in awakening, alertness, and behavioral and motor expressions (avoidance reactions, taking flight, muscle tone adaptation, etc.) which are linked to the nociceptive component.

The trigemino-collicular projections[6] and the **trigemino-diencephalic projections**[7] [14, 18, 26–29, 43, 52, 54, 64, 80, 81, 91, 115–118].

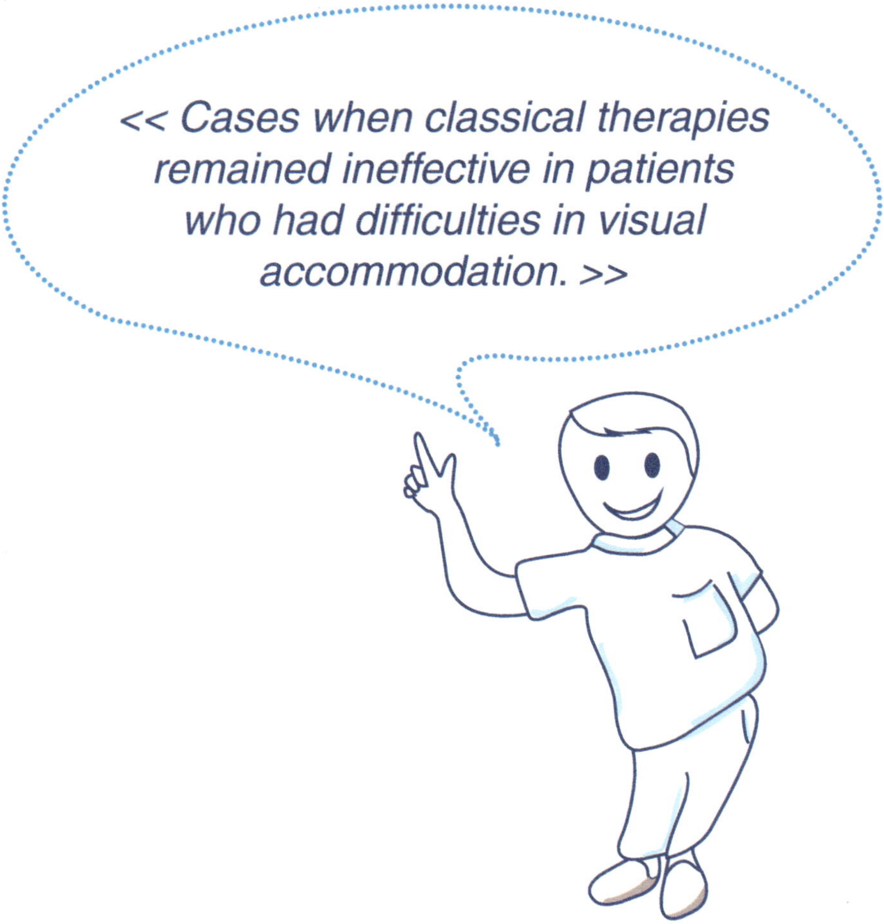

[6]They terminate at the level of the controlateral superior colliculus [6, 31, 40, 52, 113, 118]: they are involved in orientation reflexes. Other studies [6, 88] have shown that some orofacial fibers relayed into the rostral part of the trigeminal SN project to the controlateral colliculus superior. This colliculus also receives visual, auditive, and somatosensory inputs. These afferents have a behavioral role in eye control, head, and body movements [23, 95]. Some EOM and nuchal muscle afferents project to the cervical chord (C1 à C3), suggesting that there are possible interactions between these two sensory afferent groups [83]. All these scientific data can shed light on clinical symptoms such as vertigo when classical investigations remain ineffective.

[7]They reach several thalamic and hypothalamic nuclei. Most somesthetic thalamus projections (ventro-posteromedial, VPM) may originate from the NP, SnO, and SnI, which corresponds to a fine localization and discrimination of the stimuli [108]. The SnC inputs have more complex thalamic projections with nociceptive integration. Trigemino-hypothalamic projections have been confirmed by some electrophysiological recordings [102–105] particularly in the ventromedial nucleus which regulates eating behavior. Ventromedial cells were activated by both periodontal and gastric stimulations. This projection can come directly from the TBNC [43] or be relayed by

The long ascending trigemino-cerebellar projection pathways.

Cerebellar projections from the TBNC [15–17] originate primarily from NP and SnI [40–42, 47, 61, 64, 80, 93, 107, 110]. Others come from NMe [11]. These secondary afferents reach the previously mentioned primary projections.[8]

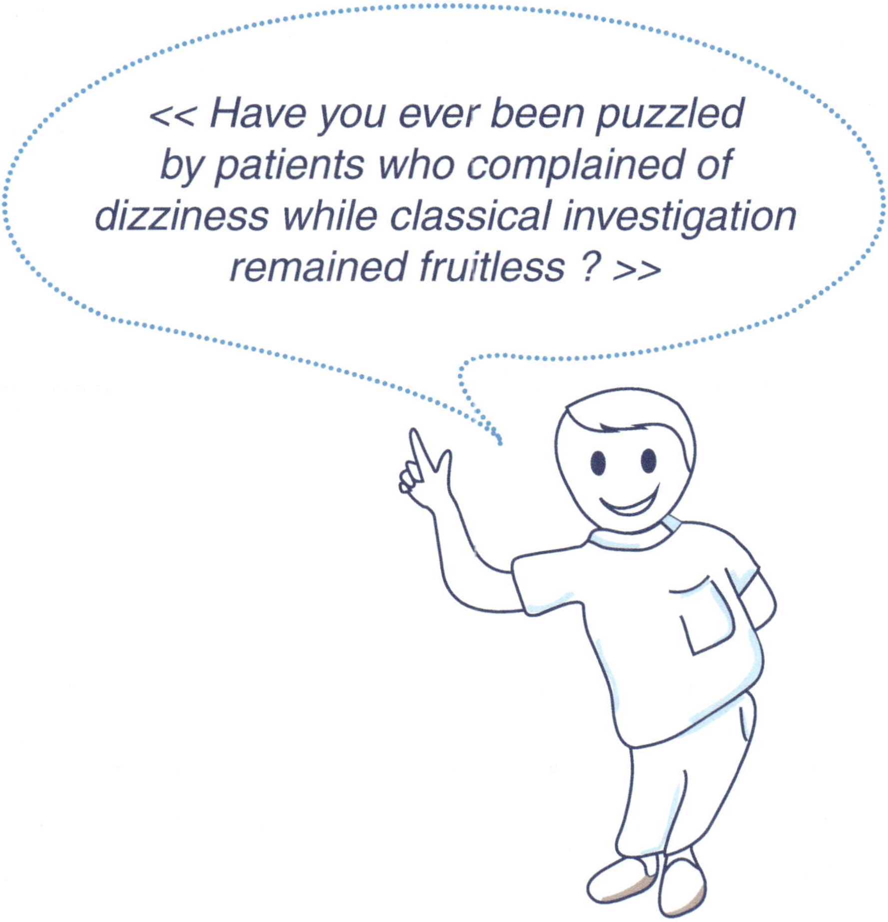

the parabrachial area [7, 20, 90, 119]. The parabrachial nucleus also receives trigeminal nociceptive inputs relayed by the SnC [55]. Just note that the parabrachial nucleus receives from the brainstem a number of inputs that project to the amygdala [73], that is, nervous center mainly implicated in aggressive behavior (see chapter "The Behavioral Side of Clenching"). There are collateral projections of the trigemino-hypothalamic tractus neurons to the colliculus [123], substantia nigra, nucleus pretectalis anterior, and hypothalamic nuclei [59]. After passing through these subcortical relays and integrations, the trigeminal inputs end in the telencephalon (cerebral cortex). The identified areas are somesthetic SI and SII [4, 7, 66, 74, 98] near the fissure of Rolando; they receive thalamic ventro-posteromedial and posterior group nuclei inputs [7]. This cortical representation participates in the somatotopic organization (body scheme) previously pointed out [78] and includes dental afferents [89].

[8]A controlateral cerebellar projection originating from the SnI and relayed in the principal and dorsal accessory subnuclei of the inferior olive was identified [40]. The periodontal inputs can inform

The outside-TBNC trigeminal projections.

It is well established that primary trigeminal afferents also extend, that is, without relays, beyond the strict neuroanatomical limits of the TBNC (Fig. 3). Studies [34, 45, 46, 62, 92, 121, 122] have shown that the recipients for these afferents include the nucleus paratrigeminalis dorsalis, nucleus supratrigeminalis, dorsal horn of the spinal cord (cervical segments C1–C7 for ipsilateral projections, C1–C5 contralateral projections), *nucleus of the solitary tact* (nucleus tracti solitarii) [97, 120], *nucleus sensorius of the vagus nerve* [99, 100], *reticular formation* (RF), *nuclei vestibulares* [62, 82], *superior colliculus* [51, 84], *and nucleus cuneatus* (relay center for body somatosensory and proprioceptive afferents)[9]. Electrophysiological [22, 32, 85] and anatomical studies [45, 46, 62] have also revealed the existence of direct projecting modes from trigeminal afferents to the cerebellum[10]. Most of them are mandibular (alveolar and lingual nerves).

---

the cerebellum about the occlusal mandibular position as they modulate stomatognathic antagonistic muscle activity. More recently, tactile cutaneous trigeminal stimulations have been found to project to deep cerebellar nuclei, inferior olive, and cerebral cortex, perhaps to control the timing of behavior [87]. The cerebellum is a major integrating and controlling center of mandibular synergical movements during mastication in mammals [44, 56, 111]. In effect the stomatognathic system must perform several complex functions about alimentary behavior from prehension to swallowing.

[9] In the vestibular nuclei, cervical proprioceptive afferents come mainly from the central cervical nucleus, but vestibular projections to TBNC and to C1–C2 medulla also exist [106]. The nucleus paratrigeminalis receives sensory inputs from trigeminal, glossopharyngeal, and vagus nerves. It projects to bulbar, pontine, and possibly thalamic structures associated with nociception, thermoregulation, and cardiovascular control. This nucleus can act as a medullar relay interposed between sensory afferents and different structures related to homeostatic functions [19]. The visceral convergence of the nucleus paratrigeminalis dorsalis can be functionally extended according to cystitis-related recorded activations [13]; it might be implicated in some TMD puzzling clinical symptoms such as unexplained prolonged fever. The projections from the trigeminal spinal subnuclei to the spinal cord [64, 65, 76, 80, 88, 109] will be described in Sect. 7 of chapter “Pathophysiological Conditions”.

[10] After crossing the superior cerebellar peduncle [45, 46, 95], they are ipsilaterally distributed to cerebellar cortex or to cerebellar subcortical nuclei (interpositus and lateralis).

References

1. Allen GV, Barbrick B, Esser MJ (1996) Trigeminal-parabrachial connections: possible pathway for nociception-induced cardiovascular reflex responses. Brain Res 715:125–135
2. Altschuler SM, Bao X, Bieger D et al (1989) Viscerotopic representation of the upper alimentary tract in the rat: sensory ganglia and nuclei of the solitary and spinal trigeminal tracts. J Comp Neurol 283:248–268
3. Anderson SA, Mahan PE (1971) Interaction of tooth pulp and periodontal ligament receptors in a jaw-depression reflex. Exp Neurol 32:295–302
4. Anderson SA, Keller O, Vylicky L (1973) Cortical activity evoked from tooth pulp afferents. Brain Res 120:221–229
5. Arvidsson J, Pfaller K (1990) Central projections of C4-C8 dorsal root ganglia in the rat studied by anterograde transport of WGA-HRP. J Comp Neurol 292:349–362
6. Auroy P, Irthun B, Woda A (1991) Oral nociceptive activity in the rat superior colliculus. Brain Res 549:575–584
7. Barnett EM, Evans GD, Sun N et al (1995) Anterograde tracing of trigeminal afferent pathways from the murine tooth pulp to cortex using herpes simplex virus type 1. J Neurosci 15:2972–2984
8. Basbaum AI, Fiels HL (1978) Endogenous pain control mechanisms: review and hypothesis. Ann Neurol 4:451–462
9. Bereiter DA (2001) Sex differences in brainstem neural activation after injury to the TMJ region. Cell Tissue Org 169(3):226–237
10. Bereiter DA, Shen S, Benetti AP (2002) Sex differences in amino acid release from rostral trigeminal subnucleus caudalis after acute injury to the TMJ region. Pain 98(1–2):89–99
11. Billig I, Yatim N, Compoint C (1995) Cerebellar afferences from the mesencephalic trigeminal nucleus in the rat. Neuroreport 6(17):2293–2296
12. Blessing WW, Yu YH, Nalivaiko E (1999) Medullary projections of rabbit carotid sinus nerve. Brain Res 816(2):405–410
13. Bon K, Lantéri-Minet M, Menétrey D (1997) Involvement of the dorsal paratrigeminal nucleus in visceral pain-related phenomena. C R Acad Sci Paris 320:607–613
14. Brodal A (1947) Central course of afferent fibers for pain in facial, glossopharyngeal and vagus nerves: clinical observations. Arch Neurol Psych Chicago 57:292–306
15. Bukowska D, Grottel K (1997) Cells in and outside the motor trigeminal nucleus projecting to the cerebellar paramedian lobule. Neuroreport 8(13):2953–2956
16. Bukowska D, Zguczynski L, Mierzejewska-Krzyzowska B, Sikora E (1998) Collateral projections of trigeminal sensory neurons to both cerebellar paramedian lobules in the rabbit: demonstration by fluorescent double labeling study. Acta Neurobiol Exp (Wars) 58(4):253–261
17. Bukowska D, Mierzejewska-Krzyzowska B, Zguczynski L (2006) Topography and axonal collaterals of trigeminocerebellar projection to the paramedian lobule and uvula in the rabbit cerebellum. Acta Neurobiol Exp (Wars) 66(2):145–151
18. Burton H, Craig AD Jr, Poulos DA, Molt JT (1979) Efferent projections from temperature sensitive recording loci within the marginal zone of the nucleus caudalis of the spinal trigeminal complex in the cat. J Comp Neur 183:753–778
19. Caous CA, de Sousa Buck H, Lindsey CJ (2001) Neuronal connections of the paratrigeminal nucleus: a topographic analysis of neurons projecting to bulbar, pontine and thalamic nuclei related to cardiovascular, respiratory and sensory functions. Auton Neurosci 94(1–2):14–24
20. Cechetto DF et al (1985) Spinal and trigeminal dorsal horn projections to the parabrachial nucleus in the rat. J Comp Neurol 22:153–160
21. Chan-Palay V (1978) The paratrigeminal nucleus. I. Neurons and synaptic organization. J Neurocytol 7:405–418
22. Cody FW, Richardson HC (1978) Mossy and climbing fibres projections of trigeminal inputs to cerebellar cortex in the cat. Brain Res 53:352–356

23. Cohen JD, Castro-Alamancos MA (2010) Behavioural State dependency of Neural Activity and Sensory (Whisker) responses in Superior Colliculus. J Neurophysiol 104:1661–1672
24. Cottle MK (1964) Degeneration studies of primary afferents of IX th and X th cranial nerves in the cat. J Comp Neurol 122:329
25. Craig AD (1992) Spinal and trigeminal lamina I input to the locus coeruleus anterogradely labeled with Phaseolus vulgaris leucoagglutinin (PHA-L) in the cat and the monkey. Brain Res 584:325–328
26. Craig AD (1995) Distribution of brainstem projections from spinal lamina I neurons in the cat and the monkey. J Comp Neurol 361:225–248
27. Craig AD Jr, Burton H (1981) Spinal and medullary lamina I projection to nucleus submedius in medial thalamus: a possible pain center. J Neurophysiol 45:443–466
28. Craig AD Jr, Dostrovsky JO (1991) Thermoreceptive lamina I trigeminothalamic neurons project to the nucleus submedius in the cat. Exp Brain Res 85:470–474
29. Dado RJ, Giesler GJ Jr (1990) Afferent input to nucleus submedius in rats: retrograde labeling of neurons in the spinal cord and caudal medulla. J Neurosci 10:2672–2686
30. Dunker E, Von Rehren D (1973) Liaisons fonctionnelles entre le système vagal et les "neurones de la douleur" du complexe nucléaire trigéminal. In: Janzen R, Keidel W, Hertz A, Steichele C (eds) La Douleur. Masson & Co (ed), Paris, pp 138–140
31. Edwards SB, Ginsburgh CL, Henkel CK, Stein BF (1979) Sources of subcortical projections to the superior colliculus in the cat. J Comp Neurol 184:309–330
32. Elias SA, Taylor A, Somjen G (1987) Direct and relayed projection of periodontal receptor afferents to the cerebellum in the ferret. Proc Roy Soc Lond B 231:199–216
33. Feil K, Herbert H (1995) Topographic organization of spinal and trigeminal somatosensory pathways to the rat parabrachial and Kölliker-fuse nuclei. J Comp Neurol 353:506–528
34. Ferr FWL (1961) Structural relation of the trigeminal tract to upper cervical roots and the solitary nucleus in the cat. Exp Neurol 4:134–148
35. Funakoshi M, Nakashima N (1980) Excitation of Masseter muscle spindle induced by Periodontal stimulation. J Dent Res Abstracts 422:992
36. Gerard MW (1923) Afferent impulses of the trigeminal nerves, the intramedullary course of the painful thermal and tactile impulses. Arch Neurol Psych 9:306–338
37. Gobel S, Purvis MB (1972) Anatomical studies of the organization of the spinal V nucleus: the deep bundles and the spinal V tract. Brain Res 48:27–44
38. Goldberg LJ (1971) Masseter muscle excitation induced by stimulation of periodontal and gingival receptors in man. Brain Res 32:369–381
39. Hathaway CB, Hu JW, Bereiter DA (1995) Distribution of Fos-like immunoreactivity in the caudal brainstem of the rat following noxious chemical stimulation of the temporomandibular joint. J Comp Neurol 356:444–456
40. Huerta M, Frankfurter A, Harting J (1983) Studies of the principal sensory and spinal trigeminal nuclei of the rat: projections to the superior colliculus, inferior olive and cerebellum. J Comp Neurol 220:147–167
41. Ikeda M (1968) Projections from the spinal and the principal sensory nuclei of the trigeminal nerve to the cerebellar cortex in the cat, as suited by retrograde transport of horseradish peroxidase. J Comp Neurol 133:71–88
42. Ikeda M (1989) Projections from the spinal and the principal sensory nuclei of the trigeminal nerve to the cerebellar cortex in the cat, as suited by retrograde transport of horseradish peroxidase. J Comp Neurol 184:567–586
43. Iwata K, Kenshalo DR, Dubner R Jr, Nahlin RL (1992) Diencephalic projections from the superficial and deep laminae of the medullary dorsal horn in the rat. J Comp Neurol 321:404–420
44. Jacquart G, Mahler P, Kachani-Mansour R (1986) Growth of trigemino-cerebellar areas in infant rat studied by micrometric and cytophometric methods. Arch Oral Biol 31(9):573–576
45. Jacquin MF, Semba K, Rhoades RW, Egger MD (1982) Trigeminal primary afferents project bilaterally to dorsal horn and ipsilaterally to cerebellum reticular formation and cuneate, solitary, supratrigeminal and vagal nuclei. Brain Res 246:285–291

46. Jacquin M, Semba K, Egger MD, Rhoades R (1983) Organization of HRP-labeled trigeminal mandibular primary afferent neurons in the rat. J Comp Neurol 215:397–420
47. Karamandilis A (1968) Trigemino-cerebellar connections in the goat studied by means of the retrograde cell degeneration method. J Comp Neurol 133:71–88
48. Kato J, Wakisaka S, Tabata MJ et al (1994) Induction of fos protein in the rat trigeminal nucleus complex during an experimental tooth movement. Archs Oral Biol 39:723–726
49. Kawamura Y (1974) Physiology of mastication. Kawamura (ed), Basel
50. Kerr WL (1962) Facial vagal and glossopharyngeal nerves in the cat. Arch Neurol 6:264–281
51. Künzle H (1998) Origin and terminal distribution of the trigeminal projections to the inferior and superior colliculi in the lesser hedgehog tenrec. Eur J Neurosci 10(1):368–376
52. Künzle H (1998) Trigeminal projections to thalamus and subthalamus in the hedgehog tenrec. Neurosci 86(2):651–661
53. Kvinnsland I, Heyeraas KJ, Byers MR (1992) Effect of traumatic occlusion on CGRP and SP immunoreactive nerve fibre morphology in rat molar pulp and periodontium. Histochemistry 97:111–120
54. Leamey CA, Ho SM (1998) Afferent arrival and onset of functional activity in the trigeminothalamic pathway of the rat. Brain Res Dev Brain Res 105(2):195–207
55. Li J, Xiong K, Pang Y et al (2006) Medullary dorsal horn neurons providing axons to both the parabrachial nucleus and thalamus. J Comp Neurol 498(4):539–551
56. Limoge A, Limoge-Lendais I (1992) Neurophysiologie générale. Régulation et comportements. Masson (éd), Paris
57. Lund JP, Lamarre Y (1973) The importance of positive feed-back from periodontal pressoreceptors during voluntary isometric contraction of jaw closing muscles in man. J Biol Bucc 1:345–351
58. Lund JP, Lavigne G, Kim JS (1987) Le rôle des récepteurs parodontaux dans le contrôle de la mastication. Symp Int Physiol Oro Fac Nancy 143–144
59. Malick A, Strassman RM, Burstein R (2000) Trigeminohypothalamic and reticulohypothalamic tract neurons in the upper cervical spinal cord and cauda medulla of the rat. J Neurophysiol 84(4):2078–2112
60. Manni E, Lucchi ML, Filippi GM, Bortolami R (1982) Area postrema and the mesencephalic trigeminal nucleus. Exp Neurol 77:39–55
61. Mantle-St John L, Tracey D (1987) Somatosensory nuclei in the brainstem of the rat: independent projections to the thalamus and cerebellum. J Comp Neurol 255:259–271
62. Marfurt CF, Rajchert DM (1991) Trigeminal primary afferent projections to "non-trigeminal" areas of the rat central nervous system. J Comp Neurol 303:489–511
63. Matsushita M, Okado N, Ikeda M, Hosoya Y (1981) Descending projections from the spinal and mesencephalic nuclei or the trigeminal nerve to the spinal cord in the cat. A study with the horseradish peroxidase technique. J Comp Neurol 196:173–187
64. Matsushita M, Ikeda M, Okado N (1982) The cells of origin of the trigeminothalamic, trigeminospinal and trigeminocerebellar projections in the cat. Neurosci 7:1439–1454
65. Matthews PBC (1972) Mammalian muscle receptors and their central-action. Arnold (ed), London
66. Melzack R, Haugen FP (1957) Responses Evoked at the Cortex by Tooth Stimulation. Am J Physiol 3(190):570–574
67. Menétrey D, Basbaum AI (1987) Spinal and trigeminal projections to the nucleus of the solitary tract: a possible substrate for somatovisceral and viscerovisceral reflex activation. J Comp Neurol 255:439–450
68. Menétrey D, Leah J, De Pommery J (1987) Efferent projections of the paratrigeminal nucleus in the rat. Neurosci Lett 73:48–52
69. Nakamura Y, Goldberg LJ, Minuzo N, Clemente CD (1970) Masseteric reflex inhibition induced by afferent impulses in the hypoglossal nerve. Brain Res 18:241–255
70. Ochardson R, Sheena H, Mac Farmale H (1980) The effect of local periodontal anaesthesia on the maximum biting force achieved by human subjects. Arch Oral Biol 25:799–804

71. Olsewski J (1950) On the anatomical and functional organization of the spinal trigeminal nucleus. J Comp Neurol 92:401–413
72. Olsson KA, Weisberg KG (1989) Interneurons in the trigeminal motor system. In: Van Steenberghe D, Delaat A (eds) Electromyography of jaw reflexes in Man. Lewen Univ Press, Lewen, p p19
73. Ottersen OP (2004) Afferent connections to the amygdaloid complex of the rat with some observations in the cat. III. Afferents from the lower brain stem. J Comp Neurol 202(3):335–356
74. Palazzi C, Paolinelli P, Adrian H, Manns A (1991) Canine Evoked Potentials in the Somatic Cortex of the Dog. J Dent Res 70(4):729
75. Panneton WM (1991) Primary afferent projections from the upper respiratory tract in the muskrat. J Comp Neurol 308:51–65
76. Panneton WM, Burton H (1985) Projections from the paratrigeminal nucleus and the medullary and spinal dorsal horns to the peribrachial area in the cat. Neurosci 15:779–797
77. Panneton WM, Johnson SN, Christensen ND (1994) Trigeminal projections to the peribrachial region in the muskrat. Neurosci 59:605–625
78. Penfield W, Rasmussen T (1950) The cerebral cortex of man. Mc Millan (ed), New York
79. Pfaller K, Arvidsson J (1988) Central distribution of trigeminal and upper cervical primary afferents in the rat studied by anterograde transport of horseradish peroxidase conjugated to wheat germ agglutinin. J Comp Neurol 268:91–108
80. Phelan KD, Falls WM (1991) The spino-trigeminal pathway and its spatial relationship to the origin of trigemino-spinal projections in the rat. Neurosci 40:447–496
81. Phelan KD, Falls WM (1991) A comparison of the distribution and morphology of thalamic, cerebellar and spinal projection neurons in rat trigeminal nucleus interpolaris. Neurosci 40:497–511
82. Pinganaud G, Bourcier F, Buisseret-Delmas C, Buisseret P (1999) Primary trigeminal afferents to the vestibular nuclei in the rat: existence of a collateral projection to the vestibulocerebellum. Neurosci Lett 264(1–3):133–136
83. Piovesan EJ, Kowacs PA, Oshinsky ML (2003) Convergence of Cervical and Trigeminal Sensory Afferents. Curr Pain Headache Rep 7:377–383
84. Rhoades RW, Fish SE, Chiaia NL et al (1989) Organization of the projections from the trigeminal brainstem complex to the superior colliculus in the rat and hamster: anterograde tracing with Phaseolus vulgaris leucoagglutinin and intra-axonal injection. J Comp Neurol 289(4):641–656
85. Richardson HC, Cody FWJ, Paul VE, Thomas AG (1978) Convergence of trigeminal and limb inputs onto cerebellar interpositus nuclear neurones in the cat. Brain Res 156:355–359
86. Rossi F, Brodal A (1957) Terminal distribution of spinoreticular fibers in the cat. Arch Physiol 37:413–429
87. Rowland NC, Jaeger D (2008) Responses to Tactile Stimulation in Deep Cerebellar Nucleus Neurons Result From Recurrent Activation in Multiple Pathways. J Neurophysiol 99: 704–717
88. Ruggiero DA, Ross CA, Reis DJ (1981) Projections from the spinal trigeminal Nucleus to the entire length of the spinal cord in the rat. Brain Res 225:225–233
89. Salenc C (1979) Projection des nerfs maxillaires et des récepteurs dentaires sur le cortex cérébral du chat. Thèse 3ème cycle Sci Odont Marseille
90. Saper CB, Loewy AD (1980) Efferent connections of the parabrachial nucleus in the rat. Brain Res 197:291–317
91. Shigenaga Y, Takabatake M, Sugimoto T, Sakai A (1979) Neurons of marginal layer of trigeminal nucleus caudalis projecting to ventrobasal complex (VB) and posterior nuclear group (PO) demonstrated retrograde labeling with horseradish peroxidase. Brain Res 166: 391–396
92. Shigenaga Y, Sera M, Nishimori T et al (1988) The central projection of masticatory afferent fibers to the trigeminal sensory nuclear complex and upper cervical spinal cord. J Comp Neurol 268(4):489–507

93. Somana R, Kotchabakdhi N, Walberg F (1980) Cerebellar afferents from the trigeminal sensory nuclei in the cat. Exp Brain Res 38:57–64
94. South EH, Ritter RC (1986) Substance P-containing trigeminal sensory neurones project to nucleus of the solitary tract. Brain Res 372:283–289
95. Strazielle C, Mahler P, Jacquart G (1987) Localisation des afférences primaires trigémino-cérébelleuses chez le rat. Wistar Symp Int Physiol Oro Fac Nancy 57–65
96. Sugimoto T, Fujiyoshi Y, Xiao C et al (1997) Central projection of calcitonin gene-related peptide (CGRP)- and Substance P (SP)-immunoreactive trigeminal primary neurons in the rat. J Comp Neurol 378:425–442
97. Sugimoto T, Fujiyoshi Y, He YF et al (1997) Trigeminal primary projection to the rat brain stem sensory trigeminal nuclear complex and surrounding structures revealed by anterograde transport of cholera toxin B subunit-conjugated and Bandeiraea simplicifolia isolectin B4-conjugated horseradish peroxidase. Neurosci Res 28(4):361–371
98. Sunakawa M (1984) Response properties of the tooth pulp-driven neurons in the primary somatosensory cortex (SI) in the cat. Kokubyo Gakkai Zasshi 51:627–640
99. Takemura M, Sugimoto T, Sakai A (1987) Topographic organization of central terminal region of different branches of the rat mandibular nerve. Exp Neurol 96:540–557
100. Takemura M, Sugimoto T, Shigenaga Y (1991) Difference in central projection of primary afferents innervating facial and intra-oral structures in the rat. Exp Neurol 111:324–331
101. Torvik A (1956) Afferent connections to the sensory trigeminal nuclei, the nucleus of the solitary tract and adjacent structures. An experimental study in the rat. J Comp Neurol 106:51–141
102. Trub M (1979) Projections hypothalamiques de la sensibilité desmodontale. Thèse 3ème Sci Odontol Marseille
103. Trub M, Mei N, Orsini JC (1991) Macro and micro-electrode study of hypothalamic projections of periodontal afferents in the rat and cat. Brain Res Bull 27:29–34
104. Trub M, Mei N (1991) Effects on periodontal stimulation on VMH neurones in anesthetized rats. Brain Res Bull 27(1):29–34
105. Trub M, Mei N, Orofino J (1996) Periodontal and gastric convergences within the hypothalamic ventromedial nucleus area - single unit study on anesthetized rats. Behav Brain Res 72:33–37
106. Valla J, Delfini C, Diagne M et al (2003) Vestibulotrigeminal and vestibulospinal projections in rats: retrograde tracing coupled to glutamic acid decarboxylase immunoreactivity. Neurosci Lett 340(3):225–228
107. Van Ham JJ, Yeo HC (1992) Somatosensory Trigeminal Projections to the Inferior Olive, Cerebellum and other Precerebellar Nuclei in Rabbits. Eur J Neurosci 4(4):302–317
108. Veinante P, Deschênes M (1999) Single- and Multi-Whisker Channels in the Ascending Projections from the Principal Trigeminal Nucleus in the Rat. J Neurosc 19(12):5085–5095
109. Vinay L, Cazalets JR, Clarac F (1995) Evidence for the Existence of a Functional Polysynaptic Pathway From Trigeminal Afferents to Lumbar Motoneurons in the Neonatal Rat. Eup J Neurosci 7:143–151
110. Watson CRR, Switzer RL (1978) Trigeminal projections to cerebellar tactile areas in the rat origin mainly from noyau interpolaris and noyau principalis. Neuro Sci Lett 10:77–82
111. Westphal A, Divry M (1991) Le comportement manducateur. Presses Univ (éd), Nancy
112. Yamoshi M, Ozawa M, Kawano J (1991) Effect of Periodontal Sensation on Masticatory Movement in Man. J Dent Res 70(4):802
113. Yasui Y, Kayahara T, Shiroyama T, Nakano K (1993) Neurons in the intertrigeminal region of the rat send projection fibers to the superior colliculus. Neurosci Lett 159(1–2):39–42
114. Yokota T, Koyama N (1981) Trigeminal nociceptive neurons in subnucleus reticularis ventralis of Caudal Medulla Oblongata. J Dent Res 60(49):1239
115. Yokota T, Matsumoto N (1983) Somatotopic distribution of trigeminal nociceptive specific neurones within the caudal somatosensory thalamus of cat. Neurosci Lett 39:125–130
116. Yokota T, Matsumoto N (1983) Location and functional organization of trigeminal wide dynamic range neurones within the nucleus ventralis posteromedialis of the cat. Neurosci Lett 39:231–236

117. Yoshida A, Dostrovsky JO, Sessle BJ, Chiang CY (1991) Trigeminal projections to the nucleus submedius of the thalamus of the rat. J Comp Neurol 307:609–625
118. Yoshida A, Sessle BJ, Dovstrovsky JO, Chiang CY (1992) Trigeminal and dorsal column projections to the anterior pretectal nucleus in the rat. Brain Res 590:81–94
119. Yoshida A, Chen K, Moritani M et al (1997) Organization of the descending projections from the parabrachial nucleus to the trigeminal sensory nuclear complex and spinal dorsal horn in the rat. J Comp Neurol 383(1):94–111
120. Zang WB, Li JS, Li HM (1991) SP-like immunoreactivity in the primary trigeminal neurones projecting to the nucleus tractus solitarii. Brain Res 558:87–89
121. Zeredo JL, Toda K, Soma K (2002) Neck motor unit activities induced by inputs from periodontal mechanoreceptors in rats. J Dent Res 8(1):39–42
122. Zeredo JL, Toda K, Soma K (2003) Nature of neck motor unit activities evoked by different trigeminal inputs in rats. J Dent Res 82(5):402–405
123. Zhou J, Shore S (2006) Convergence of spinal trigeminal and cochlear nucleus projections in the inferior colliculus of the guinea pig. J Comp Neurol 495(1):100–112

Useful Physiological Reminders

Human adaptation to permanent stressors (paratypical factors) involves sensitivity, integration, and motivity as part of a very complex set including metabolism, psyche, and memory (Fig. 1). All these behavioral units work together according to each person's genotype with the purpose of maintaining living, growing, and developing conditions. In order to have influence over their surroundings, humans and animals have to control their muscular contractions precisely [22]. The motor activity exercised by the central nervous system (CNS) integrates afferents. Then, through the motor neurons, it transmits motor efferents to muscular fibers (responses). According to some embryologic data, the *stomatognathic muscles* are special skeletal muscles because they are involved in postural activity and also participate in a digestive function. Some authors even suggest that they have characteristics largely similar to those of digestive muscles [10]. In humans their fascia and bundles are both penniform and half penniform [6], which gives these muscles very fine-motor precision. Moreover, with the exception of muscular proprioception (jaw and tongue muscles), the orofacial sphere benefits from a rich and various sensory equipment – occlusal, lingual, articular, mucosal, cutaneous, and autonomic. For occlusal proprioceptive afferents, general operation is governed by laws of *global balanced volume* between the right and left sides of the dental arches. This helps organize functional swallowing and side alternating mastication. But some painful or uncomfortable conditions (occlusal troubles, lingual dysfunctions, etc.) create abnormal reflex motor responses. They facilitate atypical swallowing or unilateral and permanent mastication. The stomatognathic system then tends to cause staggering with a *spastic tendency*. Therefore, under unfavorable physiological conditions some disorders can develop [8, 9] in relation to each patient's adaptive ability. In effect the body keeps using some adaptive mechanisms to maintain functions such as mastication, deglutition, posture, or locomotion in non-algic conditions, owing to some buffer zones as TMJ, shoulders, rachis, pelvis, knees, etc.

F. Hartmann, G. Cucchi, *Stress and Orality*,
DOI 10.1007/978-2-8178-0271-8_8, © Springer-Verlag France 2014

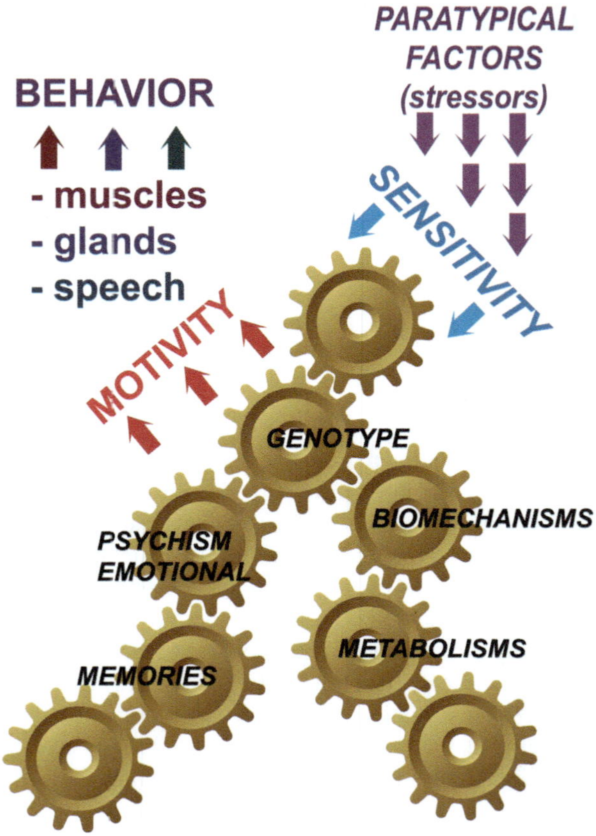

Fig. 1 Human adaptation units to stress

The sensory-motor innervation of the skeletal muscle[1]

[1]It concerns different elements including the neuromuscular spindle (NMS), both a sensory and motor set, and the Golgi tendon organ (GTO) that plays only a sensory role. Some special receptors (type III and IV) are present in muscular tissues for recording stressing nociceptive conditions as internal overpressure or abnormal histochemical values. They most certainly supply a large amount of the trigeminal overstimulation and nociception observed in those TMD spastic conditions (clenching) responsible for referred tension-type pain. Some motor neurons (β and γ) regulate the level of reactivity of NMS towards muscular internal tensions and muscular length variations. These β and γ motor neurons are tightly involved in neuromuscular pathophysiological closed circles called β–γ *loops*, responsible for spastic phenomena. The extrafusal fibers which receive the skeleto-motor innervation (α motor neuron) are of three functional types [4]: the *fast-fatigable type* whose phasic modality is involved in rapid movements, the *slow type* whose tonic modality is involved in maintaining posture and attitude, and the *fast-resistant type* whose tonico-phasic modality is involved in sustained movements. Two types of muscular contractions are typically identified: isotonic contractions with movement (phasic) and isometric contractions with no movement (tonic). For example, mastication essentially follows an isotonic mood; jaw posture is more of an isometric function. Under TMD pathophysiological conditions (parafunctions), grinding is a phasic activity, whereas clenching is an isometric sustained activity without excursive lateral movements, that is, the most deleterious working mood for the muscular tissue because of the high persistent level of tension.

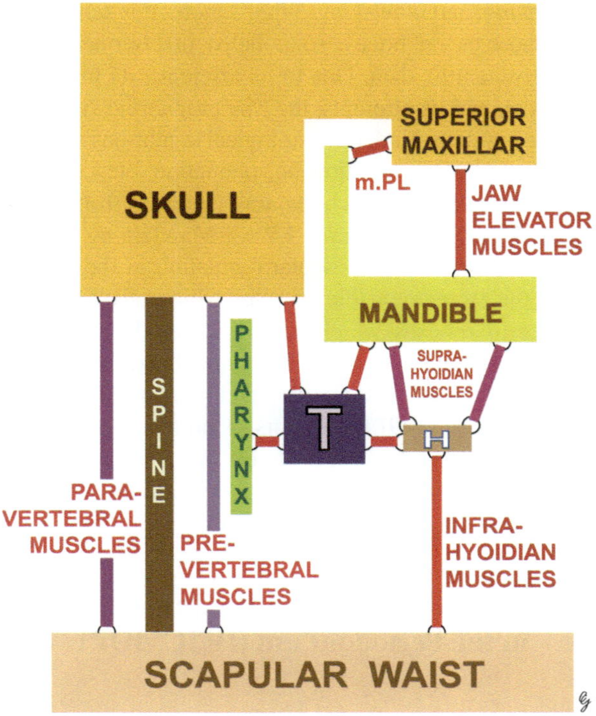

Fig. 2 Brodie's scheme. *m.PL* musculus pterygoideus lateralis (= lateral pterygoid muscle), *H* hyoidian bone, *T* tongue (Modified from Brodie [3])

1 The Rest Position of the Jaw

Brodie's scheme (Fig. 2) sets the mandibular posture in the global postural system [3]. This shows functional connections between the stomatognathic system and its surroundings, that is, particularly the scapular waist and cervical rachis [5, 17, 27]. An important and too often forgotten set was added: **the tongue**[2]. Through its multiple insertions, it plays a major operational role in one's *posture*, *breathing*, *eating*,

[2] Figure 2 schematizes the functional mechanical links between the tongue and the mandible, the soft palate, the skull, and the hyo-thyro-sternal set. Through these links, the tongue may be affected by disturbances occurring in these areas. But its role is not only passive; indeed, as a very complex unit of 17 muscles, the tongue also reacts to psycho-emotional factors from the brain. Therefore, it too is capable of disturbing the above-mentioned areas. Problems with mastication, swallowing, speaking, breathing, posture, etc. can arise when the lingual physiology goes wrong. An insufficiently functioning area between the oral floor, dental arches, and palate vault may be one of the primary etiologies generating such lingual dysfunctions and possible outcomes. Therefore, the tendency in reduced size maxillas in children is still a misunderstood factor of stomatognathic and other dysfunctions in adults [12, 20].

speaking, and *mimicking*. What's more, this scheme emphasizes the essential impact of muscles on bones, so it helps practitioners make better clinical use of new neuroscientific data. Due to its afferents, its integrating, analyzing, and controlling system, and its efferents, the *stomatognathic system* may be compared to a self-regulated system. Under physiological conditions and without any specific motor activity (mastication, swallowing, phonation, etc.), the jaw's balance remains unstable. The inferior dental arch remains separated from the superior dental arch by a space called the *freeway space* (FWS). Maintaining the FWS into a physiological value depends on a neuromuscular regulation of the postural tone in the tongue muscles and the stomatognathic muscles which position the jaw. Such regulation involves different reflexes which remain under the influence of superior nervous centres (suprasegmental control). There are also reciprocal repercussions between the regulation of the jaw rest position and breathing [23]. The hyolingual set (especially m. genioglossus) [19] through its mandibular insertions (spina mentalis) must remain far from the pharyngeal posterior wall to allow sufficient breathing flow. In this postural regulation the lateral pterygoid muscles seem to play a major role [24].

2 Inhibition Reflex of the Jaw-Closing Muscles Originating in the Periodontium (IRJCMOP)

At the end of mouth closing, the contacts between the teeth determine an inhibition of the activity of jaw-closing muscles (Fig. 3).

3 Phasic Activity of the Stomatognathic Muscles

Stomatognathic muscles participate in phasic motor functions such as *mastication*, *swallowing*, and *phonation* [1, 25, 26]. Voluntary or automatic superior nervous circuits intervene, especially for motor memorization [21]. For instance, food in the mouth activates infracortical nervous circuits by stimulating receptors (periodontal, lingual, mucosal). Then follows a motor activation of jaw-closing muscles (food crushing) which initiates an automatic mastication period [13, 15, 16]. During mastication the PR sensory threshold greatly increases [14] making them less excitable during the physiological activity. Their protective role towards masticatory excessive biting forces, particularly at the end of the movement, was confirmed by tests [18] done with suppression of periodontal perception by local anesthetics.

About swallowing, let us recall that in physiological conditions periodontal inputs contribute to guide the CNS for an accurate motor sequence. This happens about 1,500–2,000 times a day for an adult and during meals. Imbalance occlusal contacts between sides of dental arches are potential factors of abnormal reflexes during deglutition. An insufficient functional space for the tongue may be an aggravating one (see before).

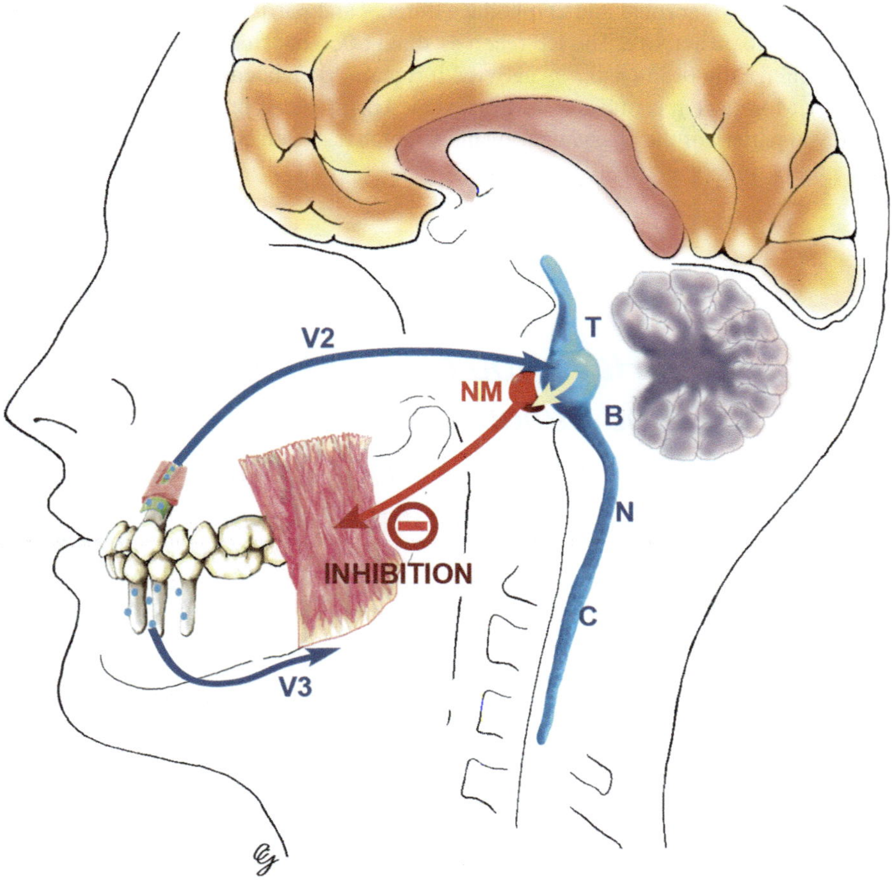

Fig. 3 Inhibition reflex of the jaw-closing muscles originating in the periodontium (IRJCMOP). The contraction of jaw-closing muscles (JCM) as the masseteris induces the dental contact. The following tactile stimulation of the periodontal receptors (PR) reaches the TBNC by V2 and V3 ways. A neural connection with the trigeminal motor nucleus of the V (MoN) makes a motor inhibition of the jaw-closing muscles (jaw relaxation)

4 The Brain Control on Muscular Activities

The physiological motor action can be regulated at two levels: the *inferior level* (bulbar or medullar) and the *superior level* (infracortical). The unit modulates the muscular tone by maintaining postural balance and making automatic movements. To achieve this regulation, several central structures operate, particularly the *reticular formation* (RF). The activating interneuron network assists with ascendant inputs to the cerebral cortex and descendant inputs to the motor nuclei of cranial nerves (tractus reticulo-nuclearis) and the spinal cord (tractus reticulospinalis). The RF seems to react to cortical and cerebellar efferents and participates in the regulation of postural tonic activity. The RF receives some afferents from other regions of the brain which calm or intensify its activity. It remains dependent on some key factors (Fig. 4). Moreover, recent EMG studies revealed that "... cerebral function influences the EMG pattern of the pharyngeal swallow which has been considered traditionally as a purely reflex pattern" [7].

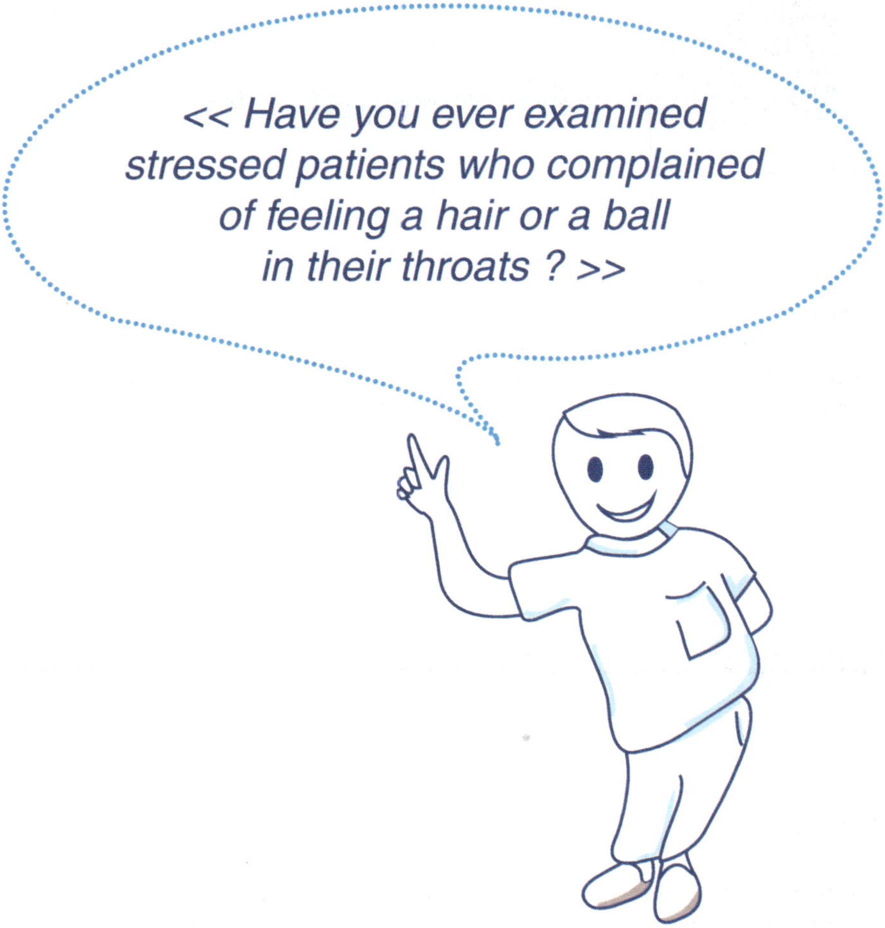

5 Other Implicated Nervous Centres

This regulation also depends on the *central gray nuclei* (CGN): the neostriatum makes it possible to sort information necessary to avoid disturbing execution of movement. The CGN also participate in controlling vigilance mechanisms [2]. Other nervous structures involved are the nuclei vestibulares, the oliva, the paleocerebellum and

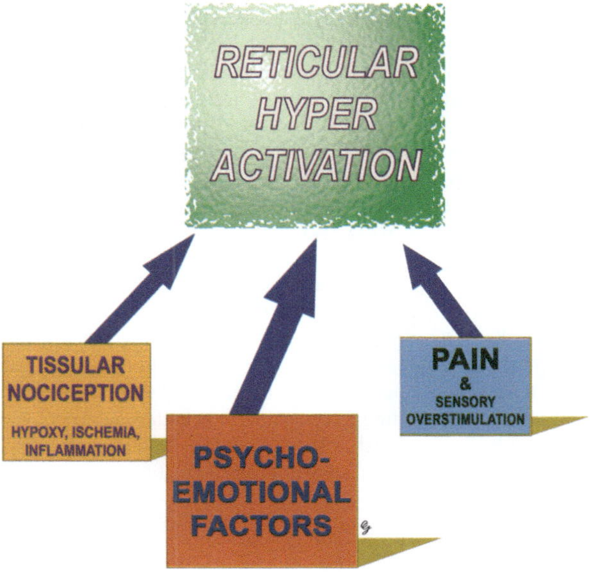

Fig. 4 Factors of reticular hyperactivity

archeocerebellum, as well as the limbic system. At the cerebellum, there is an input projection of the deep conscious sensibility from the sensory cranial nuclei, particularly of the V [11] at the level of the paleocerebellum. Furthermore, the *cerebellum* is able to memorize motor program sequences thanks to the nucleus dentatus and the nucleus interpositus.

References

1. Azerad J (1991) Physiologie de la manducation. Masson (éd), Paris
2. Bonvallet M (1966) Système nerveux et vigilance. La Science vivante, Press Univ France (ed), Paris
3. Brodie AG (1941) Croissance de la tête du 3ème mois à la 8ème année de la vie. Am J Anat 68:209–262
4. Burke RE (1981) Motor units: anatomy, physiology, and functional organization. In: Brooks VB (ed), Handbook of physiology – the nervous system. Am Physiol Soc, Washington, pp 345–422
5. Gangloff P, Perrin PP (2002) Unilateral trigeminal anaesthesia modifies postural control in human subjects. Neurosci Lett 330(2):179–182
6. Gaspard M, Laison F, Mailland M (1973) Organisation architecturale et texture des muscles ptérygoidiens chez les Primates supérieurs. J Biol Bucc 1:215–233
7. German RZ, Crompton AW, Thexton AJ (2009) Integration of the reflex pharyngeal swacllow into rhythmic oral activity in a neurologically intact Pig model. J Neurophysiol 102:1017–1025
8. Hartmann F, Cucchi G (1986) Rôle du muscle ptérygoïdien latéral dans la phase de début du SADAM. Cah Proth 56:125–144
9. Hartmann F, Cucchi G (1987) Muscle ptérygoïdien latéral et SADAM: diagnostic précoce et traitement. Rev Odont Stomatol 16(3):209–218

10. Jacquart G, Mentre C, Nicolas R (1978) Algies du Trijumeau: aspect fondamental de leur pathogénie. Encycl Med Chir Stomato 6:22041 A10
11. Jacquart G, Mahler P, Kachani-Mansour R (1986) Growth of trigemino-cerebellar areas in infant rat studied by micrometric and cytophometric methods. Arch Oral Biol 31(9):573–576
12. Jeanmonod A (1988) Occlusodontie. Applications cliniques. Cah Proth (éd), Paris
13. Kawamura Y (1974) Physiology of mastication. Kawamura (ed), Basel
14. Kiliardis S, Tzakis M, Carlsson S (1990) Short-term and long-term effects of chewing training on occlusal perception of thickness. Scand J Dent Res 98:159–166
15. Lund JP, Sessle BJ (1974) Oral-facial and jaw muscle afferent projections to neurons in cat frontal cortex. Exp Neurol 45:314–331
16. Lund JP, Lavigne G, Kim JS (1987) Le rôle des récepteurs parodontaux dans le contrôle de la mastication. Symp Int Physiol Oro Fac Nancy 143–144
17. Mc Kay DC, Christensen LV (1999) Electrognathographic and electromyographic observations on jaw depression during neck extension. J Oral Rehabil 26:865–876
18. Ochardson R, Sheena H, Mac Farmale H (1980) The effect of local periodontal anaesthesia on the maximum biting force achieved by human subjects. Arch Oral Biol 25:799–804
19. Otsuka R, Ono T, Ishiwata Y, Kuroda T (2000) Respiratory-related genioglossus electromyographic activity in response to head rotation and changes in body position. Angle Orthod 70(1):63–69
20. Planas P (1992) La réhabilitation occlusale. (Traduction: Chateau M, Kolf J) Masson (éd), Paris
21. Renaud J (1984) La mémoire passe par le cervelet. Sci & Vie 799:37–43
22. Schmidt RF, Dudel J, Janig W, Zimmermann M (1984) Neuro-physiologie. Lib Le François (éd), Paris
23. Takahashi S, Ono T, Ishiwata Y, Kuroda T (1999) Effect of changes in the breathing mode and body position on tongue pressure with respiratory-related oscillations. Am J Orthod Dentofacial Orthop 115(3):239–246
24. Talmant J (1976) Introduction à l'étude de la statique céphalique. Rev Orthop Dent Fac 3:321–334
25. Woda A (1983) Abrégé de physiologie oro-faciale. Masson (éd), Paris
26. Woda A, Fontenelle A (1975) Activité tonique et posture de la mandibule. Mastication Déglutition. In: Chateau M (ed) Orthopédie dento-faciale, vol 1. J Prélat (éd), Paris, p 244
27. Zafar H (2000) Integrated jaw and neck function in man. Studies of mandibular and head-neck movements during jaw opening-closing tasks. Swed Dent J Suppl 143:1–41

Pathophysiological Conditions

Foreword

All data mentioned and even more so the theory suggested in this chapter must be positioned in relation with the well-known neuroendocrinal data about classical stress mechanisms. The little known parafunctional oral habit called *clenching* will be presented as a possible awkward mode of response to stress. Based on its deleterious clinical outcomes, it calls for a close investigation by all clinicians.

F. Hartmann, G. Cucchi, *Stress and Orality*,
DOI 10.1007/978-2-8178-0271-8_9, © Springer-Verlag France 2014

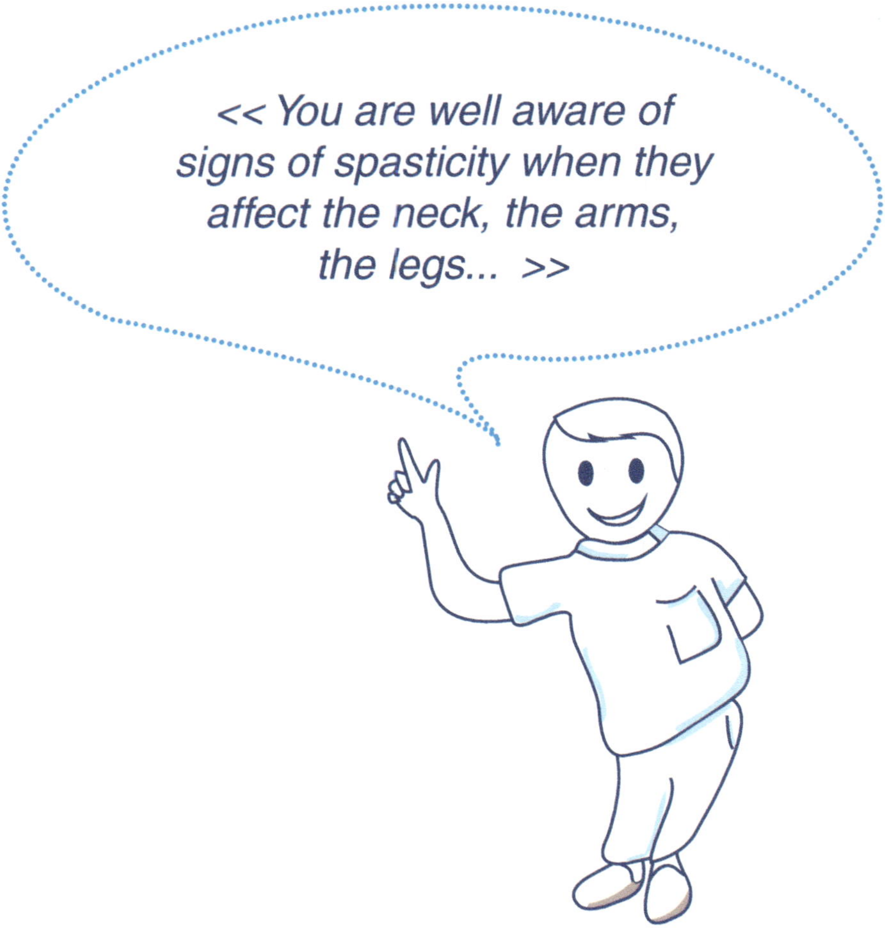
<< You are well aware of signs of spasticity when they affect the neck, the arms, the legs... >>

1 Skeletal Muscular Spasticity

Spasticity is defined as the more or less apparent predisposition to be contractured or the range of elevation of muscle tone, with a relation to a stretch reflex. When they are subject to nociceptive stimulations such as mechanical, emotional, infective, metabolical, thermic, or nutritional stimulations, muscles respond with spasms or shortenings. They lose their ability to relax by intention [82]. In contractured muscles, some points become sensitive to palpation (tender points).[1] The RF plays a major role in the mechanism of spasticity (Fig. 1) by facilitating the induction of the famous muscular $\beta - \gamma$ *loops*.

[1] At this level a tissue anoxic phenomenon might be responsible for this objectified sign [72]. Quarti and Renaud [61] explain the problem as follows: "All encapsulated receptors, including the NMS, have double innervation: beside their specific sensory fiber there exists at least one non-myelinated

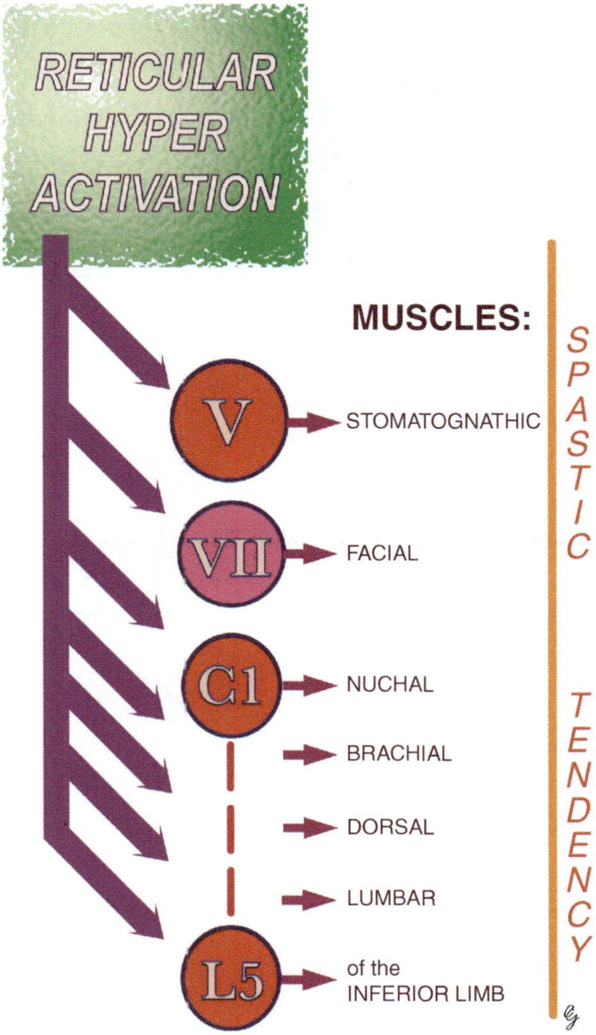

Fig. 1 Spastic influence of reticular hyperactivity at several muscular levels

ending which functions as a free-ending, as in any tissue. Biochemical conditions of stimulation may be similar for all nociceptive fibers. This would act as an internal alert system reacting to a stimulation overload on physiological limits. When reacting to a supraliminary stimulation the specialized cells of the specific receptors produce nociceptive enzymes which remain inactive towards specific endings but inflame thin non-myelinated fibers." Thus, non-myelinated fibers, those connected to type IV receptors, are strongly activated during prolonged muscular contraction under ischemic conditions [4]. Acidosis-induced vasoconstriction [17] and free radical production

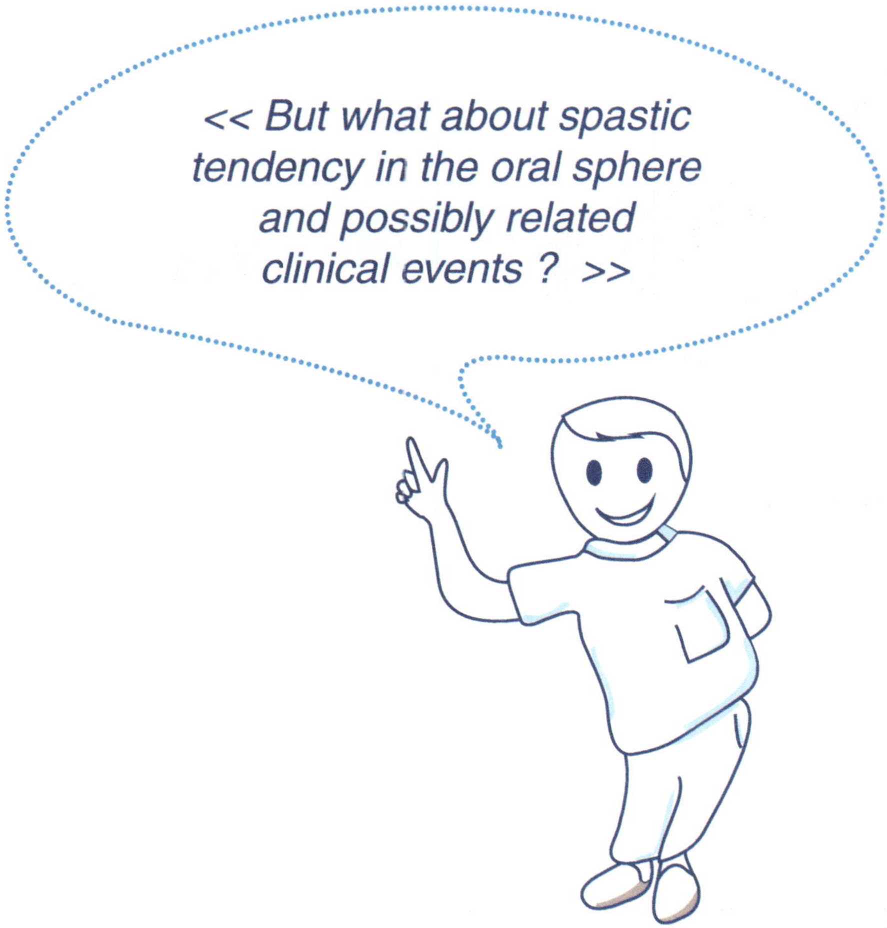

2 Stomatognathic Muscular Spasticity

In most cases, TMD are caused by several factors including *muscular overtension*, the most frequent, most important, and most misunderstood cause [54]. Overtension is all the more powerful since it results from both *peripheral* and *central factors*

rate increase are the elective stimuli to previous receptors which are connected to nociceptive muscular fibers. Such nociceptive inputs, coming from little affected tissues, are themselves reticular activating factors [5]. In this way, some factors could trigger vigilance intensification and sometimes pain from sensory overstimulation, acidosis, and hypoxia from ischemia in contractured muscle tissue [17, 50, 63, 77]. The central afferents such as limbic and hypothalamic (those linked to emotional phenomena), subcortical, and cerebellar (those linked to automatic muscular activity) may help trigger such a vascular reflex of proprioceptive origin (overstimulation).

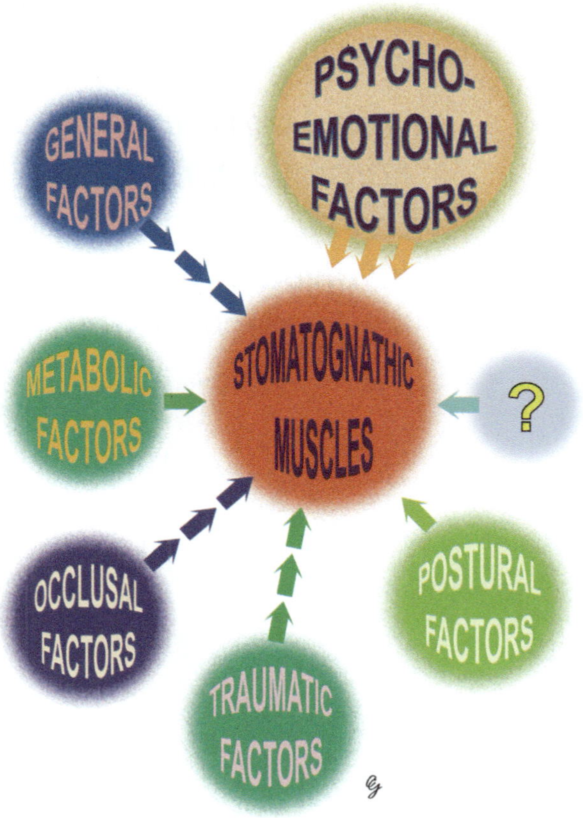

Fig. 2 Stomatognathic muscles and various spastic factors

(Fig. 2). Thoughts and emotions have been suspected to have highly direct impacts on trigeminal motor structures such as stomatognathic muscles. What's more, biochemical and metabolic factors in TMD [82] receive more attention from experts. The trigeminal system is acutely sensitive to changing levels of norepinephrine, serotonin, glutamate, and acetylcholine produced in the brain.[2] More generally, the neuromuscular disorders of the stomatognathic system may affect three levels: the *afferents*, the *central nervous system*, and the *efferents*. In cases of TMD, the most involved elements should be considered. Central overactivity is related to psycho-emotional factors (cortical, infracortical, and limbic). The overexcitability of proprioception could add to nociceptive overstimulation.

When vigilance levels rise, the RF increases the inputs coming from the muscular spindle receptor. This elevates the extensor postural tone and helps position most

[2]Thus the jaw-closing reflex is considered as the most norepinephrine-induced reflex particularly as a behavioral response to stressors.

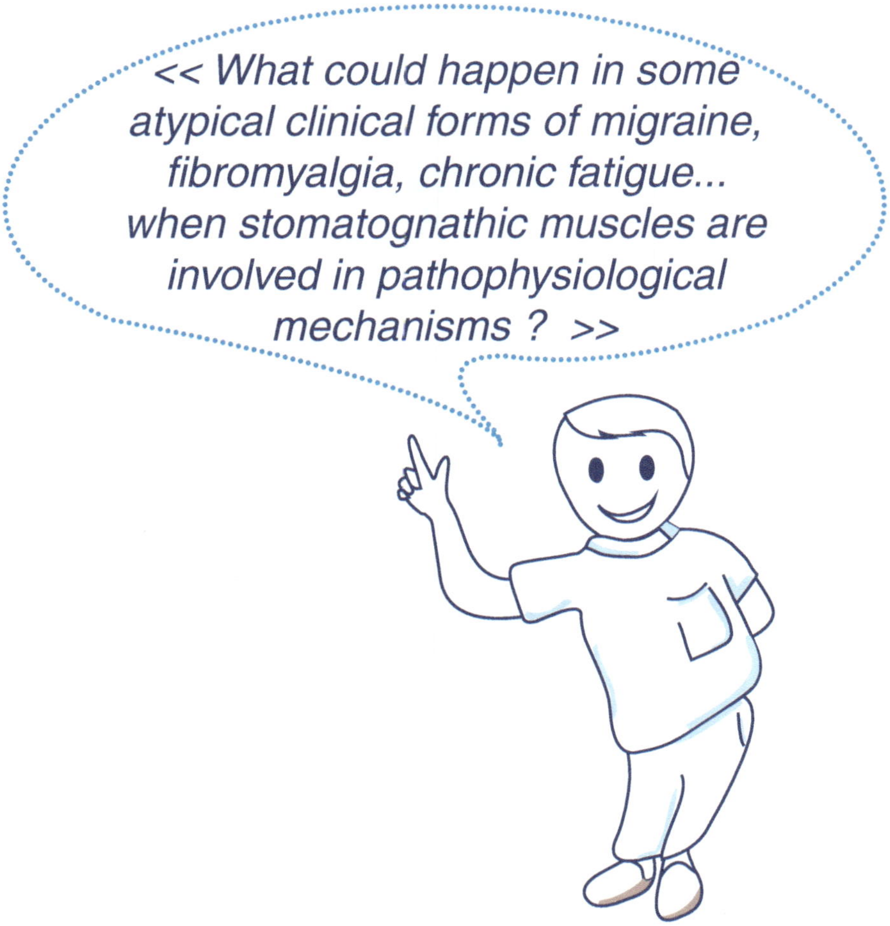

motor actions suitably. Secondly, the reticular inputs facilitate all voluntary movements (flexion or extension) by increasing the excitability of the motor neurons which receive orders directly from the cerebral cortex. Under physiological conditions, trigeminal inputs are generally accepted by the CNS and involved in protective reflex circuits. However, these circuits tend to be inhibited by a central overactivity particularly under the influence of psycho-emotional factors. So by blocking the nociceptive input transmission, the RF influx represses the flexion reflex. Such reflex would normally protect the organism at rest but would disorganize voluntary motor activity [5] (Fig. 3). In the stomatognathic system, this type of reflex (flexion) is generally represented by the *inhibition reflex of the jaw-closing muscles originating in the periodontium* (IRJCMOP). Reticular overactivity usually tends to produce muscular spasticity which initiates acute persistent pain. Consequently,

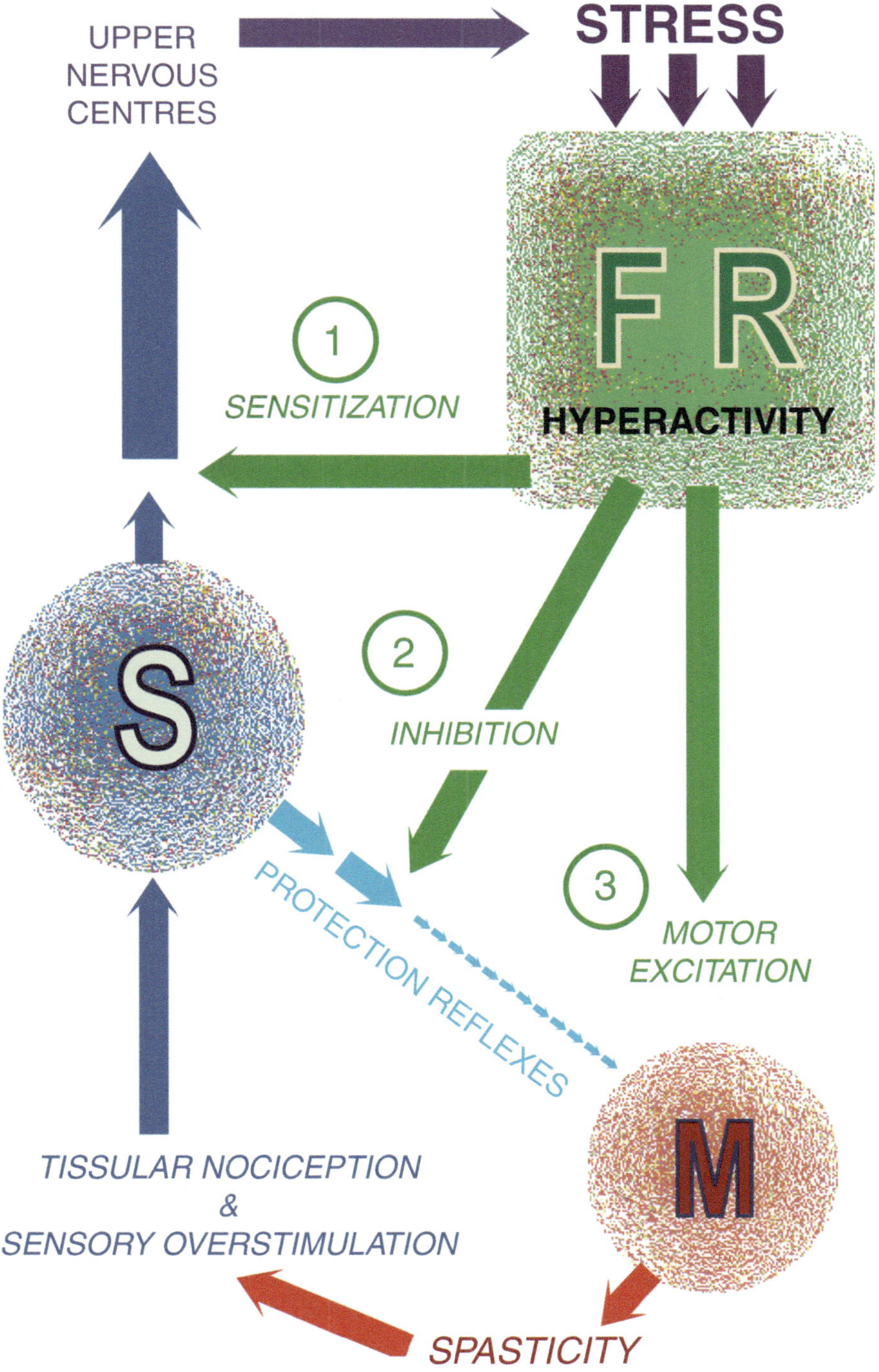

Fig. 3 Outcome of reticular hyperactivity at three levels: sensory, reflex, and motor (From Bonvallet [5])

pathophysiological conditions can activate reticular factors and inhibit protective reflexes such as the IRJCMOP. Furthermore, proprioceptive overstimulation and/or nociception occur in spasmed muscles.[3] The whole process triggers local metabolic troubles and spastic symptoms. Ischemia in the stomatognathic muscles may constitute one of the major causes of persistent pathophysiological conditions present in TMD. In the stomatognathic area, central overactivity facilitates the activity of jaw-closing muscles. This tends to make the freeway space (FWS)[4] disappear. Among the stomatognathic muscles, the thin weak *lateral pterygoid muscles* (LPMs) seem to have the capacity to develop a state of spasm or contracture [3, 16, 20, 22, 26, 46, 48, 53] perhaps due to its important physiological role [2, 23, 24, 29, 39, 51, 52, 55, 60, 66, 86, 88]. It is worth noting that some studies have shown the surprising role of vagal afferents inhibiting the oral opening reflex [8, 40].

3 Oral Parafunctions

Parafunction is defined as an abnormal activity. It's a sequence of motor activity leading to the satisfaction of a need in the oral sphere. But its inadequate implementation activates the compensation and assistance of muscles or muscular groups (supra- and infrahyoidean muscles, muscles responsible for head posture, etc.).[5] Among stomatognathic muscles, the parafunction essentially involves extensor muscles that is to say *jaw-closing muscles*.

3.1 Familiar Grinding

Dentists have long observed that occlusion disturbances were frequently accompanied by grinding. Grinding has been considered as a response from the organism to problems resulting from flawed physiological abrasion [12] or atypical wear. The

[3]More recent data have shed light on the possible role of free radicals associated with oxidative stress in TMD [65].

[4]FWS = normal space between upper and lower dental arches with jaws at rest (see before Part I, chapter "Symptoms").

[5]Movements of the limbs can in fact be divided into two categories. Flexion movements are brought about through a sense of gravity and generally result in a closing or a reduction of the angle of the joint. Extension movements tend to counter gravity and usually result in an opening of the angle made by the joint. While lowering the jaw is an action performed with the force of gravity, it is a flexion movement which opens the angle of the TMJ; the opposite occurs when the jaw is lifted and the angle of the joint is closed as the jaw works against gravity which implies that the joint is in extension [92].

parafunction has been the object of adequate clinical studies [18, 62, 64, 68, 69, 89, 93]; it does not appear to be a major alarming parafunction.

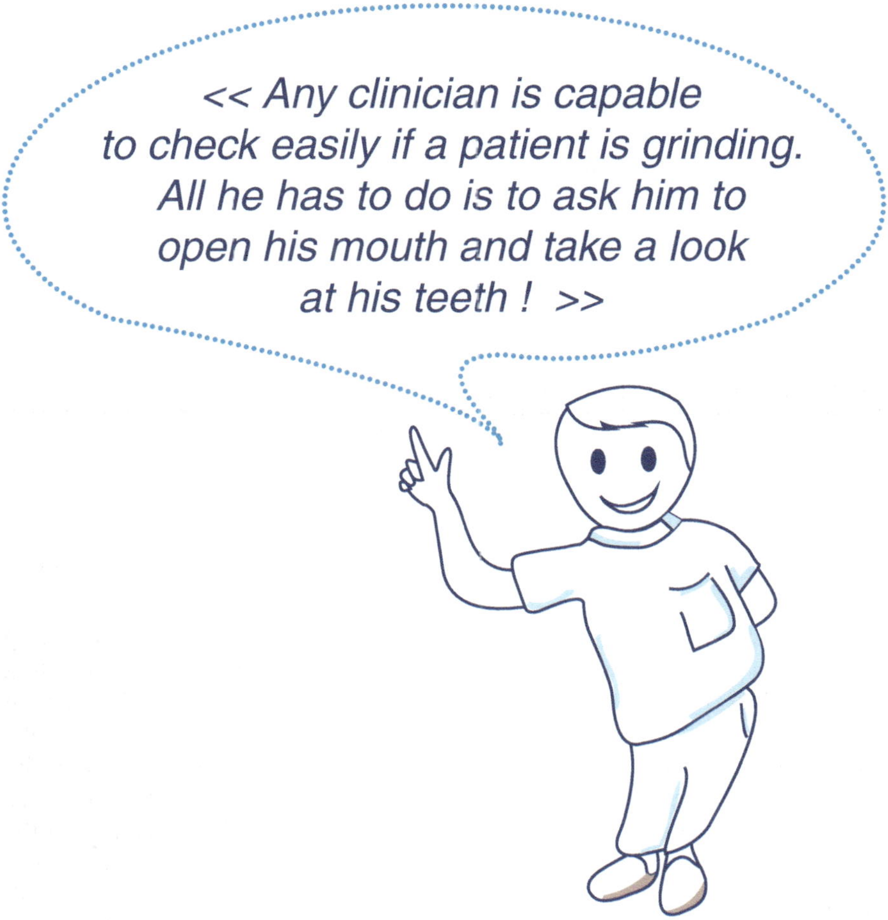

3.2 *Clenching: A Misunderstood Condition*

Let us start with the example of a trapeze artist. Through strong contraction of his masticatory muscles, he hangs from the trapeze by his teeth. To do so, he imposes mechanical forces on the above-mentioned muscles. These forces are indeed very intense but always under his control. The same type of strength – at least as intense and/or prolonged – is precisely what some patients use on their teeth. But those patients act involuntarily, even unconsciously. *Excessive clenching* shows the tendency of the masticatory muscles to contract under particular conditions of *stress* in subjects prone to certain pathologies. Indeed, like in many diseases, two conditions must be combined. The first is the general state of the patient at the moment. The brain fixes the levels of sensitivity and neuroendocrinal responses permanently. Therefore, *psycho-emotional factors* usually lead to mechanisms of adaptation to stressors. However, they are conditioned by the individual genetic background and correlated immune defenses.[6] This condition frequently affects patients with anxious, introverted psychological profiles who find it difficult to handle stressful situations (Fig. 4). The second event is an acute or chronic peripheral imbalance (i.e., too much or not enough stimulation) acting as a *disturbing stressor*. With a parafunctional tendency (such as severe clenching), reticular overactivity preferentially affects elevator fibers (extension) with an increase in the β–γ loops' activity (Fig. 5). Thus, the muscular overtension involves jaw-closing muscles (masseter, temporalis, lateral pterygoid, medial pterygoid). In these pathophysiological conditions, tensions can be considered as a biting action which goes on abnormally [35, 74]. It looks as if the CNS, after starting a biting movement, initiates tonic motricity, that is, clenching with a loss of the physiological freeway space (FWS). In clenching, the overstimulated and nociceptive trigeminal inputs represent an abnormally excessive sensory volume sent to the CNS. While diurnal less intense though durable or frequent clenching may also be observed, the *nocturnal forms of clenching* seem to be the strongest as EMG responses can exceed those from maximal voluntary clenching [10]. Moreover, all these excessive and/or frequent parafunctional stimulations are themselves a major factor of central nociceptive activation. These excessive levels of inputs (duration, intensity, frequency) are potentially aggravating for a stressed CNS. According to current clinical data, forms of tight clenching may not be predominant: less intense clenching may affect some patients who clench more frequently or durably. Another theory is based on concomitant alternate tight/ lighter clenching phases in a same patient. Regardless, clenching is not an isolated component. It is integrated into complex neuroendocrine physiopathological circuits related to a spastic phenomenon in stressed subjects. In that respect, the *reticular formation* plays its role in the hypothalamic-pituitary-adrenal axis (HPAA) during stress. It retains the essential ability to set up the loops between the CNS and the musculature.

[6]For many years, improvement of immunity and sociopsychological adaptation has been observed thanks to meditation practices [28, 38, 43, 57–59, 73].

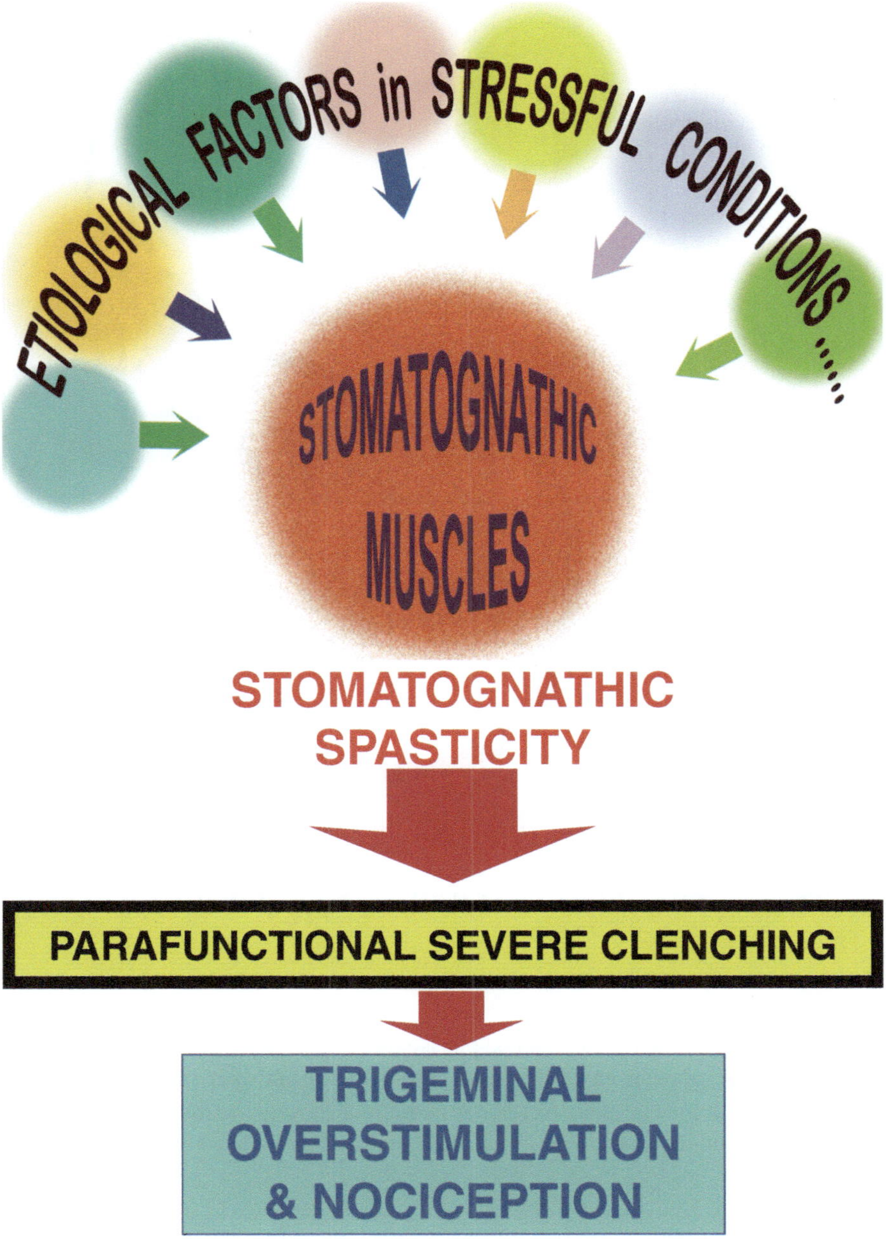

Fig. 4 Stomatognathic spasticity

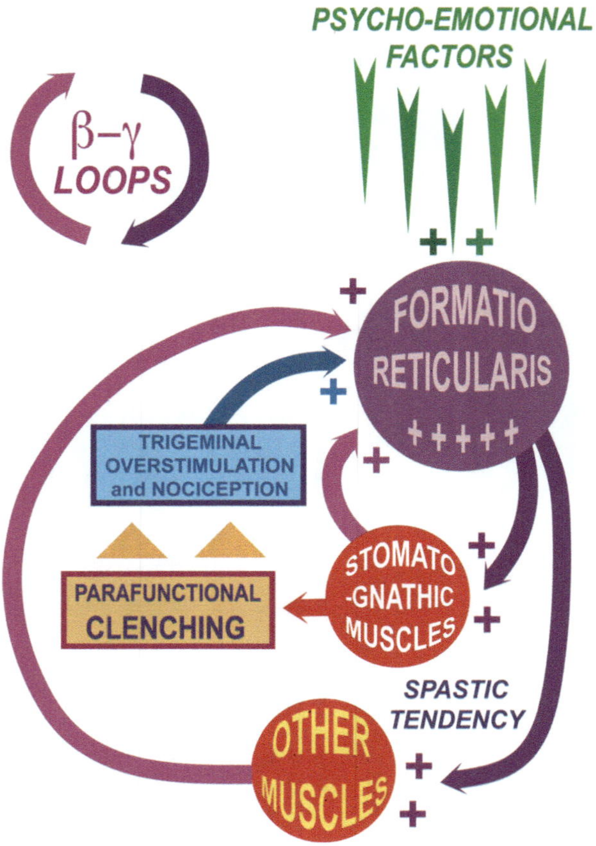

Fig. 5 Reticular hyperactivity, spastic tendency in muscles (stomatognathic and others) under the influence of central and peripheral factors

4 Theory of Sensitization of the Low Neural Pathways

Sensitization is a well-known nervous phenomenon: through innumerable connections, intense or repetitive *parafunctional afferents* can excite the adjacent neurons (Figs. 6, 7, and 8). Each reflex can be plurisegmental. **When sufficiently intense or repetitive, stimulation can diffuse all along the spinal medulla**. The diffusion can reach the subjacent and overjacent metamera through a funicular cell system [14]. Some cranial nerves (VII, IX, X, XII) and first cervical roots (C1-C2-C3) are

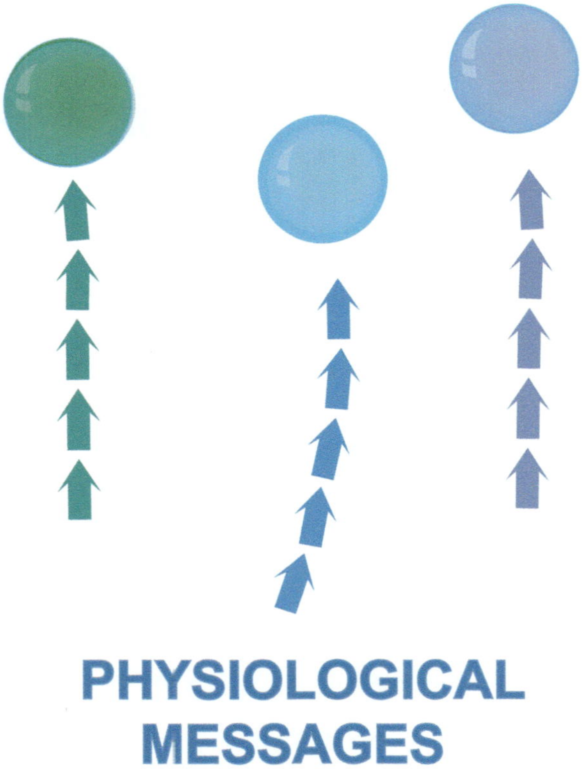

Fig. 6 Physiological messages

known to project to the trigeminal SN [15, 32]. In addition, it may explain some patients' suffering from *pain in areas distant from the trigeminal territory.* Two elements of neuroscientific data really help understand. The first one is the configuration of the trigeminal SnC at the level of the posterior horn of spinal cord C1, C2, C3, and even C4 [31]. The second one is the projections from V to the cervical roots [75, 76, 78, 79] until C7 [1], until T7 [45], all the way to the sacral levels[7] [67, 87].

[7]Projections from both rostral and caudal divisions of the nucleus spinalis (NS) go down the entire length of the spinal cord [67]: some are direct as revealed by the horseradish peroxidase retrograde technique. Other studies based on electrical stimulations confirmed the supposed polysynaptic pathways from trigeminal afferents to lumbar medulla [87].

Fig. 7 Parafunctional afferents creating a possible *overflow phenomenon*

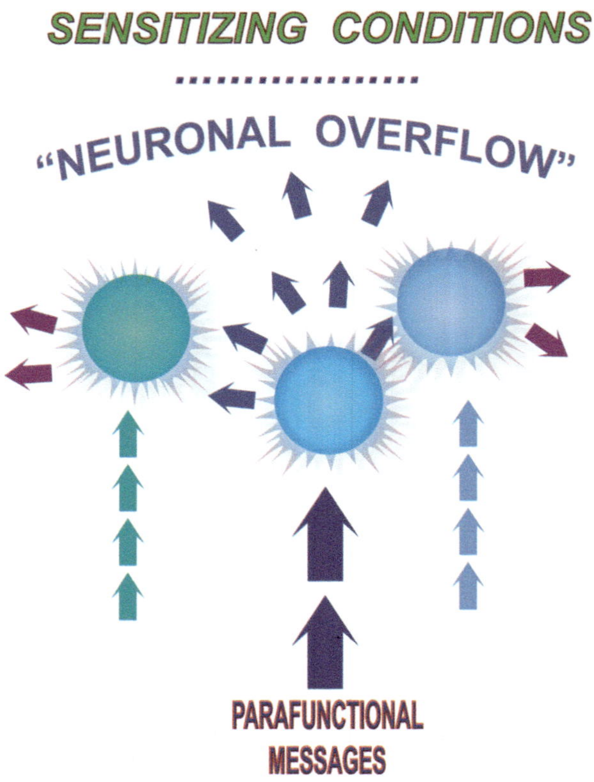

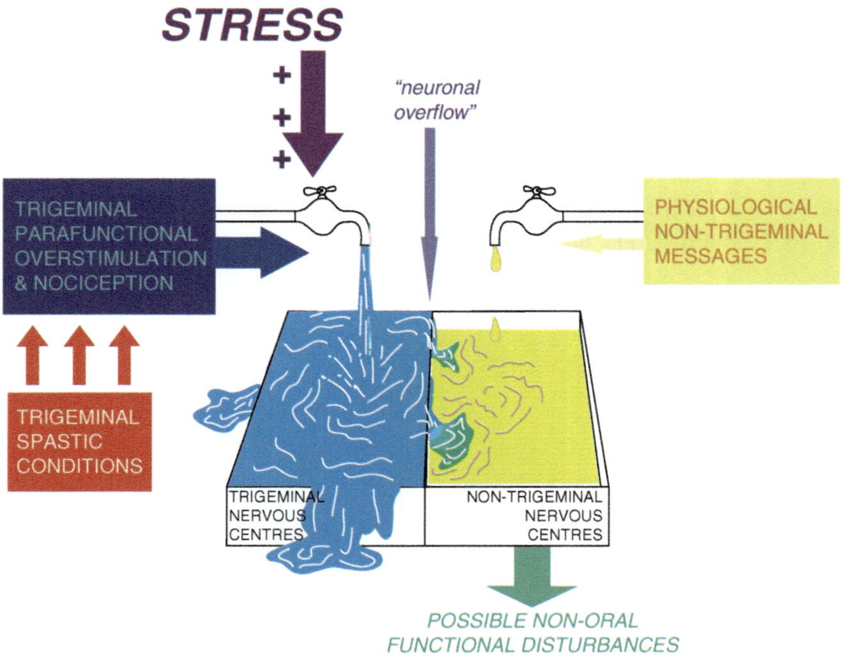

Fig. 8 Trigeminal overflowing

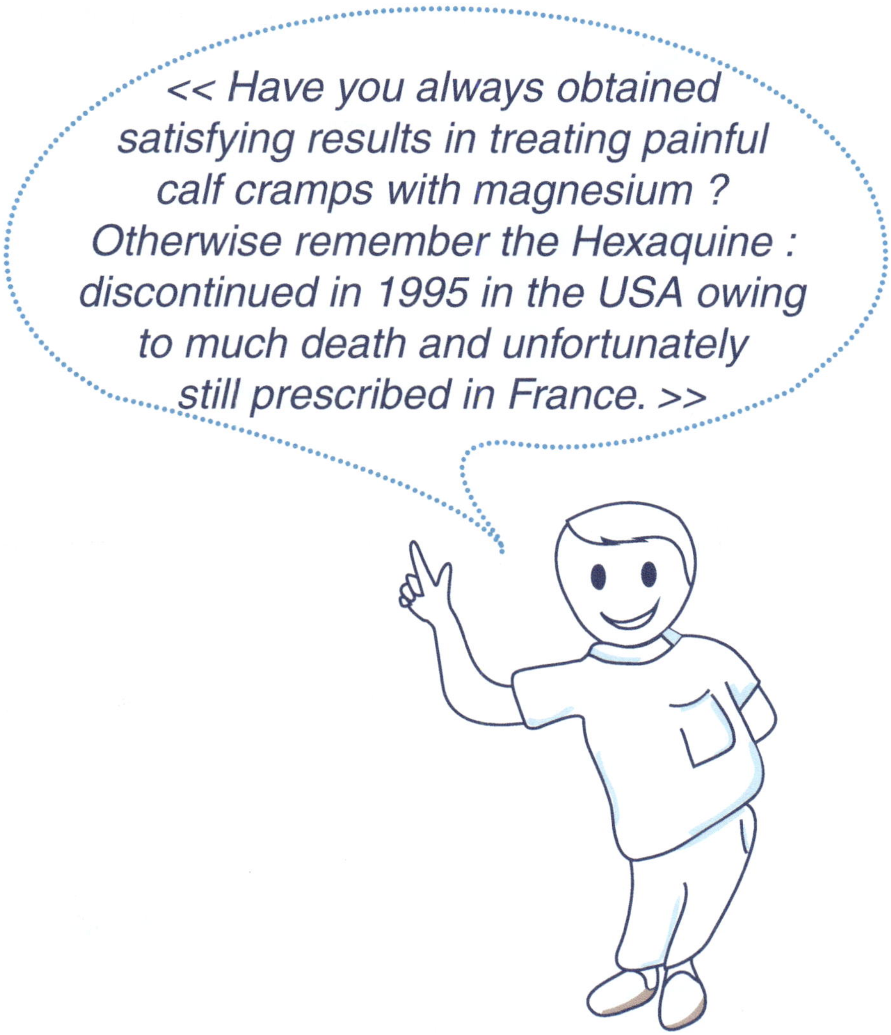

Stomatognathic spastic conditions generate trigeminal overstimulation and nociception in the TBNC (Fig. 9). This possible neural extension may correspond to a **trigeminal overstimulation phenomenon**, that is, sufficiently intense and/or durable excitation or nociception.[8] It can be described as a spatial-temporal warning in

[8]Muscular receptors are known to participate in the famous pathophysiological *β–γ loops*, but their integration depends on the CNS receptivity (stress conditions). In effect, the ascending reticular system filters the sensory inputs before they reach the thalamus, the limbic system, and finally the somatosensory cerebral cortex. Global trigeminal overactivation, often exaggerated by limbic influences, results in a rupture of the physiological *contraction-relaxation* cycle [21] and in maintaining a state of overtension leading to muscular fatigue [6]. Dysfunctional swallowing is also considered as a possible factor in the lack of relaxation of the stomatognathic muscles [27]. As for trigeminal receptors, whether or not articular (i.e., TMJ) and periodontal receptors intensely react to severe clenching phases is still unknown (see chapter "Characteristics of Periodontal Proprioception").

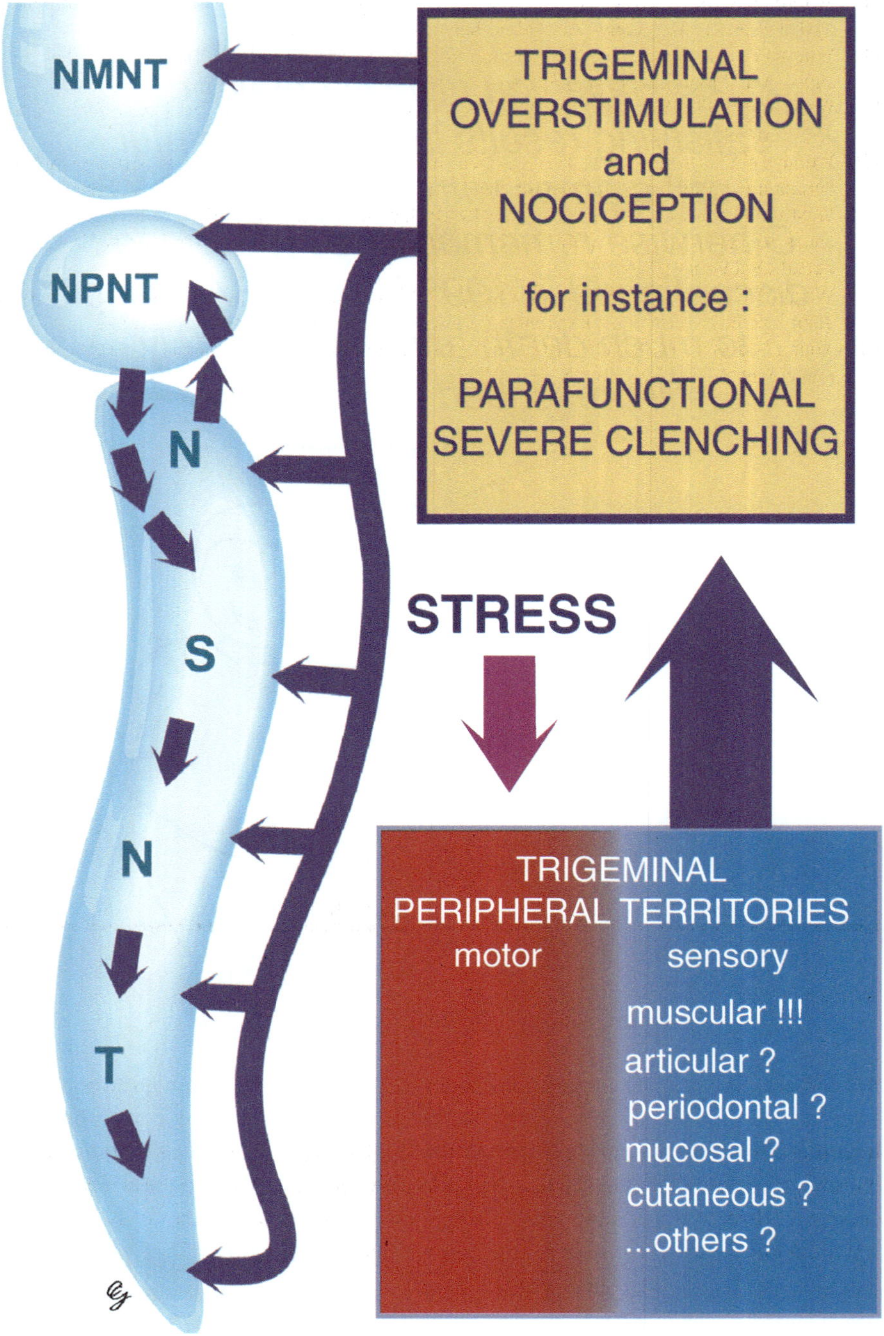

Fig. 9 Trigeminal overstimulation and nociception

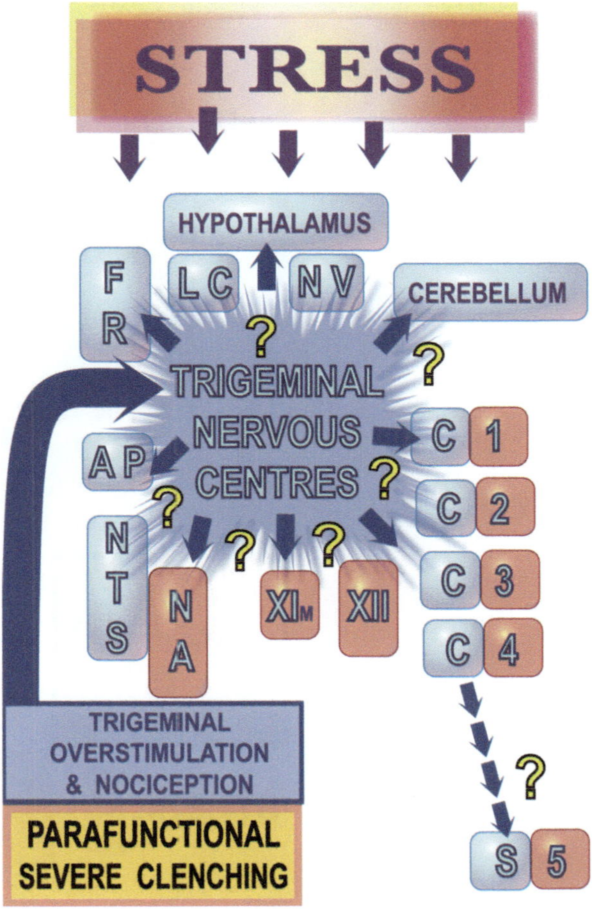

Fig. 10 Trigeminal overstimulation to several non-trigeminal centres during severe clenching. *AP* area postrema, *FR* formatio reticularis, *LC* locus coeruleus, *NA* nucleu ambiguus, *NTS* nucleus tracti solitarii, *NV* nuclei vestibulares. A pathophysiological model

the trigeminal sensory territory when spastic conditions endure, that is, strong, durable, and/or frequent **clenching:** AP area postrema, FR formatio reticularis, LC locus coeruleus, NA nucleu ambiguus, NTS nucleus tracti solitarii, NV nuclei vestibulares (Figs. 10 and 11). Recent data revealed *long-term potentiation* (LTP) in the trigeminal spinal nucleus [36]. Does the phenomenon of neural *sensitization* or *overflowing*, for example, in parafunctional conditions, explain some remote clinical signs or symptoms? Are intense and/or durable and/or repeated trigeminal overstimulation and nociception (from severe clenching) able to generate or amplify some disturbances due to stress? Lingual dysfunction is known to have repercussions on ventilatory physiology [13, 27, 80, 82]. Moreover, some trigeminal (SN) neurons and some trigeminal primary afferents project to the nucleus of the solitary tract (nucleus tracti solitarii) [44, 47, 91] especially to the vagus area which is a major relay for vegetative functions (cardiac,[9] ventilatory, digestive, etc.).

[9]For many years trigeminocardiac reflexes have been described, but they seem to be physiological entities [34, 70, 71].

Fig. 11 Trigeminal overstimulation from the TBNC to nuclei vestibulares (*NV*) and Nucleus Tracti Solitarii (*NTS*)

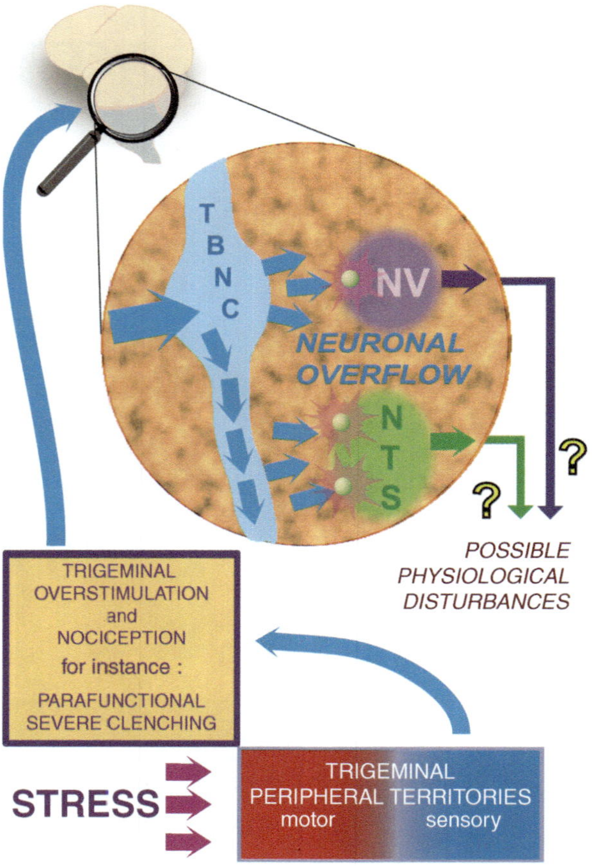

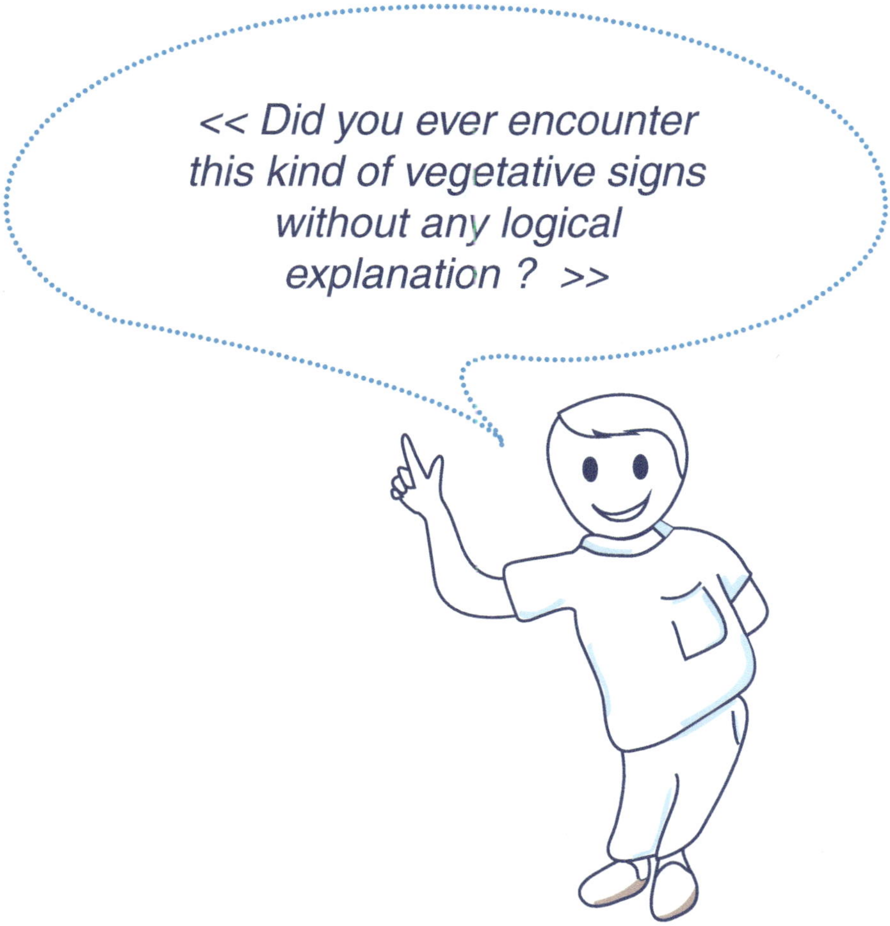
<< Did you ever encounter this kind of vegetative signs without any logical explanation ? >>

For instance, some TMD patients show a higher ventilatory rhythm at rest than control subjects [11]. Could the nearby neural relationship between V and X nuclei explain these amazing clinical facts? A close similarity was established between results from Swedish and American research teams about the two recognized phenomena of somatization in TMD patients [37] complaining of *cardiac rhythm* symptoms. Also noted is a connection between TMD and cardiac signs,[10] for instance, a heart rate increase during phases of nocturnal bruxism as compared to non-bruxism sleep phases [56].

[10]Noxious stimulation of orofacial areas (innervated by the paired V) could produce reflex increases both in cardiac rhythm and blood pressure, via a secretion of vasopressin from the pituitary gland [25]. A possible implication of the vagus nerve (X) may be considered in some clinical disturbances [47] especially in TMD patients.

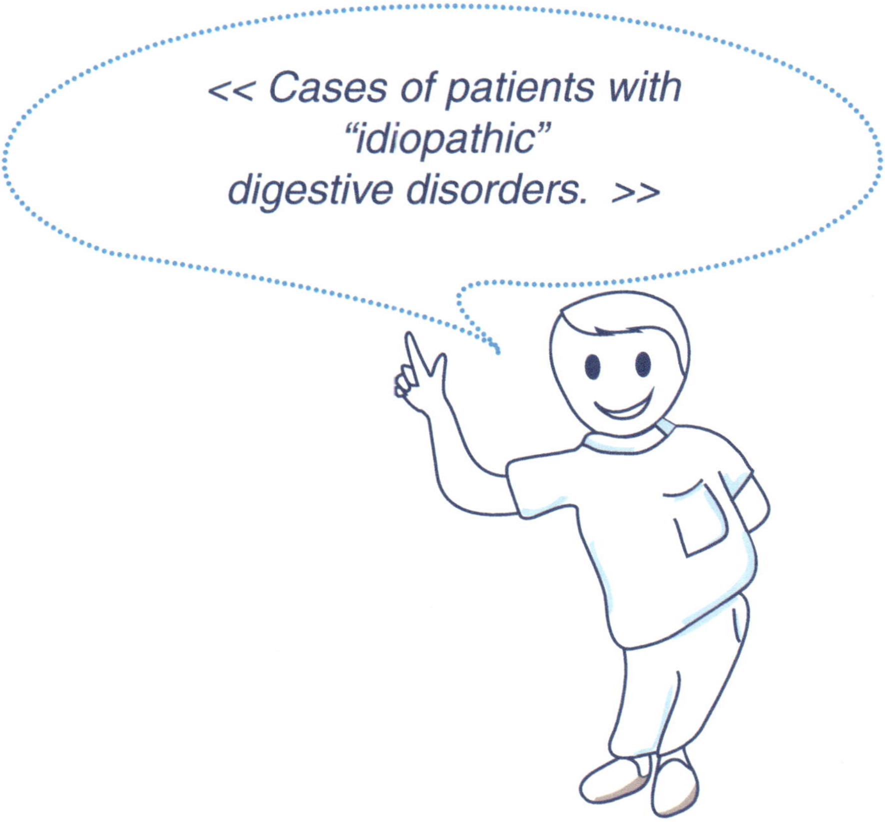

5 Theory of the *High Association Pathways*

High association pathways are identified between the hypothalamus and the brainstem as the **fasciculus longitudinalis medialis** (FLM) formerly called *Schütz fasciculus* [19]. It begins at the tuber cinereum and the corpi mamillares and divides into different nuclei of cranial nerves [30] (Fig. 12). It ends at the level of the fasciculi proprii (anterior fundamental fasciculus of the medulla) [49]. The FLM represents a vector of nervous reciprocal influences between the **hypothalamus** and the **RF**. Therefore, it can play a role in TMD pathophysiological mechanisms and their possible unexpected symptomatology. Neurons project from the

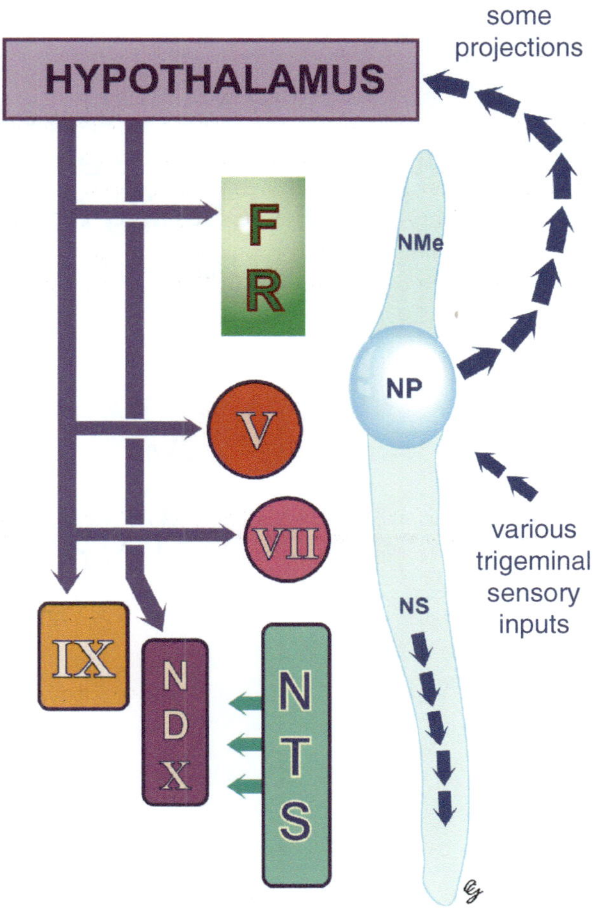

Fig. 12 Fasciculus longitudinalis medialis (*violin arrows*) and trigeminal afferents. Neurophysiological hypothesis. *FR* formatio reticularis, *NTS* nucleus tracti solitarii, *NDX* nucleus dorsalis nervi vagii, *NMe* nucleus mesencephalicus nervi trigemini, *NP* nucleus principalis nervi trigemini, *NS* nucleus spinalis nervi trigemini, *IX* nucleus nervi glossoparyngei

upper cervical spinal level and from the trigeminal sensory nuclei to the hypothalamic posterior nucleus [7, 41]. Another most interesting and unknown fact is that *the periodontal physiological afferents project to the hypothalamus* which controls food mechanisms.[11] These experimental afferents could excite or inhibit the hypothalamic cells [83, 84].

Stress has an irritating action on the hypothalamus, illustrated by Chauchard as "*the center of harmony that becomes the great master of disorder*." Under parafunctional

[11]Based on current data we do not know if excessive trigeminal afferents (clenching) reach the hypothalamus and if they do, what trigeminal tissues they originate from (periodontium, muscles, TMJ or others).

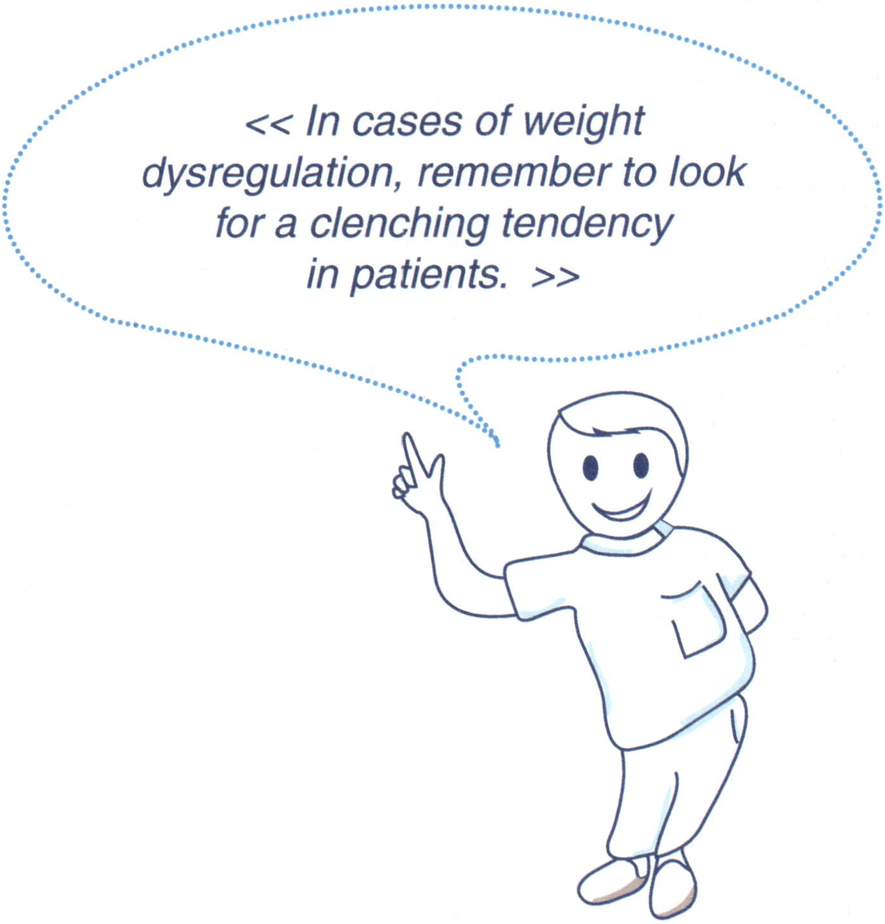

spastic conditions, can excessive and/or nociceptive trigeminal stimulations disturb the harmonious hypothalamic function? (Fig. 13) Neuroanatomical connections between the limbic system and the RF may intensify such closed pathophysiological circuits. They may have peripheral sensory and nociceptive implications (severe clenching) and central psycho-emotional influences on the behavioral dimension of stomatognathic muscle spasticity.[12] According to Landgren and Olsson theory,

[12]The trigemino-hypothalamic pathways to the lateral hypothalamus have been identified in rats [42]. Some electrophysiological study established a link between emotional behaviors induced by the hypothalamus and the activity level of the stomatognathic muscles [90]. Another interesting fact: out of 16 sites identified in the hypothalamus, 6 were reported as provoking an affective defense behavior under stimulation [33]; out of these 6 sites, 5 were located in the ventromedial hypothalamus uVMH). It is amazing that epicritic sensibility from periodontal inputs be projected at the level of the VMH [84, 85].

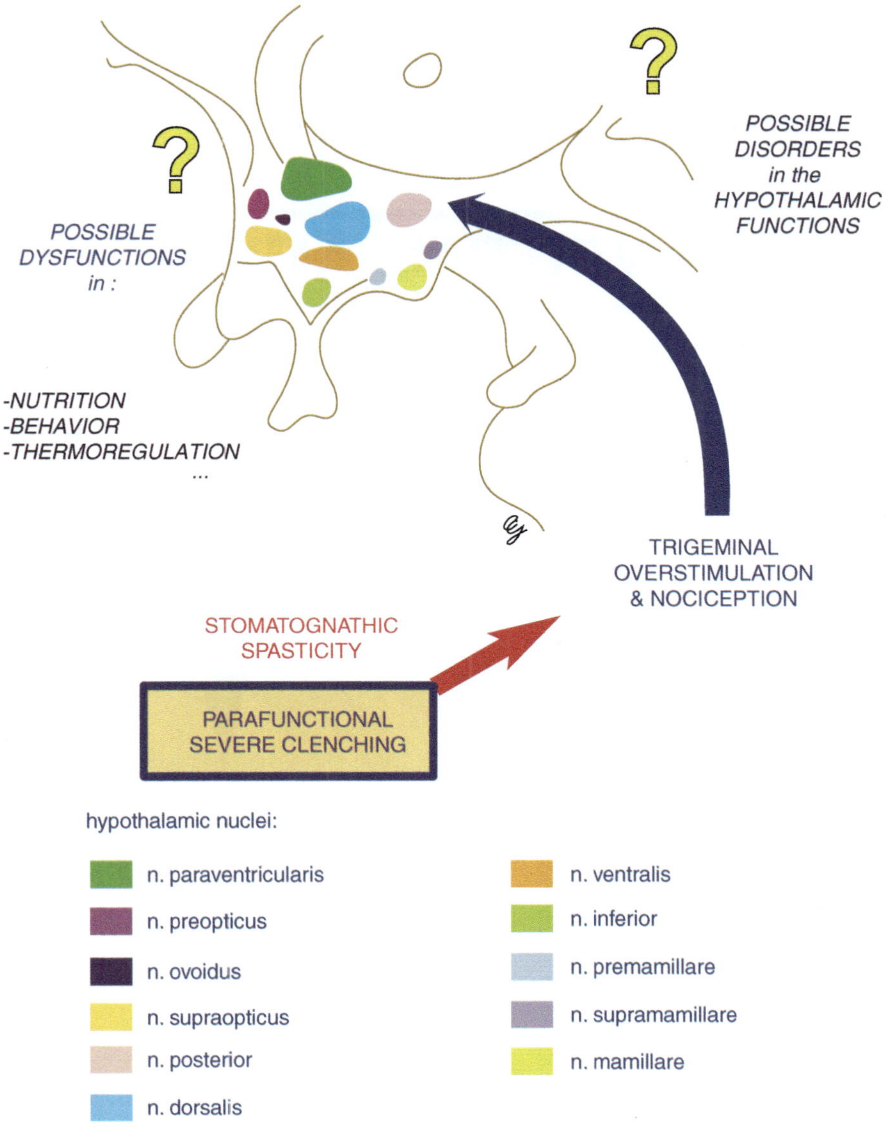

Fig. 13 Possible implication of trigeminal afferents at the hypothalamic level into the stomatognathic spasticity with parafunctional severe clenching. A simplified hypothetic model

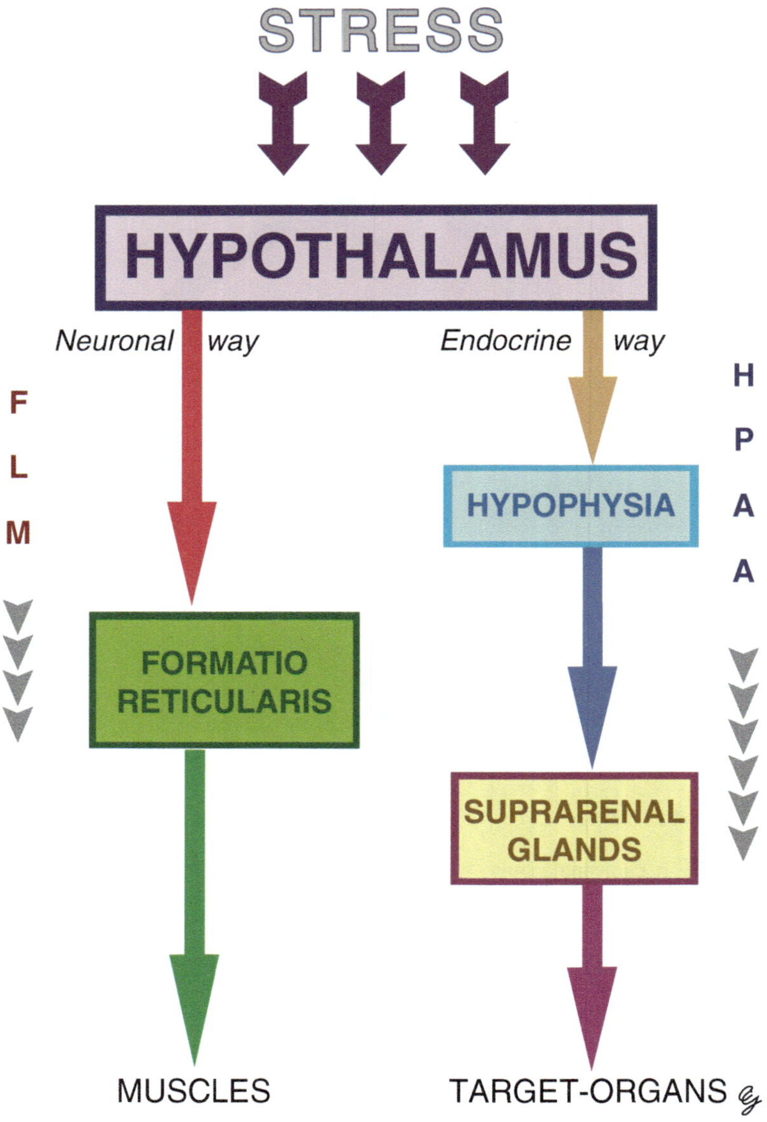

Fig. 14 The FLM and the HPA axes

"*...mental stress can change the balance of motor control towards an increased activity in the jaw closing muscles*"[33]. Does the hypothalamus really play a role in influencing emotional factors to determine the stomatognathic muscle tone, possibly through connections with the RF via the FLM and the trigeminal motor nucleus? The question remains open. The hypothalamus is more classically involved in stress

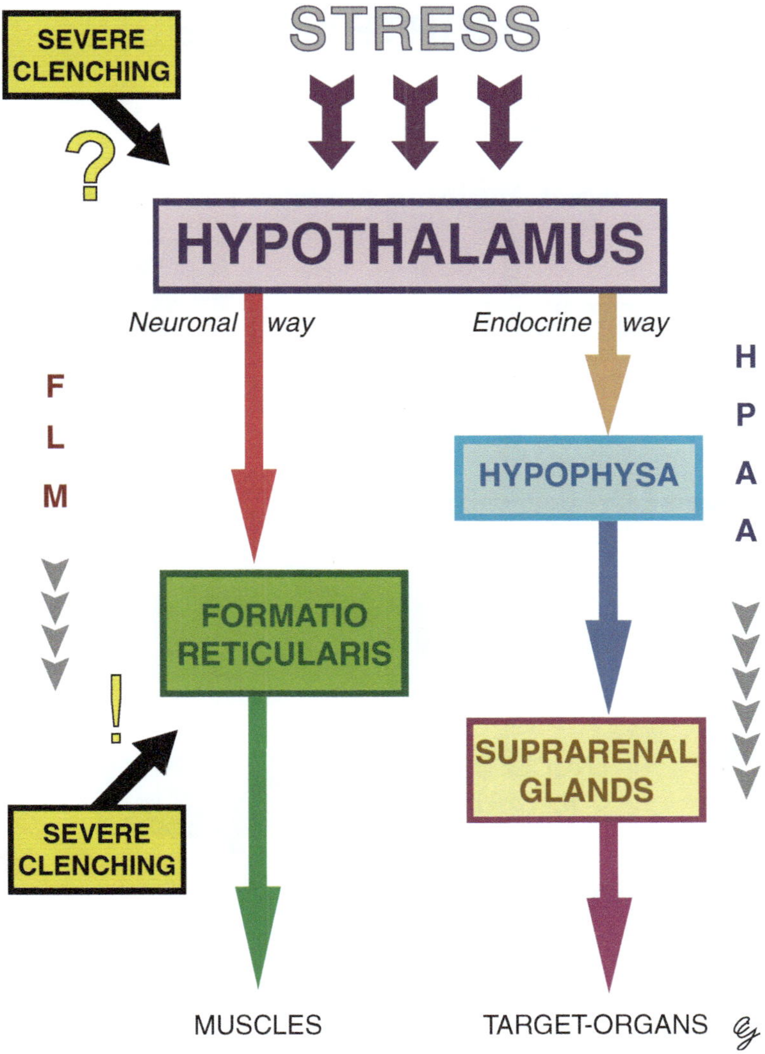

Fig. 15 The FLM and the HPA axes during severe clenching. Do clenchers unconsciously inhibit the physiological HPA axis responses and favor the FLM axis?

mechanisms through the hypothalamic-pituitary-adrenal axis (HPPA)[13] (Figs. 14 and 15). When compared with clinical facts, all these data tend to assimilate parafunctional clenching with a deleterious self-ruling system. Based on several central projections of trigeminal afferents, it may also perpetuate or even amplify some

[13]Please note that for many years, a lower impact on the HPA axis has been cited by experts on the pathogeny of fibromyalgia.

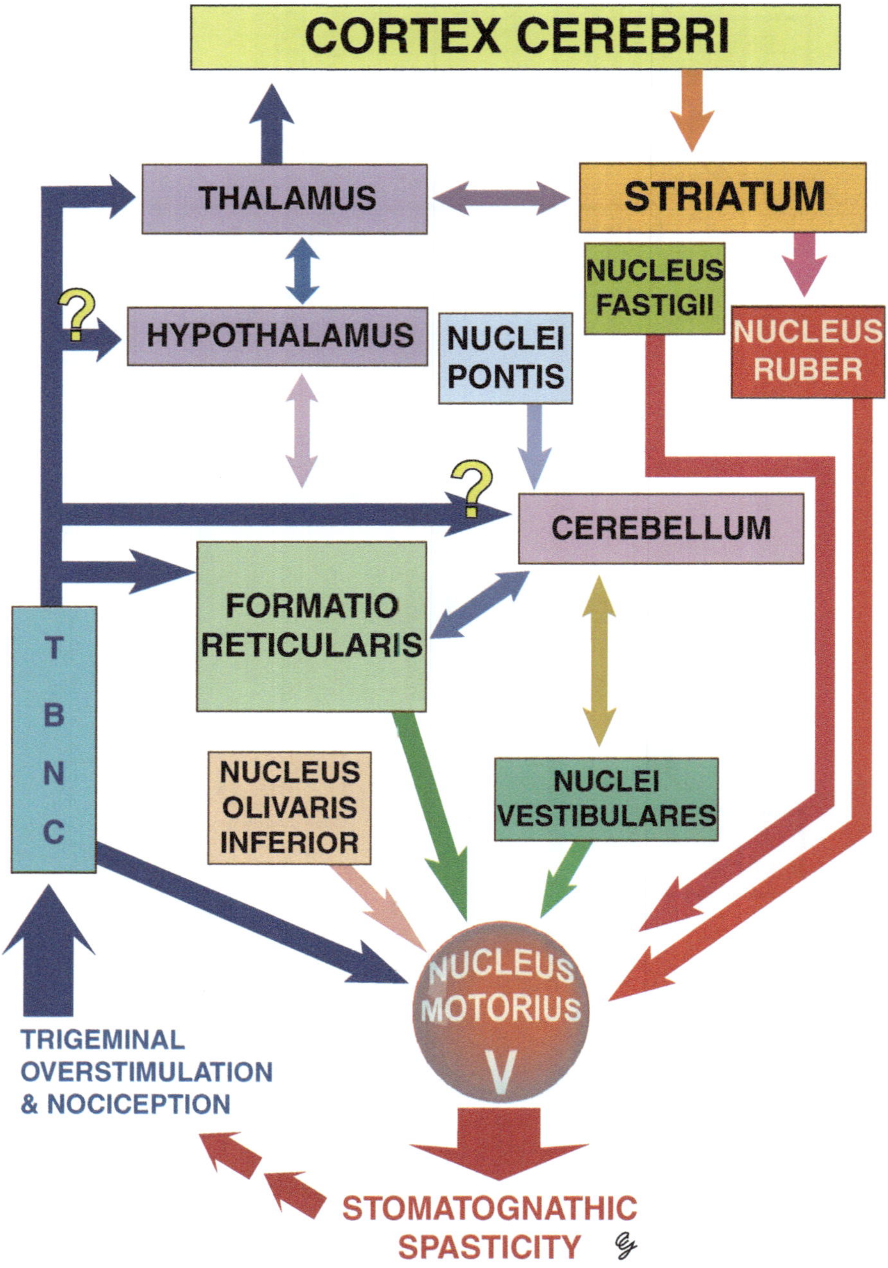

Fig. 16 Nervous structures and pathways involved in parafunctional clenching. A pathophysiological theory

pathophysiological mechanisms under stress conditions (Fig. 16). Therefore, it is not surprising that some authors lay emphasis on emotional factors as the source and persistence of TMD neuromuscular disease [9, 81].

References

1. Arvidsson J, Pfaller K (1990) Central projections of C4-C8 dorsal root ganglia in the rat studied by anterograde transport of WGA-HRP. J Comp Neurol 292:349–362
2. Aziz MA, Cowie RJ, Skinner CE et al (1998) Are the two heads of the human lateral pterygoid separate muscles? A perspective based on their nerve supply. J Orofac Pain 12(3):226–239
3. Bell WH (1989) Orofacial pains: classification, diagnosis, management, 3rd edn. Year Book Medical Pub, Inc, Chicago, p 420
4. Bessou P, Emonet-Denand F, Laporte Y (1965) Motor fibres innervating extrafusal and intrafusal muscle fibres in the cat. Physiol (London) 180:649–672
5. Bonvallet M (1966) Système nerveux et vigilance. La Science vivante, Press Univ France, Paris
6. Burke RE (1981) Motor units: anatomy, physiology, and functional organization. In: Brooks VB (ed), Handbook of physiology – the nervous system. Am Physiol Soc, Washington, pp 345–422
7. Cavdar S, Onat F, Aker R et al (2001) The afferent connections of the posterior hypothalamic nucleus in the rat using horseradish peroxidase. J Anat 198(4):463–472
8. Chase MH, Torii S, Nakamura Y (1970) The influence of vagal afferent fibre activity on masticatory reflexes. Exp Neurol 27:545–553
9. Choi JK, Kim CH, Ku SJ et al (1997) Stress and psychometric profiles of TM disorder patients according to diagnostic subgroups. 22nd annual meeting on orofacial pain and temporomandibular disorders. J Orofac Pain 11(2):abstract 184
10. Clarke NG, Towsend DGC, Carrey SE (1986) Bruxism patterns in man during sleep. J Oral Rehabil 11:123
11. Curran SL, Carlson CR, Okeson JP (1996) Emotional and physiologic response to laboratory challenges: patients with temporomandibular disorders versus matched control subjects. J Orofac Pain 10(2):141–150
12. Dawson PE (1977) Les problèmes de l'occlusion. Evaluation diagnostique et traitement. (Traduction: de Perelmuter S, Liger F) J Prélat (éd), Paris, 352p
13. Delaire J (1980) Essai d'interprétation des principaux mécanismes liant la statique à la morphogenèse céphalique. Actual Odont Stomatol 130:189–219
14. Delmas A (1975) Voies et centres nerveux. 10ème éd, Masson (éd), Paris
15. Denny-Brown D, Yanagisawa N (1973) The function of the descending root of the fifth nerve. Brain 96:783–814
16. Dœrfler LF, Rugh JD (1984) Voluntary mandibular retrusion exercises and facial pain. J Dent Res Abstr 63:288
17. Eriksson PE (1989) Blood flow regulation in masticatory muscles. Proc Finn Dent Soc 85(4–5):273–277
18. Funch DP, Gale EN (1980) Factors associated with nocturnal bruxism and its treatment. J Behav Med 3:385–397
19. Garnier M, Delamare V (1975) Dictionnaire des termes techniques de Médecine. Lib Maloine (éd), Paris
20. Grant PG (1973) Lateral pterygoid, two muscles? Am J Anat 138:1–10
21. Hartmann F, Vedel JP, Mei N (1982) Physiologie et physiopathologie de la mastication. Encycl Med Chir Paris Stomato 22008:A15
22. Hartmann F, Cucchi G (1993) Les dysfonctions cranio-mandibulaires (SADAM). Nouvelles perspectives médicales. Springer-Verlag (éd), Paris, 176p

23. Hiraba K, Hibino K, Hiranuma K, Negoro T (2000) EMG activities of two heads of the human lateral pterygoid muscle in relation to mandibular condyle movement and biting force. J Neurophysiol 83(4):2120–2137
24. Huang BY, Whittle T, Murray GM (2005) Activity of inferior head of human lateral pterygoid muscle during standardized lateral jaw movements. Arch Oral Biol 50(1):49–64
25. Ideguchi S, Hotta H, Suzuki A, Umino M (2000) Trigeminally induced cardiovascular reflex responses in spinalized rats. J Auton Nerv Syst 79(2–3):129–135
26. Janda V (1986) Some aspects of extracranial causes of facial pain. J Prosthet Dent 56(4):484–487
27. Jeanmonod A (1988) Occlusodontie. Applications cliniques. Cah Proth (éd), Paris
28. Jones BM (2001) Changes in cytokine production in healthy subjects practicing Guolin Qigong: a pilot study. BMC Complement Altern Med 1:8
29. Juniper RP (1984) Temporomandibular joint dysfunction: a theory based upon electromyographic studies of the lateral pterygoid muscle. Br J Oral Maxillofac Surg 22:1–8
30. Kahle W, Leonhardt H, Platzer W (1981) Anatomie. Tome 3: système nerveux et organes des sens. Flammarion (éd), Paris
31. Kawamura Y (1974) Physiology of mastication. Kawamura (ed), Basel
32. Kerr WL (1962) Facial vagal and glossopharyngeal nerves in the cat. Arch Neurol 6:264–281
33. Landgren S, Olsson KA (1980) The effect of electrical stimulation in the hypothalamus on the monosynaptic jaw closing and the disynaptic jaw opening reflexes in the cat. Exp Brain Res 39:389–400
34. Lang S, Lanigan DT, van der Wal M (1991) Trigeminocardiac reflexes: maxillary and mandibular variants of the oculocardiac reflex. Can J Anaesth 38(6):757–760
35. Lent C, Dickinson M (1988) Neurobiologie et alimentation de la sangsue. Pour la Science 130:82–87
36. Liang YC, Huang CC, Hsu KS (2005) Characterization of long-term potentiation of primary afferent transmission at trigeminal synapses of juvenile rats: essential role of subtype 5 metabotropic glutamate receptors. Pain 114(3):417–428
37. List T, Dworkin SF (1996) Comparing TMD diagnosis and clinical findings at Swedish and US TMD Center using research diagnostic criteria for temporo-mandibular disorders. J Orofac Pain 10(3):240–253
38. Lush E, Salmon P, Floyd A et al (2009) Mindfulness meditation for symptom reduction in fibromyalgia: psychophysiological correlates. J Clin Psychol Med Settings 13(2):200–207
39. Mahan PE, Thomas PD, Wilkinson M et al (1983) Superior and inferior bellies of the lateral pterygoid muscle EMG activity at basic jaw positions. Res Educ 50(5):170–178
40. Maixner W (1989) Autonomic and somatosensory interactions: physiological and pathophysiological implications. Proc Finn Dent Soc 85(4):395–407
41. Malick A, Burstein R (1998) Cells of origin of the trigeminohypothalamic tract in the rat. J Comp Neurol 400:125–144
42. Malick A, Strassman RM, Burstein R (2000) Trigemiohypothalamic and reticulohypothalamic tract neurons in the upper cervical spinal cord and cauda medulla of the rat. J Neurophysiol 84(4):2078–2112
43. Manzaneque JM, Vera FM, Maldonado EF et al (2004) Assessment of immunological parameters following a qigong training program. Med Sci Monit 10(6):CR264–CR270
44. Marfurt CF, Rajchert DM (1991) Trigeminal primary afferent projections to "non-trigeminal" areas of the rat central nervous system. J Comp Neurol 303:489–511
45. Matsushita M, Okado N, Ikeda M, Hosoya Y (1981) Descending projections from the spinal and mesencephalic nuclei or the trigeminal nerve to the spinal cord in the cat. A study with the horseradish peroxidase technique. J Comp Neurol 196:173–187
46. Mc Namara JA Jr (1973) The independent functions of the two heads of the lateral pterygoid muscle. Am J Anat 138:197–205
47. Menétrey D, Basbaum AI (1987) Spinal and trigeminal projections to the nucleus of the solitary tract: a possible substrate for somatovisceral and viscerovisceral reflex activation. J Comp Neurol 255:439–450

48. Mongini F (1986) An index system to quantify etiopathogenetic factors in oral dysfunction. Cranio 4(2):180–189
49. Monod C, Duhamel B (1960) Schémas d'anatomie, fasc 9. Système nerveux central. Gilbert & Co (éd), Paris
50. Monteiro AA, Kopp S (1989) The sufficiency of blood flow in the intercuspidal position and on a force transducer. Pro Finn Dent Soc 85(4–5):261–272
51. Murray GM, Phanachet I, Uchida S, Whittle T (2004) The human lateral pterygoid muscle: a review of some experimental aspects and possible clinical relevance. Aust Dent J 49(1):2–8
52. Murray GM, Bhutada M, Peck CC (2007) The human lateral pterygoid muscle. Arch Oral Biol 52(4):377–380
53. Nozaki S, Iriki A, Nakamura Y (1985) Trigeminal mesencephalic neurons innervating functionally identified muscle spindles and involved in the monosynaptic stretch reflex of the lateral pterygoid muscle in the Guinea pig. J Comp Neurol 236(1):106–120
54. Ogus HD, Toller PA (1981) Common disorders of temporomandibular joint. J Wright & Sons limited (ed), Bristol, 150p
55. Ogutsen-Toller M, Juniper RP (1994) The development of the human lateral pterygoid muscle and the temporomandibular joint and related structures: a three-dimensional approach. Early Hum Dev 39(1):57–68
56. Okeson JP, Philips BA, Berry DTR, Baldwin RM (1994) Nocturnal bruxing events: a report for normative data and cardiovascular response. J Oral Rehabil 2(1):623–630
57. Olivo EL (2009) Protection throughout the life span: the psychoneuroimmunologic impact of Indo-Tibetan meditative and yogic practices. Ann N Y Acad Sci 1172:163–171
58. Pace TW, Negi LT, Adame DD et al (2009) Effect of compassion meditation on neuroendocrine, innate immune and behavioral responses to psychosocial stress. Psychoneuroendocrinology 34(1):87–98
59. Pace TW, Negi LT, Sivilli TI et al (2010) Innate immune, neuroendocrine and behavioral responses to psychosocial stress do not predict subsequent compassion meditation practice time. Psychoneiroendocrinology 35(2):310–315
60. Phanachet I, Whittle T, Wanigaratne K et al (2003) Functional heterogeneity in the superior head of the human lateral pterygoid. J Dent Res 82(2):106–111
61. Quarti C, Renaud J (1972) Neurophychologie de la douleur. Hermann (éd), Paris
62. Rao SM, Glaros AG (1979) Electromyographic correlates of experimentally induced stress in diurnal bruxists and normals. J Dent Res 58:1872–1878
63. Rasmussen OC, Bonde-Petersen F, Christensen LV, Moller E (1977) Blood flow in human mandibular elevators at rest and during controlled biting. Arch Oral Biol 22:539–543
64. Reding GR, Zepelin H, Robinson JE et al (1968) Nocturnal teeth-grinding: all night psychophysiologic studies. J Dent Res 47:786–797
65. Richards RS, McGregor NR, Roberts TK (2005) Association between oxidative damage markers and self-reported temporomandibular dysfunction symptoms in patients with chronic fatigue syndrome. J Chr Fatig Synd 12:3
66. Ruangsri S, Whittle T, Murray GM (2007) Superior head of human lateral pterygoid muscle: single motor unit firing rates during isometric force. Arch Oral Biol 52(10):995–1001
67. Ruggiero DA, Ross CA, Reis DJ (1981) Projections from the spinal trigeminal nucleus to the entire length of the spinal cord in the rat. Brain Res 225:225–233
68. Rugh JD, Solberg W (1976) Psychological implications in temporomandibular pain and dysfunction. Oral Sci Rev 1:3–30
69. Satoh T, Hadara Y (1973) Electrophysiological study on tooth-grinding during sleep. Electroencephalogr Clin Neurophysiol 35:267–275
70. Schaller B (2004) Trigeminocardiac reflex. A clinical phenomenon or a new physiological entity? J Neurol 251(6):658–665
71. Schaller B, Cornelius JF, Prabhakar H et al (2009) The trigemino-cardiac reflex: an update of the current knowledge. J Neurosurg Anesthesiol 21(3):187–195
72. Sjoogard G, Savard G, Juel C (1988) Muscle blood flow during isometric activity and its relation to muscle fatigue. Eur J Appl Physiol 57:327–335

73. Solberg EE, Halvorsen R, Sundgot-Borgen J et al (1995) Meditation: a modulator of the immune response to physical stress? A brief report. Br J Sports Med 29(4):255–257
74. Strand FL, Kenneth JR, Zuccarelli LA et al (1991) Neuropeptides hormones as neurotrophic factors. Physiol Rev 71(4):1034–1035
75. Strassman AM, Vos BP (1993) Somatotopic and laminar organization of fos-like immunoreactivity in the medullary and upper cervical dorsal horn induced by noxious facial stimulation in the rat. J Comp Neurol 331:495–516
76. Strassman AM, Mineto Y, Vos BP (1994) Distribution of fos-like immunoreactivity in the medullary and upper cervical dorsal horn produced by stimulation of dural blood vessels in the rat. J Neurosci 14:3725–3735
77. Ström D, Holm S, Carlsson GE (1989) Blood-flow and metabolic response in a contracting canine masticatory muscle. Proc Finn Dent Soc 85(4–5):251–260
78. Sunakawa M, Yamamoto H, Ikeda H et al (1989) Response properties of the neurons in the cervical cord to stimulation of the inferior alveolar nerve in the cat. Kokubyo Gakkai Zasshi 56:486–493
79. Sunakawa M, Yamamoto Y, Ikeda H et al (1989) Inferior alveolar nerve - driven neurons in cervical spine. J Dent Res Abstr 68:884
80. Talmant J, Rouvre M, Thibult JL, Turpin P (1982) Contribution à l'étude des rapports de la ventilation avec la morphogenèse cranio-faciale. Déductions thérapeutiques concernant l'O.D.F. Orthod Franç 53(1):7–181
81. Thomass LJ, Tiber N, Schireson S (1973) The effects of anxiety and frustration on muscular tension related to the temporomandibular joint syndrome. J Dent Res 36(5):763–768
82. Travell JG, Simons DG (1983) Myofascial pain and dysfunction. The trigger-point manual. Williams & Wilkins, Baltimore, 713p
83. Trub M, Mei N, Orsini JC (1991) Macro and micro-electrode study of hypothalamic projections of periodontal afferents in the rat and cat. Brain Res Bull 27:29–34
84. Trub M, Mei N (1991) Effects on periodontal stimulation on VMH neurons in anesthetized rats. Brain Res Bull 27(1):29–34
85. Trub M, Mei N, Orofino J (1996) Periodontal and gastric convergences within the hypothalamic ventromedial nucleus area - single unit study on anesthetized rats. Behav Brain Res 72:33–37
86. Ushida S, Whittle T, Wanigaratne K, Murray GM (2002) Activity in the inferior head of the human lateral pterygoid muscle with different directions of isometric force. Arch Oral Biol 47(11):771–778
87. Vinay L, Cazalets JR, Clarac F (1995) Evidence for the existence of a functional polysynaptic pathway from trigeminal afferents to lumbar motoneurons in the neonatal rat. Eur J Neurosci 7:143–151
88. Wang MQ, Yan CY, Yuan YP (2001) Is the superior belly of the lateral pterygoid primarily a stabilizer? An EMG study. J Oral Rehabil 28(6):507–510
89. Weideman CL, Bush DL, Yan-Go FL et al (1996) The incidence of parasomnias in child bruxers versus non-bruxers. Pediatr Dent 18(7):456–460
90. Weiner S, Shaikh MJ, Siegel A (1993) Electromyographic activity in the masseter muscle resulting from stimulation of hypothalamic behavioral sites in the cat. J Orofac Pain 7:370–377
91. Whitehead MC, Bergula A, Holliday K (2000) Forebrain projections to the rostral nucleus of the solitary tract in the hamster. J Comp Neurol 422(3):429–447
92. Woda A, Fontenelle A (1975) Activité tonique et posture de la mandibule; Mastication Déglutition. In: Chateau M (ed) Orthopédie dento-faciale, vol 1. J Prélat (éd), Paris, pp 244–280
93. Wruble MK, Lumley MA, Dudley MC, Mc Glynn FD (1989) Sleep-related bruxism and sleep variables: a critical review. J Craniomandib Disord Facial Oral Pain 3:152–158

The Behavioral Side of Clenching

When patients become aware of their oral parafunction, they often call upon the sagacity of the clinician and ask the key question: *Why do I constantly clench my teeth*? Therefore, it is interesting to tackle the problem of this oral parafunction from a behavioral point of view. Any aggressive alarming process of the CNS, whether external (nociception or sensory overstimulation) or internal (psycho-emotional problems), initiates an increase in vigilance and calls for an individual adaptive response. Through reticular influence, the response involves the effectors (muscles and glands), a reaction commonly known as the *fight or flight response*. In these conditions, a phasic-type muscle response occurs (different movements including speaking). This refers to a larger problem of necessary adaptation to stressors and to a more specific problem, that is, **verbal expression**. It involves the oral sphere and the stomatognathic system as parts of the main interhuman communication process. Some experts [8, 9, 15, 21, 22, 30, 36, 39, 41, 43, 44, 46–48, 50] emphasize the links between TMD and disturbed psychopathological states (anxiety, frustration, depression) and even psychosocial factors [2, 25, 26, 30, 45]. *Grinding* may be considered mainly as an adaptive effort – even if a parafunctional response (hyper-phasic mood) especially to dental occlusion disorders, a factor we wish to discuss now. *Clenching* may instead correspond with an isometric contracture state (hypertonic mood) under the influence of non-adjusted psycho-emotional stress. It generates a situation of *acting inhibition* towards one's surroundings [13]. In humans, the famous *fight or flight response* becomes *fight, flight, or speech*.

Clenching may be a substitute for a phasic action such as verbal expression which implicates the same oral structures [37]. It seems that in many patients, a tonic-type response is elicited, that is, without movement. This procedure prevents clenching. The pressure of socio-professional and family surroundings is such a heavy load of stress that compensation often results in a parafunctional activity of the stomatognathic system [42]. **Parafunctional clenching** appears as a **derived**

F. Hartmann, G. Cucchi, *Stress and Orality*,
DOI 10.1007/978-2-8178-0271-8_10, © Springer-Verlag France 2014

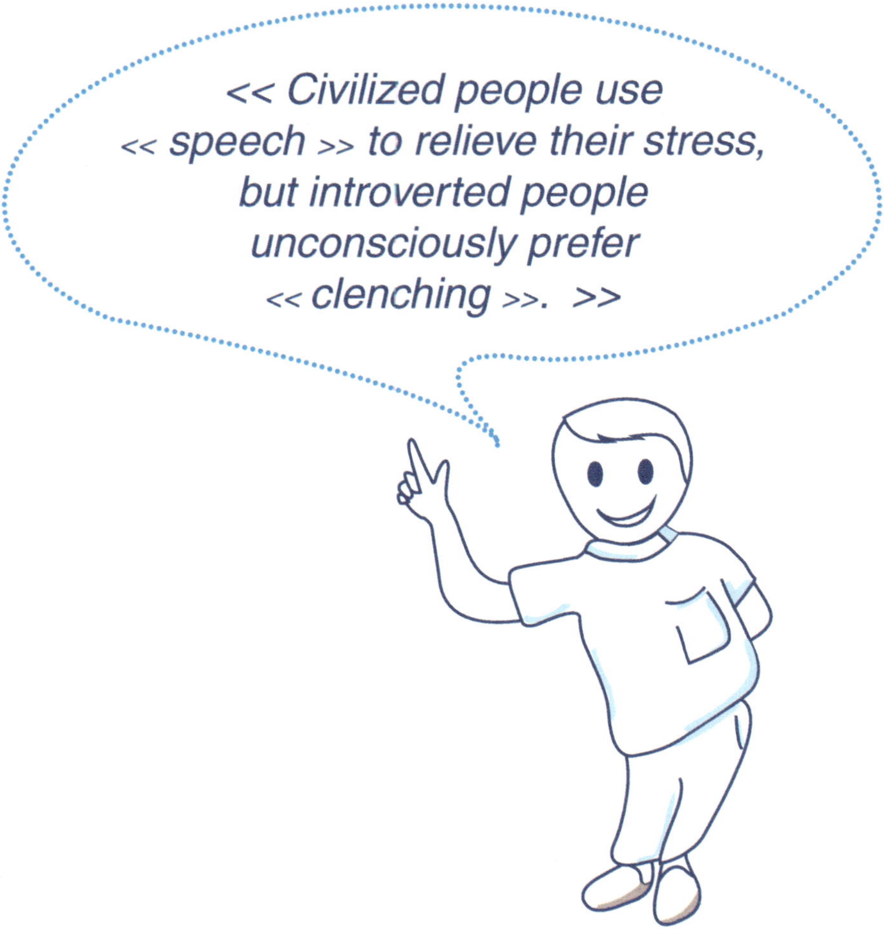
<< Civilized people use << speech >> to relieve their stress, but introverted people unconsciously prefer << clenching >>. >>

solution in conflictual situations when oral expression remains inhibited[1]. Clinicians speak of *alexithymia* [41], that is, the inability to verbalize emotions and feelings. This is a link to Watson concept of the *verbo-viscero-motor* organization of human beings. Repressed verbal responses are diverted to other effectors, that is, muscles and glands (Fig. 1). Unspoken feelings and non-dispelled emotional tensions may generate behavioral disturbances and/or physiological dysfunctions (Figs. 2 and 3). Then, a tonic muscular mood such as *fright* may unconsciously

[1]The periaqueducal grey (PAG) matter serves as a link between sensory and motivation-controlling structures on the one hand and the periambigual reticular formation coordinating the activity of the different phonatory muscles on the other. The PAG matter receives a glutamatergic input from several sensory areas, such as the mediofrontal cortex, amygdala, hypothalamus, locus coeruleus, vestibular nuclei, superior and inferior colliculi, nucleus tracti solitarii, nuclei nervi trigemini (n. mesencephalicus, n. spinalis) [7, 11]. In introverted persons, is there an inhibiting phenomenon at the (PAG) level under psycho-emotional influences (Fig. 7)? Are women more sensitive to these disturbances since higher glutamate sensitivity was noted in females' TMJ receptors [14]?

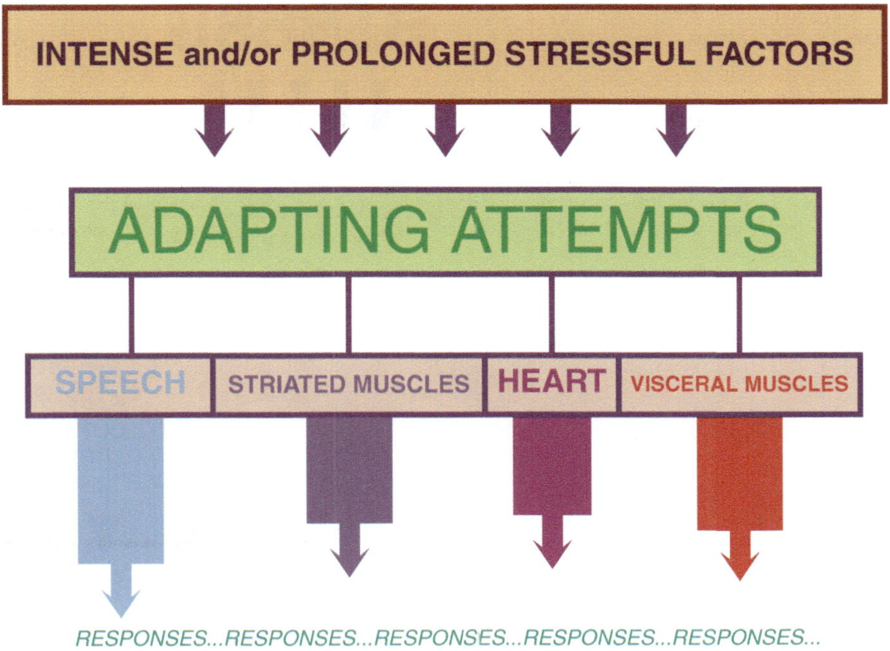

Fig. 1 Normal adapting attempts to stressors

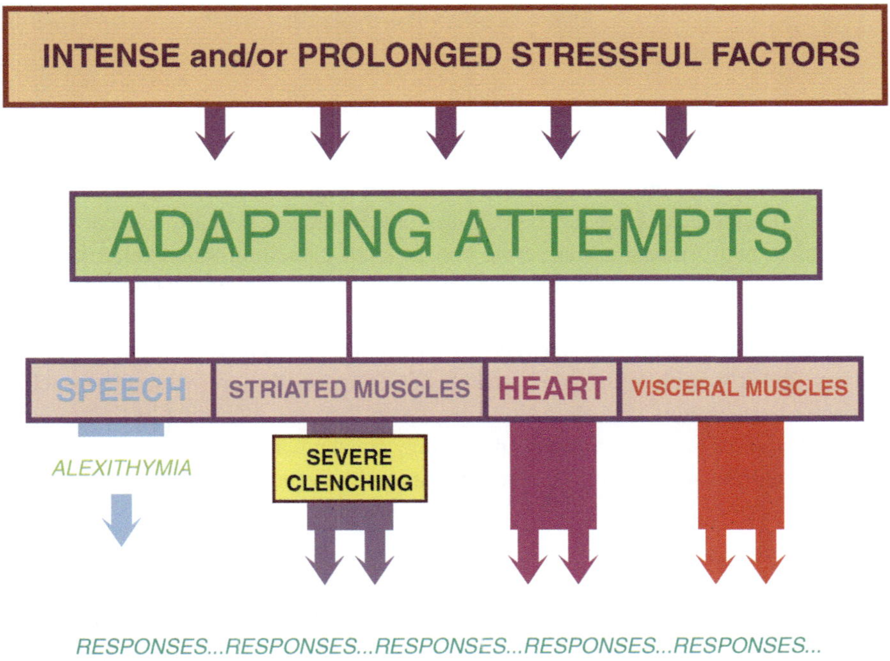

Fig. 2 Abnormal adaptation when verbalization is inhibited

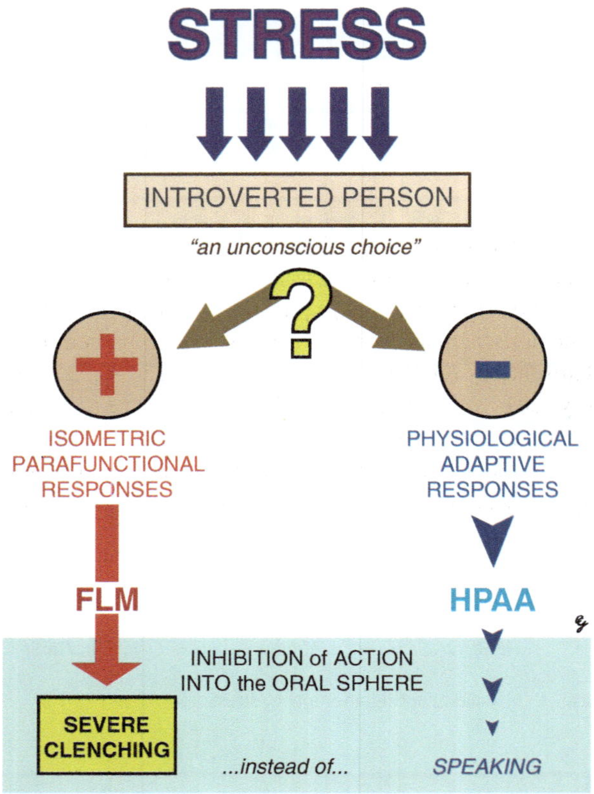

Fig. 3 Stress, introversion, and clenching. Model

triumph over phasic muscular moods such as *fight, flight, or speech*. In these conditions, TMD emerges as a major type of oral psychosomatic disease. Once aware of the clinical neuro-musculo-endocrine outcomes of clenching, one cannot be only consider the parafunction as a possible subterfuge for reducing stress. In effect, clenching itself can cause severe and detrimental stress to the CNS. It is really important to identify the link between the parafunction and its psychophysiological factors. Yet it would be dangerous to play it down and ignore its somatopsychic impacts. Due to their key physiological role in the oral sphere's physiology, the *paired V nerves* seem to make some strong, constant, frequent impacts through overstimulation and nociception to the *central trigeminal and non-trigeminal*

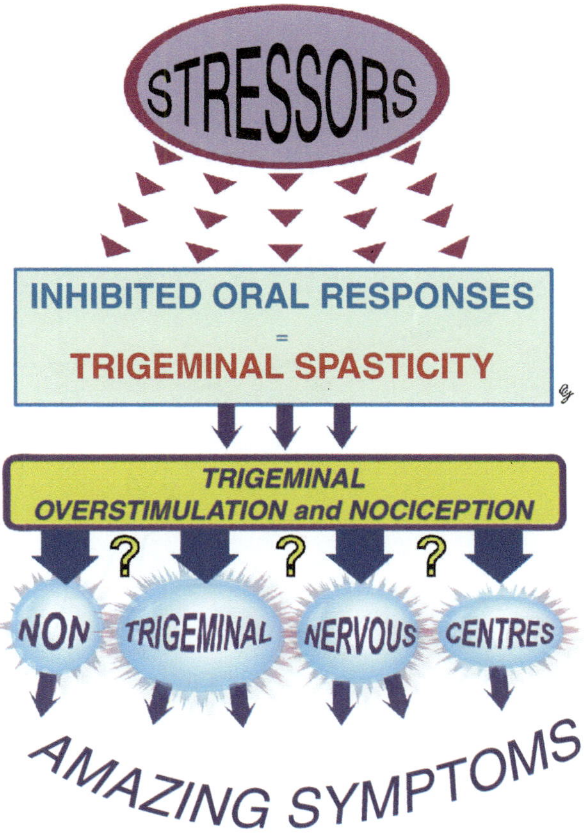

Fig. 4 Inhibited oral response and stomatognathic spasticity

nervous structures (Fig. 4). Therefore, it is important to offer help to patients who try to reduce or even manage the parafunction – and then look for better adaptive procedures to the individual's constraints and necessary social principles through relational and psycho-emotional tactics. Finally, the patient should be encouraged to diversify, enrich, and expand his or her personal modes of creative expression.

As revealed by clinical observation, this situation usually affects rather introverted individuals who are self-effacing and afraid to express their feelings. Possible links with clinical signs and symptoms may be observed in stressed clenching

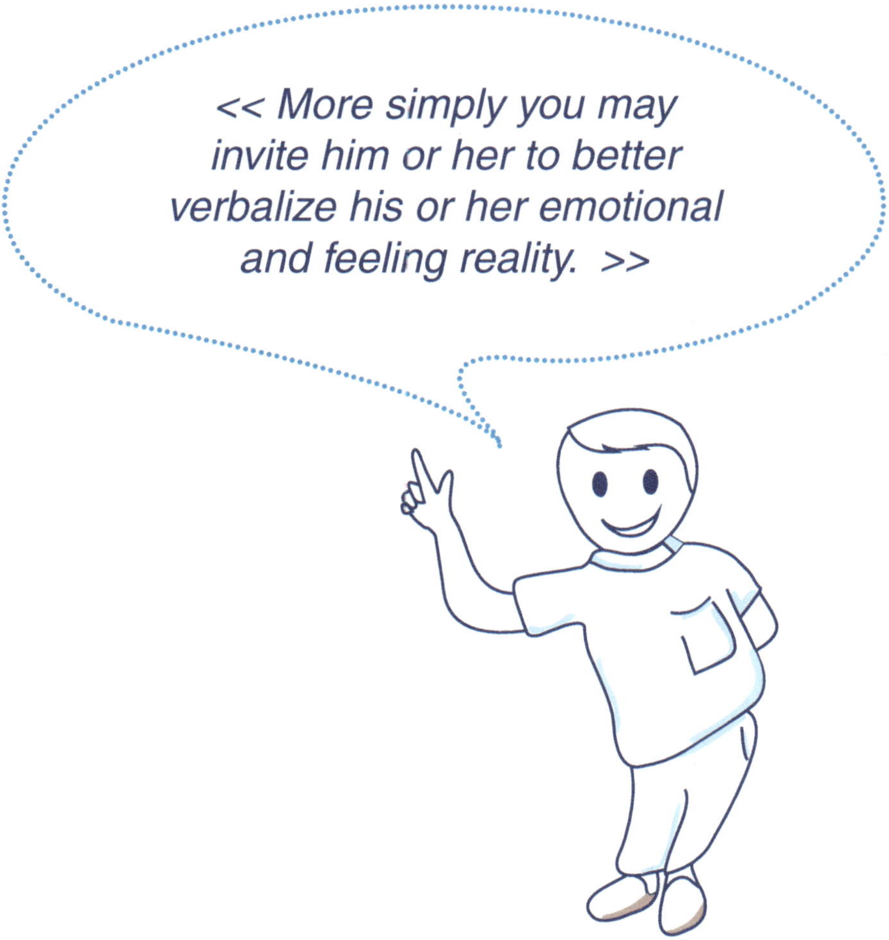
<< More simply you may invite him or her to better verbalize his or her emotional and feeling reality. >>

patients (Figs. 5, 6, and 7). Excessive exactingness towards themselves or others, that is, too much perfectionism can also easily lead patients to frustration. Nevertheless *action inhibition* does not prevent some rare and episodic phases of aggressiveness towards surroundings [25] which patients often seem to be aware of. In spite of their lucidity about behavioral troubles, patients rarely think of parafunctional habits as a cause of aggressiveness. **Amygdala** is known as a major nervous center responsible for aggressive behavior. Physical responses come through the amygdalian-reticular connections. Is the special role played by the trigeminal territory underestimated (Figs. 8, 9, 10, and 11)? When responding to math stressors, TMD patients reacted with more anger than control subjects [6].

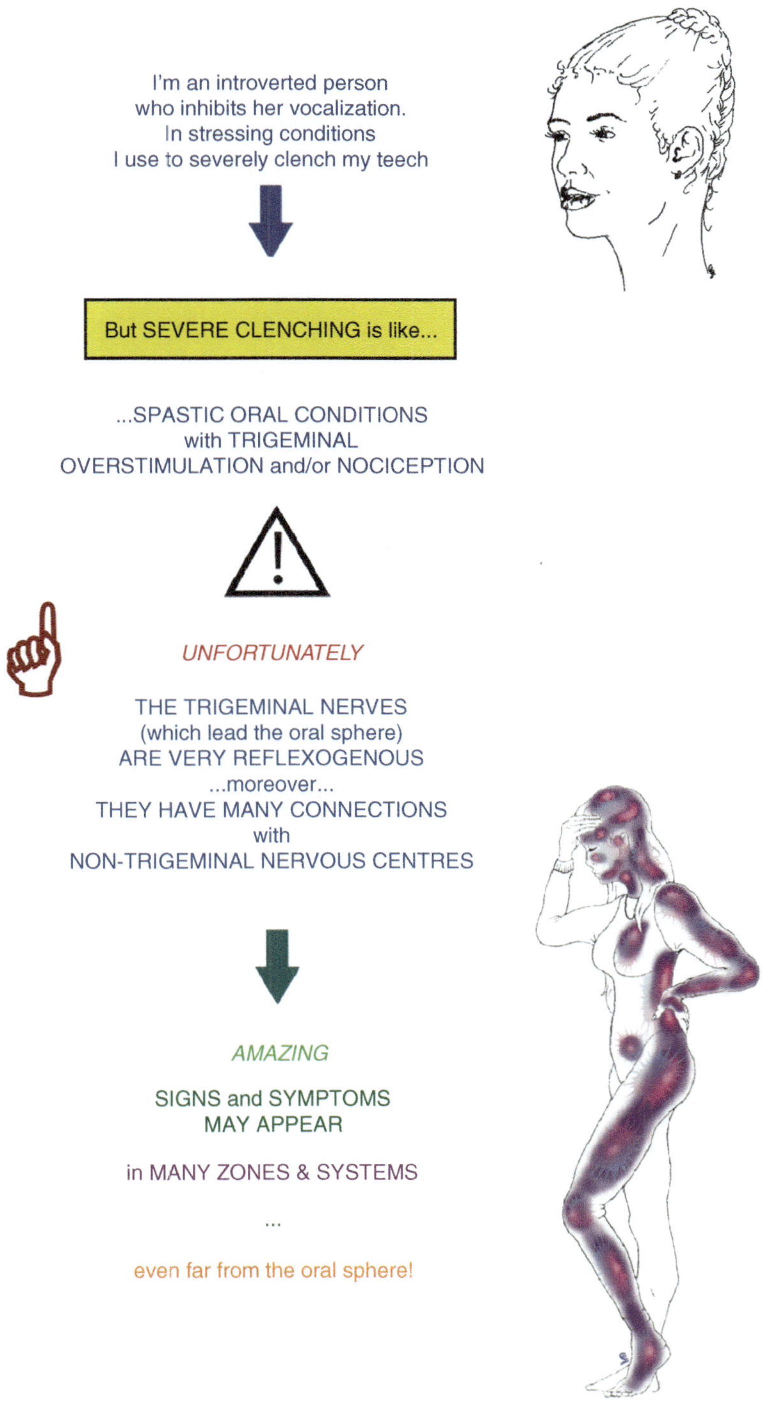

Fig. 5 Introversion as a source of clinical signs and symptoms

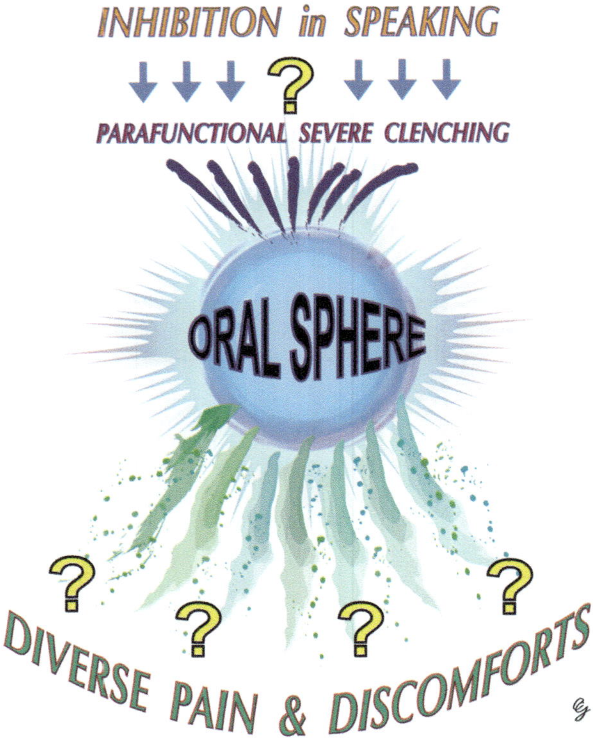

Fig. 6 The oral sphere as a relay from vocal inhibition and diverse pain or discomforts. Model

Furthermore, they expressed high levels of anxiety and sadness and a strong feeling of guilt. Some neuroanatomical data may explain these clinical facts[2]. A recent fMRI study shed some light on the converging roles of clenching, occlusal

---

[2]Some central nervous structures, particularly limbic structures, add an emotional impact to the adaptive system between information analysis and elaboration of response. The limbic system receives two kinds of immediate information: the first kind concerns the external environment (sensory afferents), the second concerns the internal environment (individual physiological parameters, those recorded by the hypothalamus). The limbic system usually compares these inputs from surroundings with the memorized data and adds its own emotional touch to the situation [32]. This phenomenon modulates the equilibrium between activation and inhibition as it exists at the hypothalamic or reticular levels. When this equilibrium is disturbed by *unpleasant* emotional factors, it affects preferentially the posterolateral hypothalamus and the corpus amygdaloideum; in this case, patients will show a rather aggressive behavior. Inversely when the ventromedial hypothalamus is affected, an *action inhibition* may occur. Those two situations (inhibition, aggressiveness) are not incompatible because they can affect the same patient at different moments. For some TMD patients, *tension caused by expectation* [13] with severe clenching may represent a behavioral starting point from which aggressive episodes occasionally occur, particularly when faced with enduring *blocked situations*. Hyperemotional and/or perfectionist patients cannot find a quick adequate solution to solve the problem they face. Frustration may constitute a *psychological ransom*, when the neocortex does not exercise its modulatory control on the limbic system and the RF. It can also be an involvement of the limbico-reticular tract: the limbic system which manages feelings and memory plays a major role in reticular activity. As for reticulo-limbic projections under

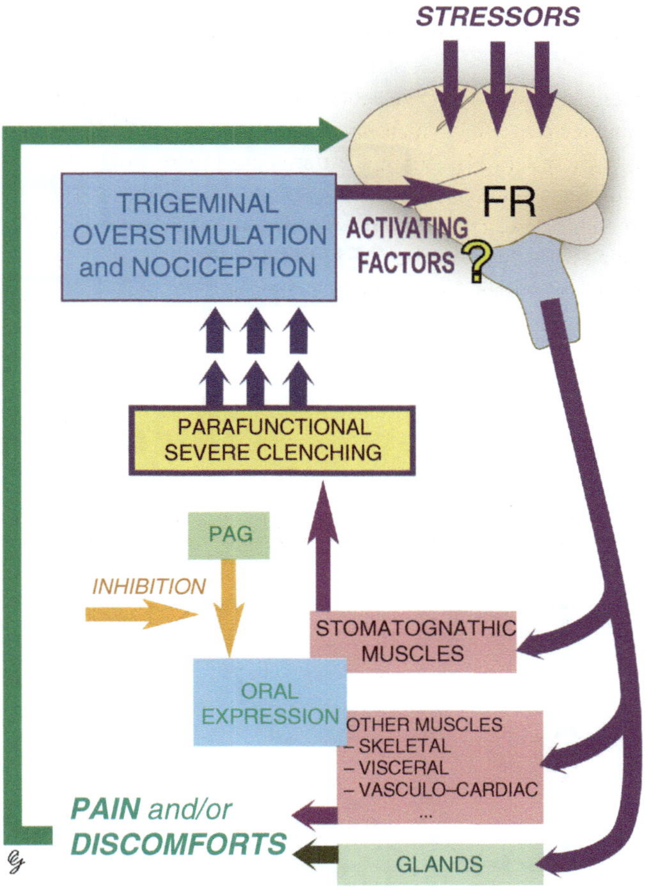

Fig. 7 Watson's concept and oral parafunctional conditions. Model. *FR* formatio reticularis, *PAG* periaqueducal grey

painful circumstances, a condition of suffering involves two types of neurons in the rostroventromedial nuclei (RVM) of the bulbar RF (Fig. 8):

- The *off-type* neurons tend to slow down the nociceptive trigeminal input from the nucleus subcaudalis; this happens with minimal or occasional input (habituation phenomena through suprasegmental pain control)
- On the contrary, the *on-type* neurons tend to amplify the nociceptive responses when severe pain persists such as in TMD; here it seems that some *closed circles* are operating with pathophysiological components such as limbic and emotional factors, trigeminal spasticity and overstimulation, and reticular overactivity [35].

Orofacial behaviors are always associated with emotions and their expression in the stomatognathic system: language, mimics, and gesture [5]. A close link must be considered between psychoemotional factors and stomatognathic behavior [53] particularly in parafunctional situations. Reciprocal connections between the hypothalamus and amygdala do exist. From a clinical point of view, it is generally admitted that complex syndromes involving emotional factors may appear [27]. Above all, the amygdala seems to represent a modulator for the hypothalamus. Furthermore, stressful situations and their memory can implicate the hippocampus through the phenomenon of *long-term potentiation* in which the hippocampic neurons have the ability to develop excitative postsynaptic potentials during very long periods of time, even several months [40]. The main interconnections between the limbic structures in the memory process are better known today. Considering their hypothalamic projections, excessive and nociceptive parafunctional trigeminal afferents (severe clenching) may well interfere in hypothalamo-hippocampic connections.

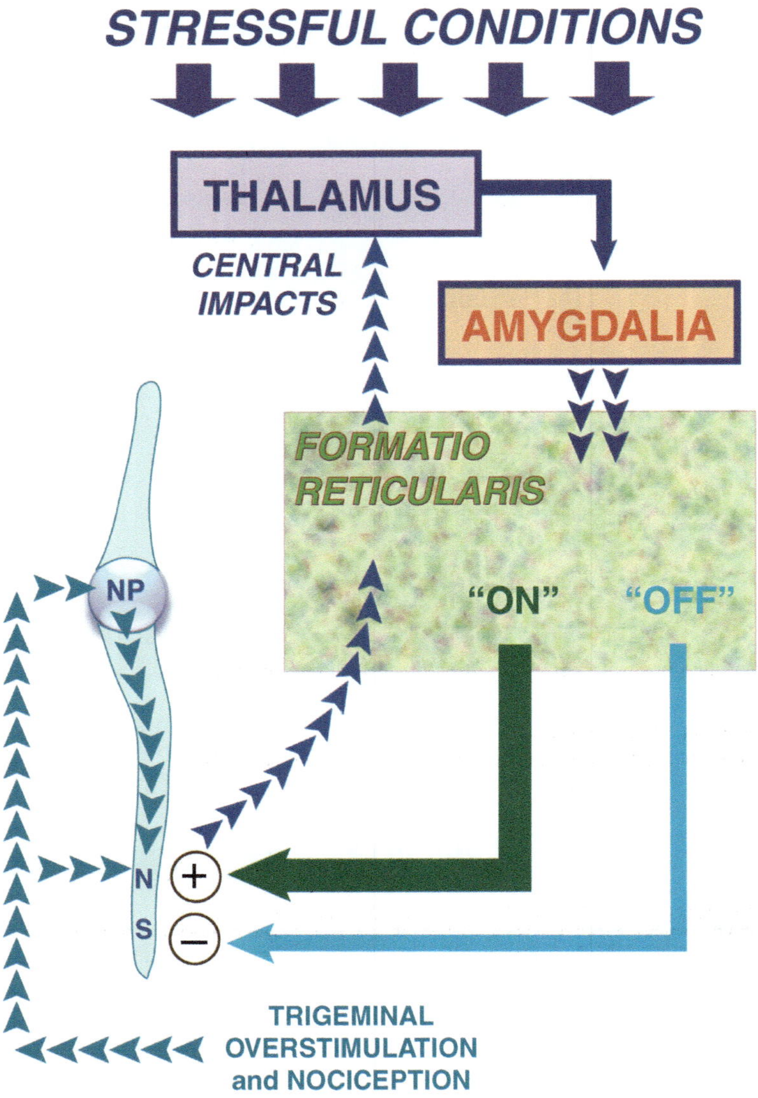

Fig. 8 Reticular and amygdalian control of the trigeminal pathways. Neurophysiological theory. *A* amygdala, *FR* formatio reticularis, *RVM* rostroventromedial nucleus, *TH* thalamus, + excitation, – inhibition. In stressed, anxious, introverted subjects, suprasegmental components (i.e., psycho-emotional factors) tend to magnify abnormal inputs and their clinical outcome, thus making them deleterious. In such cases, the reticular influence works through its *on-type* receptors. It results in a strengthening of the central impacts of nociception and overstimulation caused by parafunctional spastic activities such as severe clenching

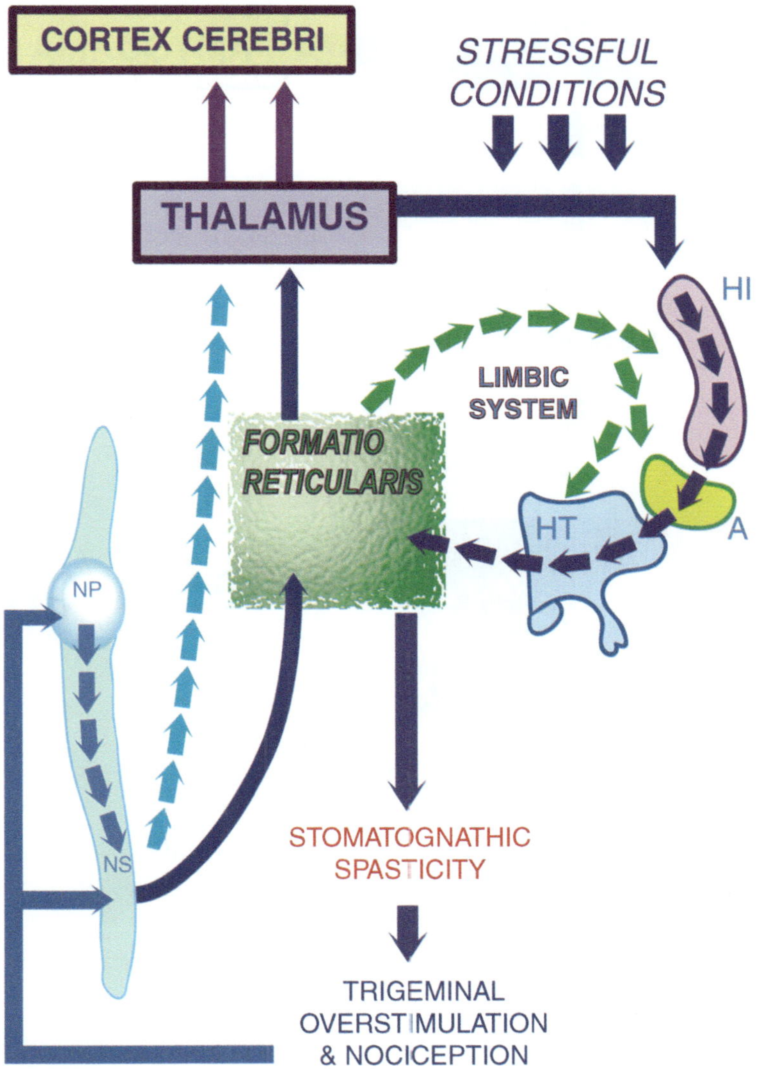

Fig. 9 Trigeminal territory and central connections in aggressiveness. Model

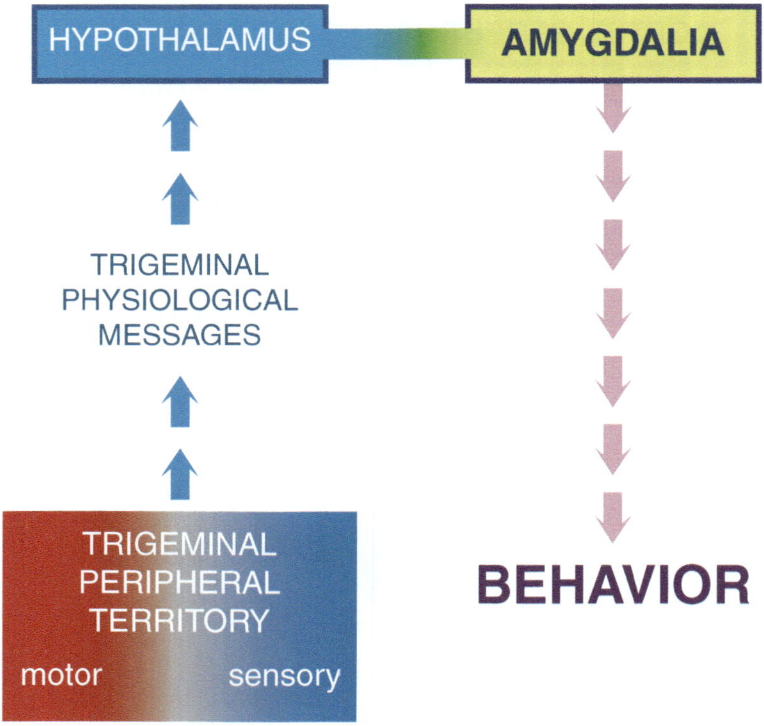

Fig. 10 Trigemino-amygdalian physiological connections

disturbances, and/or pain-related emotions in the increase of neural activity in the anterior cingulate cortex and amygdala [31].

1 Biochemical Data

1.1 Serotonin

Serotonin (5-HT) is involved in the regulation of cerebral vascularization, sleeping, inhibition of cardiovascular spinal centers, excitation of motor neurons, and suprasegmental pain control. In leeches, 5-HT triggers salivation, biting, and laryngeal contraction [17]. In rats, 5-HT agonists increase the clenching tendency, while 5-HT antagonists decrease it. 5-HT may be largely involved in *action inhibition* behaviors [13]. Whether or not 5-HT is clearly involved in tonic muscular parafunctional tendencies such as clenching is still unknown. Figure 12 recalls some conditions involving the 5-HT.

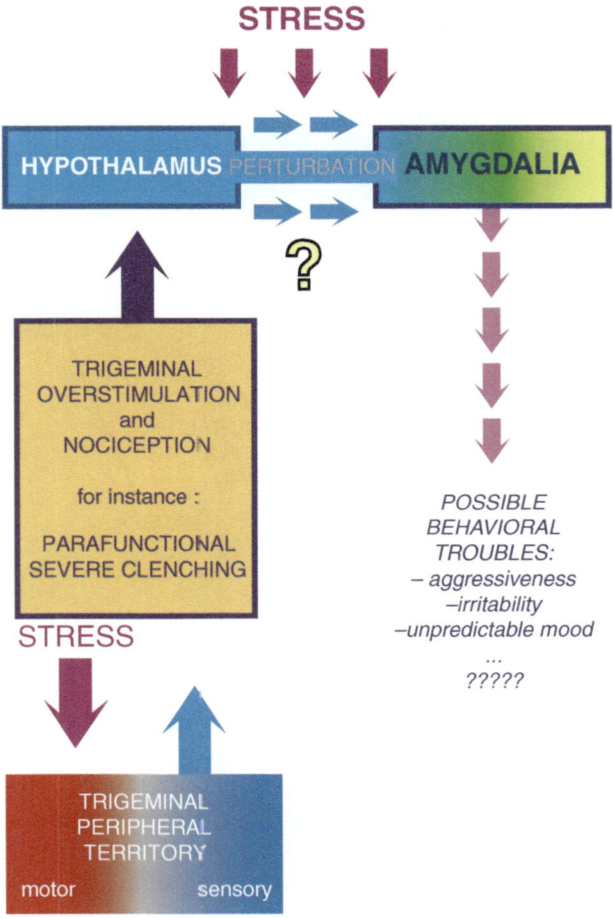

Fig. 11 Trigemino-amygdalian pathophysiological connections. Model

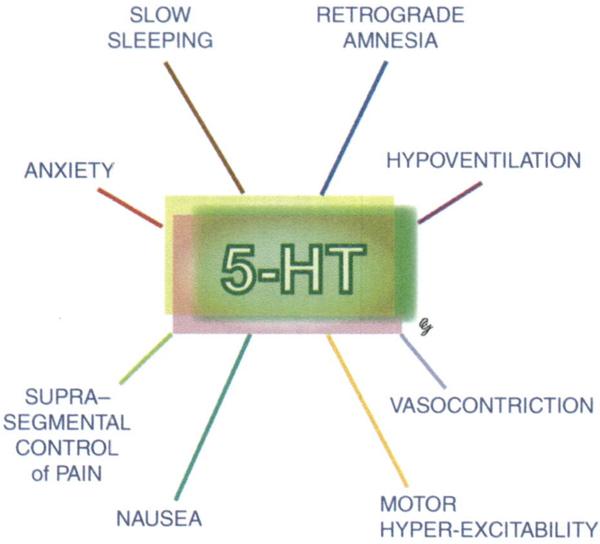

Fig. 12 Principal conditions involving the 5-HT

1.2 Dopamine

Dopamine (Dopa) activates the nigrostriatal pathway called *the medial forebrain bundle* (MFB). Nigrostriatal projections intervene in the behavior and normal use of peripheral inputs [4]. Areso et al. suggested that "...the possibility that alterations in occlusion, which would alter oral sensory inputs to the Central Nervous System through the trigeminal pathway, can modify central dopaminergic neurotransmission." [3]. Therefore, excessive sensory stimulation, such as trigeminal stimulation during clenching phases, may facilitate a dysfunction in the CGN and disturb the subcortical control of the stomatognathic muscle tone. This may be a neural support of the pathophysiological trigeminal sensitivo-motor *closed circle*. Some CGN inputs project to limbic structures, particularly the corpus amygdaloideum [4]. In animals, the amygdalian stimulation initiates mandibular movements that resemble grinding [38, 49], chewing, swallowing, salivation, and vomiting efforts. Projections to the anterior cingular gyrus initiate complex movements of chewing, licking, swallowing, and vocalization [4]. In addition, estradiol has an effect on the Dopa transmission with possible endocrine and behavioral disturbances [16]. These data can explain the high percentage in female TMD subjects [1] and the correlation between TMD and premenstrual syndrome [29]. It has been determined that disharmonious contact between upper and lower teeth could disturb central catecholaminergic activity in rats [3]. Previous data showed that monoamines (Dopa and 5-HT) were involved in a behavioral syndrome which may well surface in the stomatognathic system through parafunctional tendencies such as clenching.

1.3 Substance P

The substance P will be evoked in Part IV about migraine.

1.4 Acetylcholine

Acetylcholine (ACh): ACh antagonists (e.g., scopolamine) may decrease uncontrolled masticatory movements in rats. Parafunctional uncontrolled masticatory movements are reinforced by ACh agonists. An ACh-5HT interaction may be needed to initiate this kind of movement. Finally, an (Ach) axis exists between the limbic system and cerebral cortex from which some fibers project to the corpus amygdaloideum which plays a role in emotion, motivation, and behavior [4].

1.5 Others

The relationship between female hormonal conditions and TMD is often discussed [23, 51] and supported by fundamental data [33, 34, 52]. The estrous cycle tends to modify the processing of deep craniofacial inputs at the spinomedullary junction, a key region for the initial integration of sensory signals from TMJ [28]. Other data tend to show that estrogen replacement treatments do not expose women to increased risk of TMD [10], but it seems that rapid estrogen change can be associated with increased pain [18, 19]. Another study shed light on the higher glutamate sensitivity of TMJ receptors in females. Cortisol secretion in TMD women is abnormal, perhaps due to orofacial pain implications [12]. Nociception was also noted with an induction of long-term potentiation (LTP): stimulation of the primary afferent nerve fibers affected glutamate receptors in the trigeminal caudal nucleus [20]. Otherwise a significant correlation has been found especially in females between cigarette smoking and the intensity of pain [24].

References

1. Abubaker AO, Wassim FR, Raslan WF, Sotereanos GC (1993) Estrogen and progesterone receptors in temporomandibular joint discs of symptomatic and asymptomatic persons: a preliminary study. J Oral Maxillofac Surg 51(10):1095–1100
2. Ahlberg J, Savolainen A, Rantala M et al (2004) Reported bruxism and biopsychosocial symptoms: a longitudinal study. Community Dent Oral Epidemiol 32(4):307–311
3. Areso MP, Giralt MT, Sainz B et al (1999) Occlusal disharmonies modulate central catecholaminergic activity in the rat. J Dent Res 78(6):1204–1213

4. Bossy J (1990) Anatomie clinique: neuro-anatomie. Springer Verlag (éd), Paris
5. Chase PF, Rosenoer L (1999) Parameters of odontostomatognathic disability: guidelines for evaluation of impaired simple complex human functions involving the odontostomatognathic functional system. Cranio 17(1):70–76
6. Curran SL, Carlson CR, Okeson JP (1996) Emotional and physiologic response to laboratory challenges: patients with temporomandibular disorders versus matched control subjects. J Orofac Pain 10(2):141–150
7. Dujardin E, Jürgens U (2005) Afferents of vocalization-controlling periaqueducal regions in the squirrel monkey. Brain Res 1034(1–2):114–131
8. Fine E (1971) Psychological factors associated with non-organic temporomandibular joint pain-dysfunction syndrome. Br Dent J 131:402–404
9. Green CS, Laskin DM (1983) Long-term evaluation of treatment for myofascial pain-dysfunction syndrome: a comparative analysis. J Am Dent Assoc 107(2):253–258
10. Hatch JP, Rugh JD, Sakai S, Saunders MJ (2001) Is use of exogenous estrogen associated with temporomandibular signs and symptoms? J Am Dent Assoc 132(3):319–326
11. Jürgens U (1994) The role of the periaqueducal grey in vocal behaviour. Behav Brain Res 62(2):107–117
12. Korszun A, Young EA, Singer K et al (2002) Basal circadian cortisol secretion in women with temporomandibular disorders. J Dent Res 81(4):279–283
13. Laborit H (1986) L'inhibition de l'action. Biologie comportementale et physiopathologique, 2nd edn. Masson (éd), Montréal
14. Lam DK, Sessle BJ, Cairns BE, Hu JW (2005) Neural mechanisms of temporomandibular joint and masticatory muscle pain: a possible role for peripheral glutamate receptor mechanisms. Pain Res Manag 10(3):145–152
15. Lautenbacher S, Spernal J, Schreiber W, Krieg JC (1999) Relationship between clinical pain complaints and pain sensitivity in patients with depression and panic disorders. Psychosom Med 61:822–827
16. Lejoyeux H (1988) Hormones et cancer. Pour une écologie sexuelle dans la vie moderne. In: Les thérapeutiques du stress. Les Entretiens de Monaco. Edit du Rocher, Monaco, p 63
17. Lent C, Dickinson M (1988) Neurobiologie et alimentation de la sangsue. Pour la Science 130:82–87
18. LeResche L, Saunders K, Von Korff MR et al (1997) Use of exogenous hormones and risk of temporomandibular disorder pain. Pain 69(1–2):153–160
19. LeResche L, Mancl L, Sherman JJ et al (2003) Changes in temporomandibular pain and other symptoms across the menstrual cycle. Pain 106(3):253–261
20. Liang YC, Huang CC, Hsu KS (2005) Characterization of long-term potentiation of primary afferent transmission at trigeminal synapses of juvenile rats: essential role of subtype 5 metabotropic glutamate receptors. Pain 114(3):417–428
21. Lupton DA (1969) Psychological aspects of TMJ dysfunction. J Am Dent Assoc 79:131
22. Marbach JJ (1978) Facial pain and anxiety levels: considerations for treatment. J Prosthet Dent 40:434–437
23. Meisler JG (1999) Chronic pain conditions in women. J Womens Health 8(3):313–320
24. Melis M, Lobo SL, Ceneviz C et al (2010) Effect of cigarette smoking on pain intensity of TMD patients: a pilot study. Cranio 28(3):187–192
25. Molina OF, Dos Santos J, Nelson SJ, Nowlin T (2000) Profile of TMD and bruxer compared to TMD and nonbruxer patients regarding chief complaint, previous consultations, modes of therapy, and chronicity. Cranio 18(3):205–218
26. Moody PM, Kemper JT, Okesson JP et al (1982) Recent life changes and myofascial pain syndrome. J Prosthet Dent 48(3):328–330
27. N'Guyen JP, Keravel Y, Poirier J (1987) Vues anatomiques commentées du rhinencéphale. Encycl Med Chir, Paris, Neurol 17001(R 10):1–22
28. Okamoto K, Hirata H, Takeshita S, Bereiter DA (2003) Response properties of TMJ units in superficial laminae at the spinomedullary junction of female rats vary over the estrous cycle. J Neurophysiol 89(3):1467–1477

29. Olson GB, Peters CJ, Franger AL (1988) The incidence and severity of premenstrual syndrome among female craniomandibular pain patients. Cranio 6(4):330–338
30. Ong KS, Keng SB (2003) The biological, social, and psychological relationship between depression and chronic pain. Cranio 21(4):286–294
31. Otsuka T, Watanabe K, Hirano Y et al (2009) Effects of mandibular deviation on brain activation during clenching: an fMRI preliminary study. Cranio 27(2):88–93
32. Paris CJ (1991) L'amineptine: effet antidépresseur et restauration de l'anticipation, vol 4. Référence (Lancet), Sympos Monte-Carlo, Monaco, pp 13–15
33. Puri V, Cui L, Liverman CS et al (2005) Ovarian steroids regulate neuropeptides in the trigeminal ganglion. Neuropeptides 39(4):409–417
34. Puri V, Chandrala S, Puri S et al (2006) Ghrelin is expressed in trigeminal neurons of female mice in phase with the estrous cycle. Neuropeptides 40(1):35–46
35. Renaud J (1991) Le cerveau exagère la douleur. Sci Vie 891:48–165
36. Rothwell PS (1972) Personality and temporomandibular joint dysfunction. Oral Surg 34:734–742
37. Rugh JD, Lemke RR (1984) Significance in oral habits. In: Matarazzo JD et al (eds) Behavioural health: a handbook of heath enhancement and disease prevention. Wiley, New York, p 947
38. Shärer P (1971) Recherches sur l'organisation des mouvements masticateurs et parafonctionnels. Rev Franç Odont Stomatol 4:75–80
39. Shipman WG, Green CS, Laskin DM (1974) Correlation of placebo responses and personality characteristics in myofascial pain-dysfunction (MPD) patients. J Psychosom Res 18:475–483
40. Shors JT, Matzel LD (1997) Long-term potentiation: what's learning got to do with it? Behav Brain Sci 20:597–655
41. Sipilä K, Veijola J, Jokelainen J et al (2001) Association of symptoms of TMD and orofacial pain with alexithymia: an epidemiological study of the Northern Finland 1966 Birth Cohort. Cranio 19(4):246–251
42. Slavicek R (1996) Reflexions sur les soi-disant parafonctions. Trad Hurez C. Rev Orthop Dentofac 30:75–88
43. Southwell J, Deary IJ, Geisler P (1990) Personality and anxiety in temporomandibular joint syndrome. J Oral Rehabil 17:239–243
44. Speculand B, Goss AN (1985) Physiological factors in temporomandibular joint dysfunction pain. Int J Oral Surg 14:131–137
45. Steed PA, Wexler GB (2001) Temporomandibular disorders-traumatic etiology vs. nontraumatic etiology: a clinical and methodological inquiry into symptomatology and treatment outcomes. Cranio 19(3):188–194
46. Stein S, Loft G, Davis H, Hart DL (1982) Symptoms of TMJ dysfunction as related to stress measured by social readjustment rating scale. J Prosthet Dent 47:545–548
47. Stockstill JW, Callahan CD (1991) Personality hardiness, anxiety, and depression as constructs of interest in the study of temporomandibular disorders. J Craniomandib Disord 5:129–134
48. Thomass LJ, Tiber N, Schireson S (1973) The effects of anxiety and frustration on muscular tension related to the temporomandibular joint syndrome. J Dent Res 36(5):763–768
49. Uursin H, Kaaba BR (1980) Functional localization within the amygdaloid complex in the cat. Electroencephalogr Clin Neurophysiol 12:1–20
50. Vimpari SS, Knuttila ML, Sakki TK, Kivela SL (1995) Depressive symptoms associated with symptoms of the temporomandibular joint pain and dysfunction syndrome. Psychosom Med 57:439–444
51. Warren MP, Fried JL (2001) Temporomandibular disorders and hormones in women. Cells Tissues Organs 169(3):187–192
52. Yamada K, Nozawa-Inoue K, Kawano Y et al (2003) Expression of estrogen receptor alpha (ER alpha) in the rat temporomandibular joint. Anat Rec A Discov Mol Cell Evol Biol 274(2):934–941
53. Yardin M (1995) Odontologie globale. Masson (éd), Paris

Painful Outcomes of Parafunctional Clenching

The following figures suggest different ways to summarize the hypothetical model about clinical outcome of *severe clenching in introverted stressed patient* (Figs. 1, 2, 3, and 4).

Severe pain has been observed in TMD patients [6, 17, 28, 53, 82]. Spasmed muscles can play an important role in initiating *tension-type headache*, especially in cases of nuchal pain [82]. Therefore, patients suffering from both tension-type headache and nuchal pain are three times more likely to experience painful palpation of the stomatognathic muscles. **Severe clenching** does seem to play a part in the most severe clinical forms of TMD [14, 19, 20, 24, 25, 27, 28, 37, 38, 50, 51, 54–56, 67, 73, 83]. When stressful situations are poorly managed, intensive and/or durable diurnal or nocturnal muscular contraction indicates a particularly deleterious parafunction for the stomatognathic system. Connections between trigeminal nuclei and some non-trigeminal nervous areas seem to validate this theory. In such cases, the pathology shows a disconcerting symptomatology with some pain that may be *remote from the oral sphere* (see Part I) [1, 3, 6, 7, 14, 15, 18, 23, 25–28, 37, 38, 40, 46, 47, 50, 53, 54, 60, 64, 65, 70–72, 77, 82–84]. Various observations have shed light on the *aggravating role of parafunctional habits* [2, 16, 21, 22, 34, 42, 48, 50, 51, 59, 80, 83] particularly with regard to craniofacial pain and feeling of *fatigued jaws*. There is increasingly clear evidence of a correlation between clenching and dysfunctional symptoms [9, 54] significantly expressed by muscular pain, even to axial musculature pain (arm, hand, calf) [83]. Some authors have even observed that voluntary clenching alone was sufficient to provoke headaches in some TMD patients [34]. The Headache Classification Committee of the International Headache Society gives some concise guidelines whose description refers to clinically observed pain.

Paragraph 2 = Tension-type headache[1]

[1]Sometimes pain originating in muscles can also be considered as nontypical facial neuralgia for which classical treatments fail. Pharyngeal [86] or lingual [87], auricular, and orbital [61] irradiations may be observed. More rarely pain is felt in the teeth [18, 53, 63, 77], although these are intact according to clinical and radiological investigations; this hyperesthesia can be explained by a lowering of sensitive threshold in nociceptive pulpo-dentinar receptors [40] under suprasegmental facilitating influences.

F. Hartmann, G. Cucchi, *Stress and Orality*,
DOI 10.1007/978-2-8178-0271-8_11, © Springer-Verlag France 2014

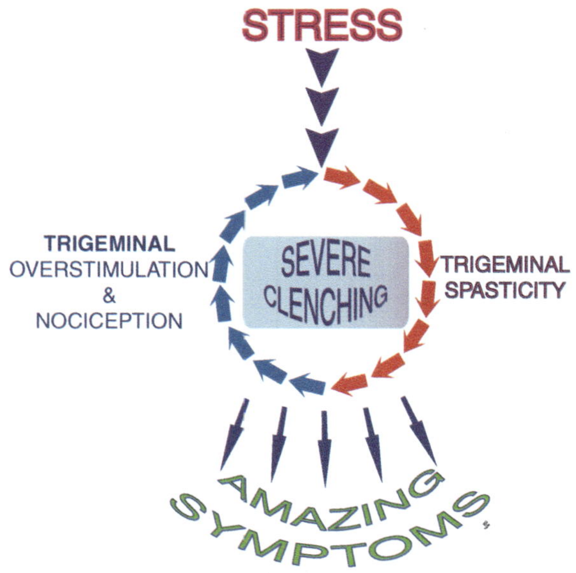

Fig. 1 Stress and severe clenching in the trigeminal area

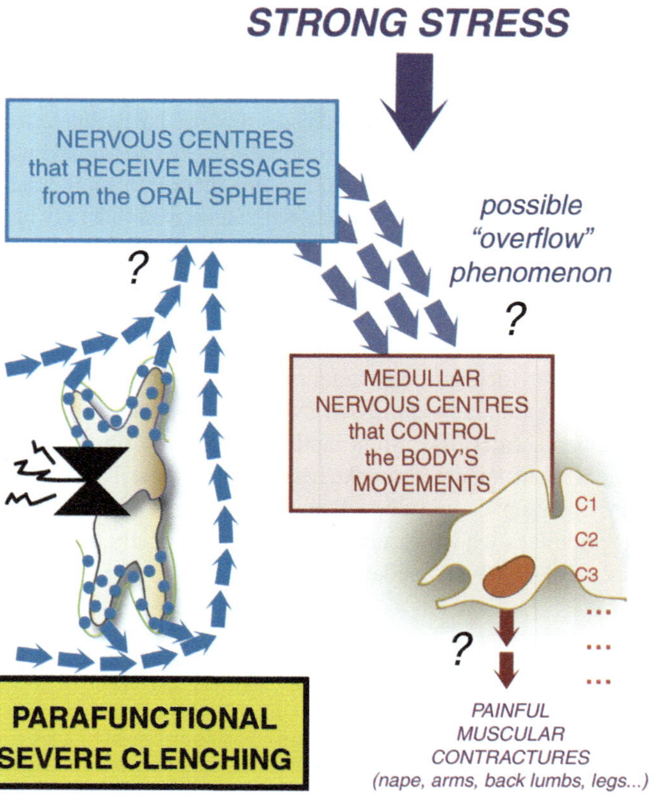

Fig. 2 Stress and severe clenching outcome on axial muscles

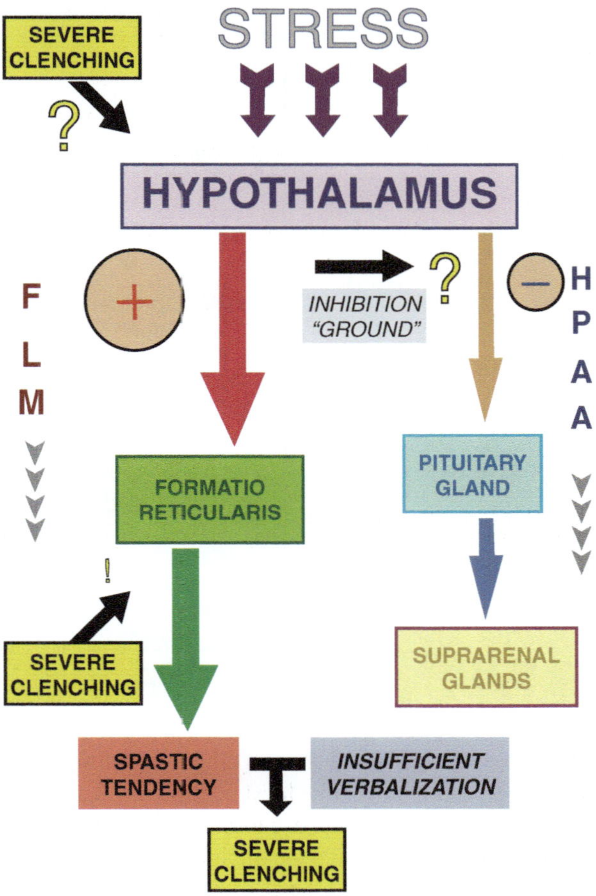

Fig. 3 Stress and severe clenching around the HPA axis

Paragraph 5 = Headache associated with head trauma[2]

Paragraph 11 = Headache and facial pain associated with dysfunction of several structures [52]: cranial, nuchal, ocular, auricular, nasal, sinusital, dental, buccal, or other

Chapter 11.2[3]

---

[2]This paragraph includes some observations on minor, acute (5.1.2.), or chronic (5.2.2) posttraumatic headaches.

[3]This chapter focuses on the nape with particular mention in Sect. 11.2.1 (cervical rachis) of occipital and nuchal headaches correlated to joint and ligament problems: a condition of muscle contraction triggering resistance or limitation in nuchal passive movements [10, 31, 32, 39, 76]. The projection of some trigeminal fibers on C1, C2, and C3 helps understand the possible presence of pain in the trapezius and the SCM in TMD when severe clenching persists [81]. Some electromyographic studies confirm that voluntary clenching tends to increase the activity of the SCM [8, 57] but also of the trapezius [89, 90]. Furthermore, increased responses of the m. rectus abdominis and paravertebral muscles [13] have been observed as well as a significant variation of the solar reflex during clenching [49]. Referred pain in the C2–C3 myotome can provide evidence of the connection between stomatognathic diseases and some minor intervertebral disorders [4, 12, 66, 74, 75, 78, 85] which need to be adequately treated together [61, 66, 79]. The trigemino-nuchal relationship will be developed in Chapter 7 in the section about *Dizziness and Visual Problems*.

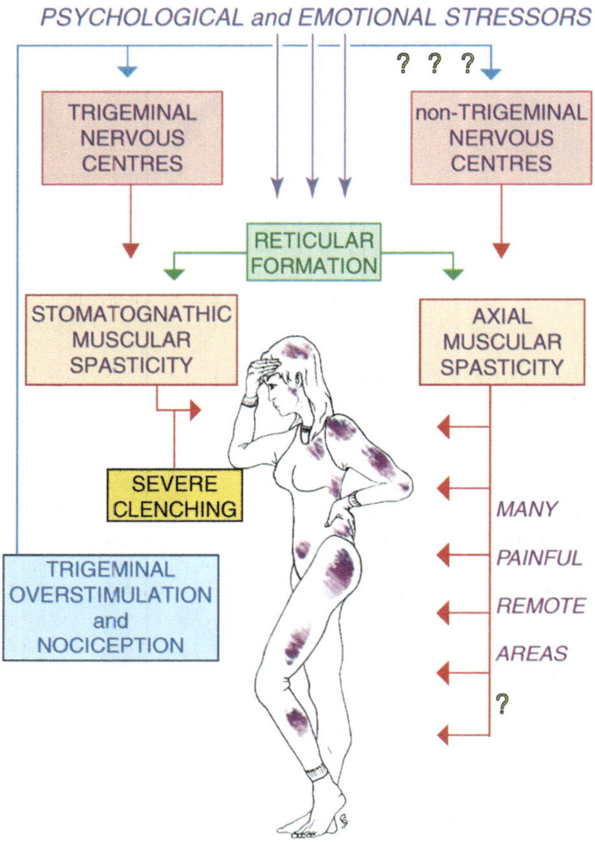

Fig. 4 Trigeminal overstimulation and possible remote signs

Chapter 11.3[4]
Chapter 11.4[5]
Chapter 11.5[6]
Chapter 11.6[7]

[4]In this chapter on eyes, Sect. 11.3.3 deals with heterophoria and heterotrophy linked to external ocular muscles (EOM), sometimes involved in TMD via the ophthalmic nerve (V1).

[5]In this chapter on ears, Sect. 12 refers to headaches due to dysafferentation, nervous trunk compressions, and cranial neuralgia. Clinical observations demonstrate the possible correlation between this pain topography and some contractured areas in the SCM and incidentally in the masseteris and the medial pterygoid muscle [77].

[6]In this chapter on sinus and nose, Sect. 11.5.2 is about sinusalgia: it is not consecutive to infection [44] or obstruction of these structures, but it results from a projected tension-type headache. Note that it is a frequent referred pain from the LP muscle [18, 27, 29, 53, 77].

[7]This chapter on teeth, maxillas, and adjacent structures explains headaches due to inflammatory processes, particularly in periodontal or pericoronary areas. Yet sometimes dental aches are due to a referred phenomenon from a contractured muscle [63] that is consistent with tension-type headache.

Chapter 11.7[8]

Brachial and antebrachial pain is often followed by vasomotor problems such as cold hand feelings [62, 69, 88] or by acroparesthesia (numbness of fingers) [36]. These symptoms are classically explained by the mechanical compression of the vasculo-nervous plexus, for instance, at the level of the scalene outlet. A possible compression by the superior tendon of m. pectoralis minor [77] may also be considered as a factor.

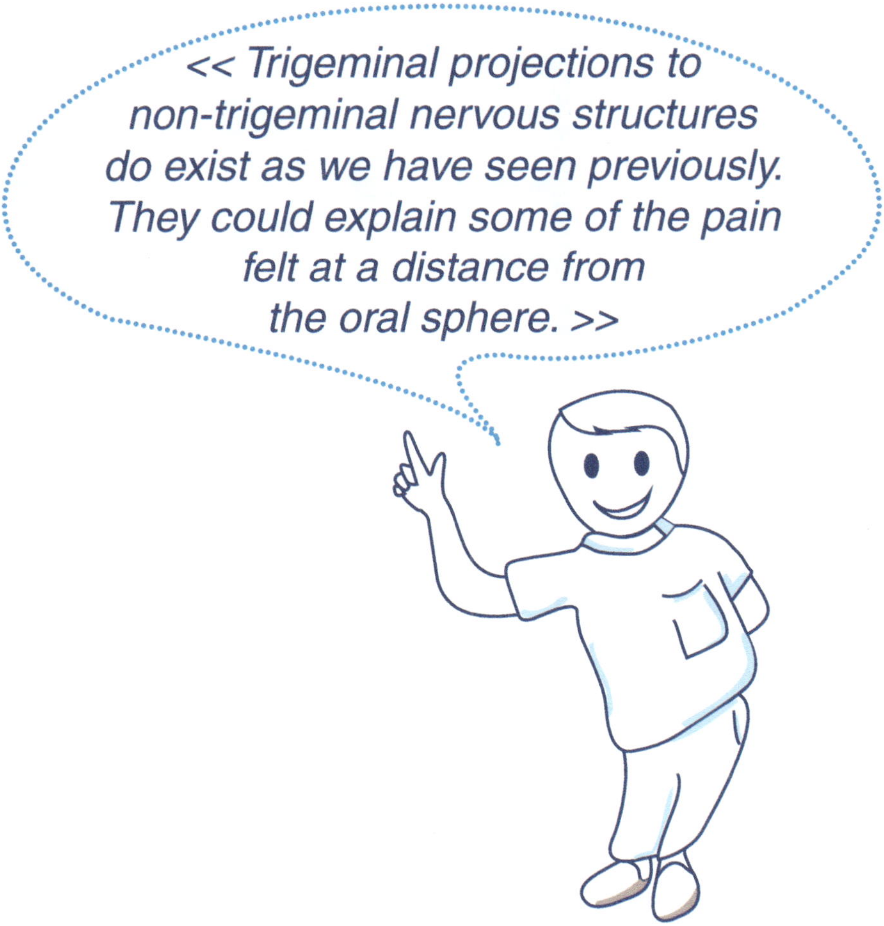

[8]This chapter on TMJ refers to headaches originating from TMJ disorders. The classification admits that this type of pain is often linked to oromandibular disorders. This view is further confirmed by literature [1, 30, 41, 46, 90]. If tendons or ligaments can trigger some muscular pain [58], articular pain is more frequently a referred pain from the spasmed lateral pterygoid m. [3, 18, 77] (when the muscle's two heads do not work in concert [35]; that pain is all the more intense since the patient

These little-known projections may prove useful to practitioners faced with uncommon clinical settings, particularly when patients complain about symptoms very remote from the oral sphere. The same is true when classical treatments have failed to get satisfying results and reduce symptoms of atypical forms of migraine, fibromyalgia, and chronic fatigue, as well as for female patients with comorbid orofacial pain conditions and other diseases or disorders whose treatment shows limited results [11].

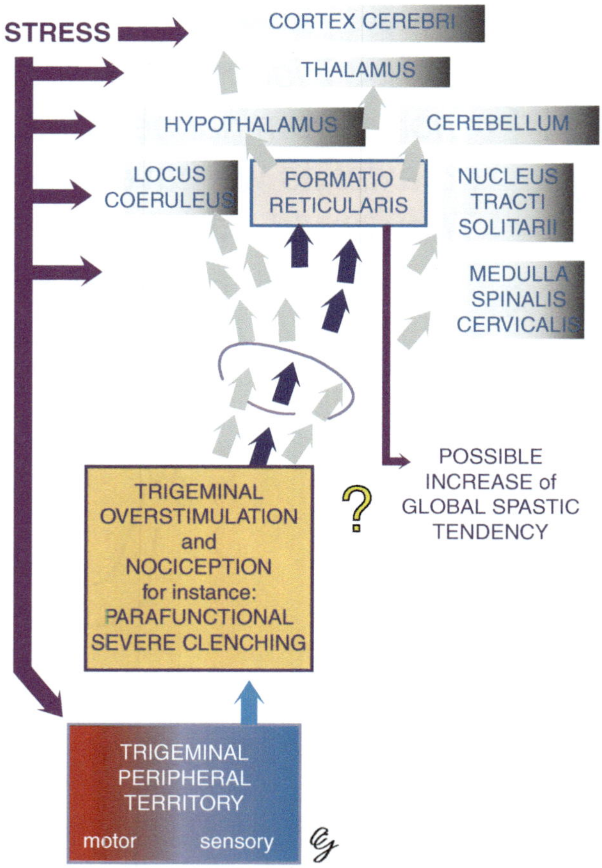

Fig. 5 Reticular projections of trigeminal parafunctional inputs

suffers from parafunctional clenching [35]). The connection is confirmed in patients suffering from TMJ clacking by the very high frequency in painful palpation of the temporalis muscles [45]. Distinctions between TMD clinical forms remain hazardous, because of different evolutions or phases of a same pathological functional unit. There were no significant symptomatologic differences between subgroups of patients with pain referred to as *muscular*, *anterior disc dislocation with reduction*, *anterior disc dislocation without reduction*, *osteoarthritis*, or *mixed* [43]. TMJs seem to be a less frequent factor of pain than stomatognathic muscles. In some cases, marrow edema and osteonecrosis of the condyle can be an etiological factor of intense pain in the TMJ [68]. Algesic phenomena can be accompanied by a feeling of *mandibular fatigue*; such sign is more frequently related to an isometric parafunction (clenching) than an isotonic parafunction (grinding).

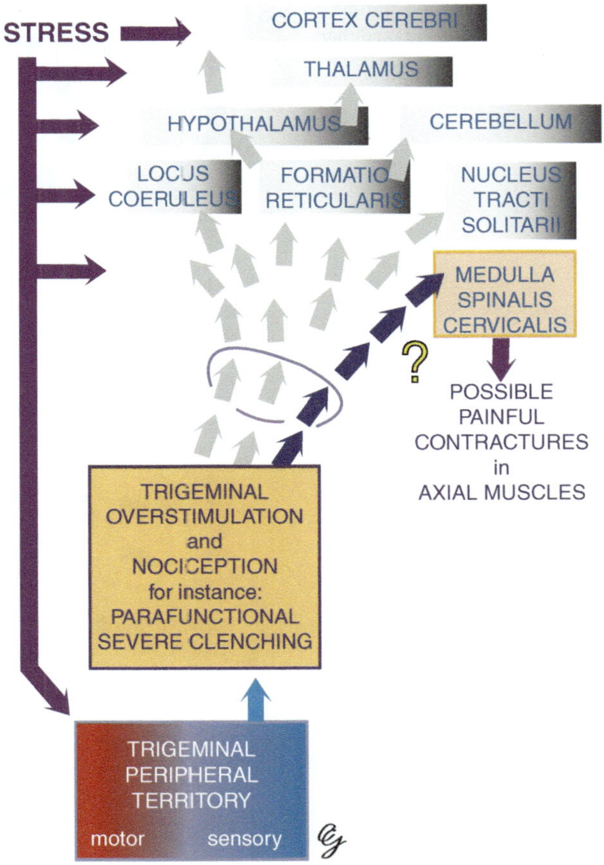

Fig. 6 Medullar projections of trigeminal parafunctional inputs

The following figures (Figs. 5, 6, 7, and 8) suggest some models about projections of trigeminal overstimulation on axial musculature in stressful conditions.

Fig. 7 Trigeminal parafunctional projections to medullar zones

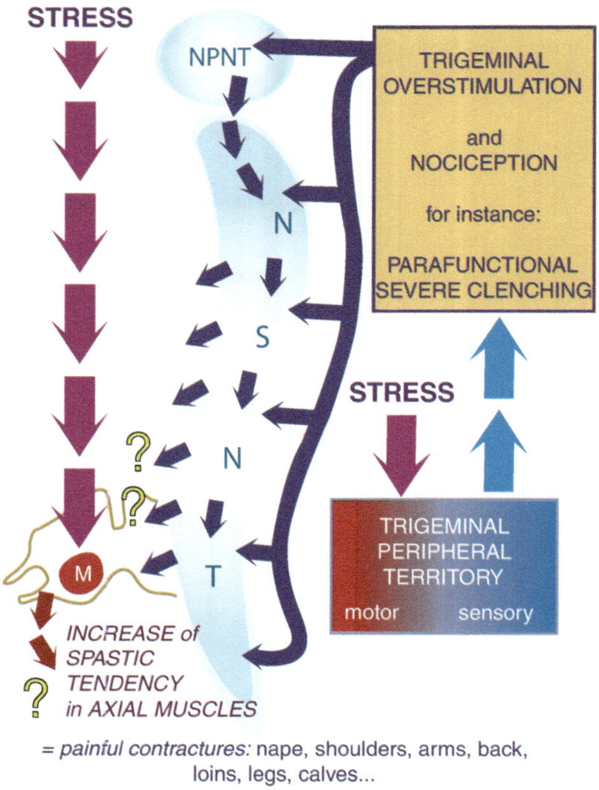

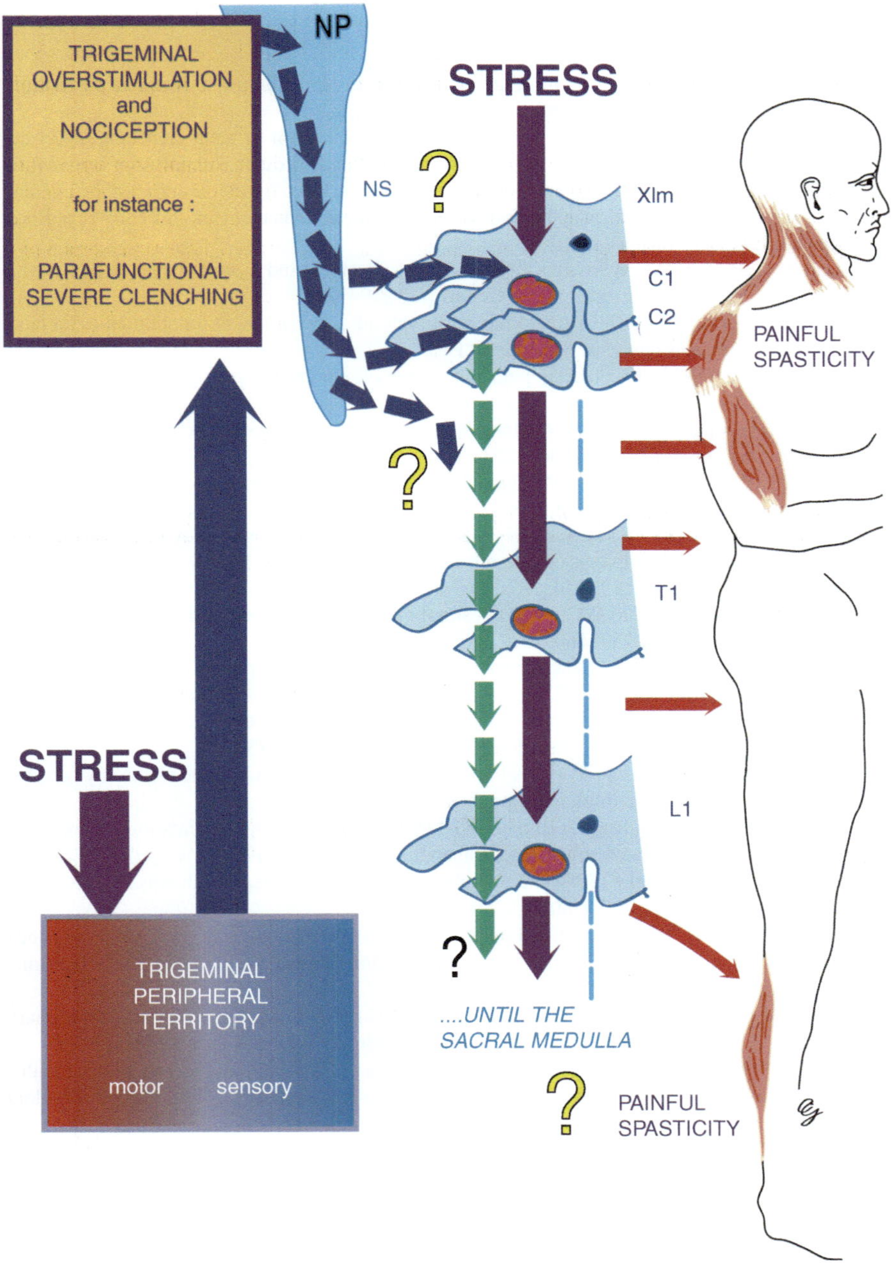

Fig. 8 Trigeminal parafunctional projections to medullar motor centers

References

1. Agerberg G, Inkapool I (1990) Craniomandibular disorders in an urban Swedish population. J Craniomandib Disord 4:154–164
2. Aydin G, Keles I, Zog G, Orkun S (2004) How does the habit of teeth clenching affect the symptoms and signs of patients with temporomandibular disorders? Kulak Burun Bogaz Ihtis Derg 13(1–2):19–24
3. Bell WH (1989) Orofacial pains: classification, diagnosis, management, 3rd edn. Year Book Medical Pub Inc, Chicago, 420p
4. Bjorne A, Berven A, Agerberg G (1998) Cervical signs and symptoms in patients with Meniere's disease: a controlled study. Cranio 16(3):194–202
5. Bouchet A, Cuilleret J (1980) Anatomie topographique, descriptive et fonctionnelle. La face, la tête et les organes des sens. Simep (ed), Paris
6. Brechner VL (1982) Myofascial pain syndrome of the lateral pterygoid muscle. Cranio 1(1):42–45
7. Büdz-Jorgensen E, Luan W (1984) Mandibular dysfunction and occlusal conditions in a group of elderly patients. J Dent Res 63(4):573
8. Clark GT, Browne PA, Nakano M, Yang Q (1993) Co-activation of sternocleidomastoid muscles during jaw clenching. J Dent Res 72(11):1499–1502
9. Conti PCR, Ferreira PM, Pegorado LF et al (1996) A cross sectional study of prevalence and etiology of signs and symptoms of temporomandibular disorders in High School and University Student. J Orofac Pain 10(3):254–262
10. Daly P, Preston CB, Evans WG (1982) Postural response of the head to bite opening in adults males. Am J Orthod 82:157–160
11. De Leeuw R, Klasser GD, Albuquerque RJC (2005) Are female patients with orofacial pain medically compromised? J Am Dent Assoc 136(4):459–468
12. De Wijer A, Steenks MH, De Leeuw J et al (1996) Symptoms of the cervical spine in temporomandibular and cervical spine disorders. J Oral Rehabil 23:742–750
13. Ehrlich R, Garlick D, Ninio M (1999) The effect of jaw clenching on the electromyographic activities of 2 neck and 2 trunk muscles. J Orofac Pain 13(2):115–120
14. Etzel KR, Stockstill JW, Rugh JD, Fisher JG (1991) Tryptophan supplementation for nocturnal bruxisms: report negative results. J Craniomandib Disord 5:115–120
15. Forssell H, Kangasniemi P (1984) Mandibular dysfunction in patients with muscle contraction headache. Proc Finn Dent Soc 80:211–216
16. Fragoso YD, Alves HH, Garcia SO, Finkelsztejn A (2010) Prevalence of parafunctional habits and temporomandibular dysfunction symptoms in patients attending a tertiary headache clinic. Arq Neuropsiquiatr 68(3):377–380
17. Franco AL, Gonçalves DA, Castanharo SM et al (2010) Migraine is the most prevalent primary headache in individuals with temporomandibular disorders. J Orofac Pain 24(3):287–292
18. Gelb H (1985) Clinical management of head, neck and TMJ pain and dysfunction: a multidisciplinary approach to diagnosis and treatment. WB Saunders Co, Philadelphia/London/Toronto
19. Glaros AG, Tabacchi KN, Glass EG (1998) Effect of parafunctional clenching on TMD pain. J Orofac Pain 12(2):145–152
20. Glaros AG, Baharloo L, Glass EG (1998) Effect of parafunctional clenching and estrogen on temporomandibular disorder pain. Cranio 16(2):78–83
21. Glaros AG, Burton E (2004) Parafunctional clenching, pain, and effort in temporomandibular disorders. J Behav Med 27(1):91–100
22. Glaros AG, Williams K, Lausten L (2005) The role of parafunctions, emotions and stress in predicting facial pain. J Am Dent Assoc 136(4):451–458
23. Gole DR (1993) A clinical observation: a relationship of occlusal contacts to distal musculature. Cranio 11(1):55–61
24. Gonçalves DA, Bigal ME, Jales LC et al (2010) Headache and symptoms of temporomandibular disorder: an epidemiological study. Headache 50(2):231–241

25. Hagberg C, Hagberg M, Kopp S (1994) Musculoskeletal symptoms and psychosocial factors among patients with craniomandibular disorders. Acta Odont Scand 52:170–177
26. Hall EH, Terezhalmy GT, Pelleu GB, Bethesda PD (1986) A set of descriptors for the diagnosis of dental pain syndrome. Oral Surg Oral Med Oral Pathol 61:153–157
27. Hartmann F, Cucchi G (1986) Rôle du muscle ptérygoïdien latéral dans la phase de début du SADAM. Cah Proth 56:125–144
28. Hartmann F, Cucchi G (1987) Muscle ptérygoïdien latéral et SADAM: diagnostic précoce et traitement. Rev Odont Stomatol 16(3):209–218
29. Hartmann F, Cucchi G (1993) Les dysfonctions cranio-mandibulaires (SADAM). Nouvelles perspectives médicales. Springer-Verlag (éd), Paris, 176p
30. Helkimo M (1974) Studies on function and dysfunction of the masticatory system. Swed Dent J 67:101–121
31. Hellsing E, Hagberg C (1990) Changes in maximum bite force related to extension of the head. Eur J Orthod 12(2):148–153
32. Huggare JA, Rausta AM (1992) Head posture and cervicovertebral and craniofacial morphology in patients with craniomandibular dysfunction. Cranio 10(3):173–177
33. Izquiedo I (1992) Trends in pharmacological. Sciences 13:7
34. Jensen R, Rasmussen BK, Pedersen B et al (1993) Prevalence of oromandibular dysfunction in a general population. J Orofac Pain 7(2):175–182
35. Juniper RP (1984) Temporomandibular joint dysfunction: a theory based upon electromyographic studies of the lateral pterygoid muscle. Br J Oral Maxillofac Surg 22:1–8
36. Kalia M, Sullivan JM (1982) Brainstem projection of sensory and motor components of the vagus nerve in the rat. J Comp Neurol 211:248–264
37. Kampe T, Hannerz H, Strom P (1991) Five-year follow-up of mandibular dysfunction in adolescents with intact and restored dentitions: a comparative anamnestic and clinical study. J Craniomandib Disord 5:121–128
38. Kampe T, Hannerz H, Strom P (1996) Ten-year follow-up study of signs and symptoms of craniomandibular disorders in adults with intact and restored dentitions. J Oral Rehabil 23(6):416–423
39. Kapandji IA (1982) Physiologie articulaire. Tome 3: tronc et rachis. Maloine (éd), Paris
40. Kleier DJ (1985) Referred pain from a myofascial trigger point mimicking pain of endodontic origin. J Endodont 11(9):408–411
41. Knutsson K, Hassrelgren G, Nilner M, Petersson A (1989) Craniomandibular disorders in chronic orofacial pain patients. J Craniomandib Disord 3(1):15–19
42. Kobs G, Bernhardt O, Kocher T, Meyer G (2005) Oral parafunctions and positive clinical examination findings. Stomatologija 7(3):81–83
43. Lobbezoo-Scholte AM, De Leeuw JRJ, Steenks MH et al (1995) Diagnostic subgroups of craniomandibular disorders. J Orofac Pain 9(1):24–43
44. Lupoli TA, Lockey RF (2007) Temporomandibular dysfunction: an often overlooked cause of chronic headaches. Ann Allergy Asthma Immunol 99(4):314–318
45. Magnusson T (1984) Patients referred for stomatognathic treatments – a survey of 282 patients. Swed Dent J 8:193–201
46. Magnusson T, Carlsson GE (1983) A 2 1/2 years follow-up in headache and mandibular dysfunction after stomatognathic treatment. J Prosthet Dent 9:398–402
47. Maixner W (1989) Autonomic and somatosensory interactions: physiological and pathophysiological implications. Proc Finn Dent Soc 85(4):395–407
48. Minagi S, Watanabe H, Takashi S, Hiromichi T (1990) The relationship between balancing side occlusal contact patterns and TMJ sounds in humans: proposition of the concept of balancing-side protection. J Craniomandib Disord 4:251–256
49. Miyahara T, Haglya N, Ohyama T, Nakamuna Y (1996) Modulations of human soleus H-reflexes in association with voluntary clenching of the teeth. J Neurophysiol 76:2033–2041
50. Molina OF, Dos Santos J, Nelson SJ, Nowlin T (2000) Profile of TMD and bruxer compared to TMD and nonbruxer patients regarding chief complaint, previous consultations, modes of therapy, and chronicity. Cranio 18(3):205–218
51. Molina OF, Dos Santos J, Mazzetto M et al (2001) Oral jaw behaviors in TMD and bruxism: a comparison study by severity of bruxism. Cranio 19(2):114–122

52. Mongini F (1996) Headache and facial pain. Pathophysiology and treatment. IEA (ed), St. Louis
53. Morgan DH, Hall WP, Vanwas SJ (1977) Diseases of the temporo-mandibular apparatus. A multidisciplinary approach. CV Mosby Co, St. Louis, 481p
54. Moss RA, Lombardo TW, Villarosa GA et al (1995) Oral habits and TMJ dysfunction in facial pain and non-pain subjects. J Oral Rehabil 22(1):79–81
55. Myers DE, Mc Call WD Jr (1983) Head pain as a result of experimental ischemic exercise of the temporalis muscle. Headache 23:113–116
56. Nilner M (1983) Relationships between oral parafunctions and functional disturbances in the stomathognathic system among 15- to 18-year-olds. Act Odont Scand 41:197–201
57. Palazzi C, Miralles R, Soto MA et al (1996) Body position effect on EMG activity of sterno-cleidomastoid and masseter muscles in patients with myogenic cranio-cervical-mandibular dysfunction. Cranio 14(3):200–209
58. Palesy PD (1997) Tendon and ligament insertions – a possible source of musculoskeletal pain. Cranio 15(3):194–202
59. Pullinger AG, Seligman DA, Solberg WK (1988) Temporomandibular disorders. Part II: occlusal factors associated with TMJ tenderness and dysfunction. J Prosthet Dent 59:363–367
60. Quemar JC, Lazard B (1992) Multivariate analysis of craniomandibular disorders. Cranio 10(2):89–95
61. Rageot E, Djenazian F (1980) Rôle du dysfonctionnement de l'articulation temporo-mandibulaire dans les cervicalgies et les céphalées. Rhumatol 32(10):253–257
62. Reding GR, Zepelin H, Robinson JE et al (1968) Nocturnal teeth-grinding: all night psychophysiologic studies. J Dent Res 47:786–797
63. Reeh ER, Eldeeb ME (1991) Referred pain of muscular origin resembling endodontic involvement. Oral Surg Oral Med Oral Pathol 71:223–227
64. Reik L (1985) Unnecessary dental treatment in headache patients for temporomandibular joint disorders. Headache 25(5):246–248
65. Rigolet D (1983) Le syndrome de dysfonctionnement des A.T.M. Ann Oto Laryngol 98:527
66. Rocabado M (1984) Diagnosis and treatment of abnormal cranio-cervical and cranio-mandibular mechanics. In: Solberg WK, Clark CT (eds) Abnormal jaw mechanics. Quintess Pub, Chicago, p 141
67. Rugh JD, Graham GS, Smith JC, Ohrbach RK (1989) Effects of canine versus molar occlusal splint guidance on nocturnal bruxism and cranio mandibular symptomatology. J Craniomandib Disord 3:203–210
68. Sano T, Westesson P-L, Yamamoto M, Okano T (2003) Differences in temporomandibular joint pain and age distribution between marrow edema and osteonecrosis in the mandibular condyle. Cranio 22(4):283–288
69. Satoh T, Hadara Y (1973) Electrophysiological study on tooth-grinding during sleep. Electroencephalogr Clin Neurophysiol 35:267–275
70. Schokker RP, Hanson TL, Ansink BJ (1989) Craniomandibular disorders in headache patients. J Craniomandib Disord 3:71–74
71. Schokker RP, Hanson TL, Ansink Ben JJ (1990) The result of treatment of the masticatory system of chronic headache patients. J Craniomandib Disord 4:126–130
72. Schwartz HC, Kendrick RW (1984) Internal derangements of the temporomandibular joint: description of clinical syndromes. Oral Surg Oral Med 58(1):24–29
73. Shankland WE (2001) Migraine and tension-type headache reduction through pericranial muscular suppression: a preliminary report. Cranio 19(4):269–278
74. Shimshak DG, DeFuria MC (1998) Health care utilization by patients with temporomandibular joint disorders. Cranio 16(3):185–193
75. Sunakawa M, Yamamoto Y, Ikeda H, Suda H, Sudana I (1989) Inferior alveolar nerve – driven neurons in cervical spine. J Dent Res Abstract 68:884
76. Talmant J (1976) Introduction à l'étude de la statique céphalique. Rev Orthop Dent Fac 3:321–334

77. Travell JG, Simons DG (1983) Myofascial pain and dysfunction. The trigger-point manual. Williams & Wilkins (ed), Baltimore, 713p
78. Urbanowicz M (1987) Alteration of vertical dimension and its effect on head and neck posture. Cranio 5:51–53
79. Van Tichelen P, Rousie-Baudry D (1989) SADAM et cervicalgies. Relations anatomo-physio-pathologiques. Aspects cliniques et thérapeutiques. Rev Med Orthop 17:11–18
80. Velly AM, Gornitsky M, Philippe P (2003) Contributing factors to chronic myofascial pain: a case–control study. Pain 104(3):491–499
81. Wajima K, Tagami A, Kogai H, Nanami T (1997) The relationship between tension-type headache and TMD. 22nd annual meeting on orofacial pain and temporomandibular disorders. J Orofac Pain 11(2):185
82. Wänman A (1995) The relationship between muscle tenderness and craniomandibular disorders: a study of 35 years old from the general population. J Orofac Pain 9(3):235–243
83. Wänman A, Agerberg G (1988) Fatigue in the jaws: a longitudinal study in adolescent. J Craniomandib Disord 2(1):29–34
84. Weed ND (1983) When shoulder pain isn't bursitis. The myofascial pain syndrome. Postgrad Med 74(3):97–104
85. Westling L, Carlsson GE, Helkimo M (1990) Background factors in CMD with special references to general joint hypermobility, parafunctions and trauma. J Craniomandib Disord 4:89–98
86. Wierzba CB, Maman L, Pham Huy D (1985) Algies buccales postérieures et algies pharyngées. Inf Dent 67(33):3371–3375
87. Woda A, Fontenelle A (1975) Activité tonique et posture de la mandibule; Mastication Déglutition. In: Chateau M (ed) Orthopédie dento-faciale, vol 1. J Prélat (éd), Paris, pp 244–280
88. Wruble MK, Lumley MA, Dudley MC, Mc Glynn FD (1989) Sleep-related bruxism and sleep variables: a critical review. J Craniomandib Disord 3:152–158
89. Yoshimatsu T, Namikoshi T, Koyama Z et al (1989) Changes of muscles activities in neck and shoulder region during sustained isometric contractions of jaw muscles. Nippon Hotetsu Shika Gakkai Zasshi 33(5):1044–1049
90. Yussuf H, Rothwell PS (1986) Temporomandibular joint pain-dysfunction in patients suffering from atypical facial pain. Br Dent J 161:208–212

Discomfort as the Outcome of Parafunctional Clenching

Based on numerous fundamental data about trigeminal connections with non-trigeminal nervous centers, Figs. 1, 2, 3, and 4 propose a common pathophysiological pattern in patients who clench their teeth firmly. Many dysfunctions may occur and endure as long as the parafunctional habit continues.

1 Auditory Problems

In the vertebra phylum, links noted between stomatognathic structures and the aural apparatus may constitute a very interesting morphological and functional set [22, 90, 103]. A close functional link between the *TMJ* and the *middle ear* is suggested [3, 81]. Histology tends to give the anterior ligament of malleus a pathophysiological involvement in the aural functional disorders sometimes observed in TMD. The richly vascularized sphenomandibular ligament may contribute to set off otalgia when stressed by excessive tensions (supraclusion, mandibular protracted position). The sphenomaxillary ligament is, through its cranial insertion, an extension of the malleus and its anterior ligament [15].

A same nervous branch of the mandibular nerve (V3) carries common motor innervation to the medial pterygoid m., TT m., and TVP m. As a result, the V intervenes, through this motor branch, in three functional activities (mastication, deglutition, hearing) which may seem distinct[2] but are always under central –particularly reticular – influences (Fig. 8). The central factors prevent from causing

[2]In fact they are closely interrelated according to phylogenetic, ontogenetic, and embryological data. In order to open the Eustachian tube, the TVP makes a lateral movement with the medial pterygoid muscle and interposed fascia. Modifications in the intratympanic pressure result from a Eustachian tube dysfunction: this can explain some hypoacousis and tinnitus observed in TMD [9].

F. Hartmann, G. Cucchi, *Stress and Orality*,
DOI 10.1007/978-2-8178-0271-8_12, © Springer-Verlag France 2014

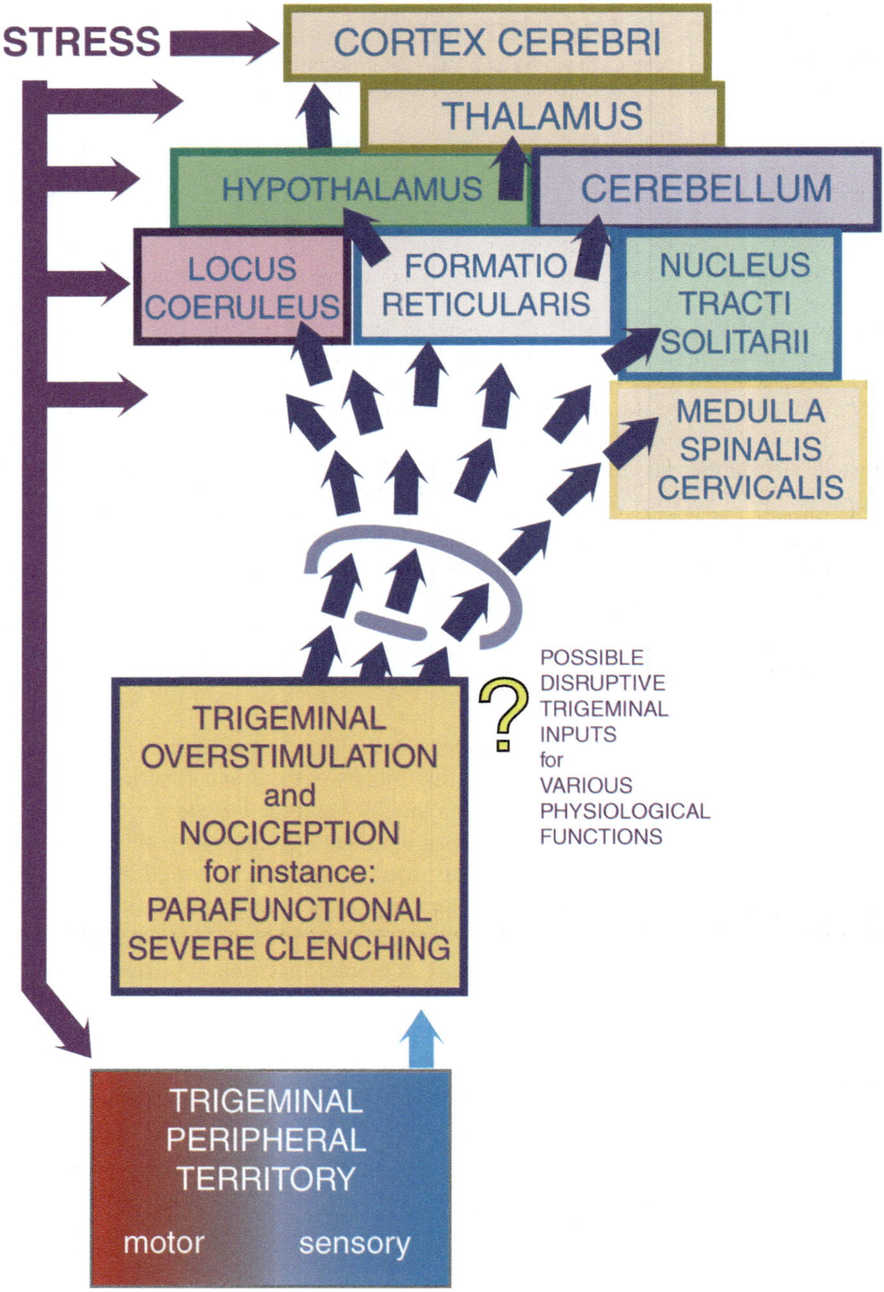

Fig. 1 Stress and possible projections of trigeminal overstimulation

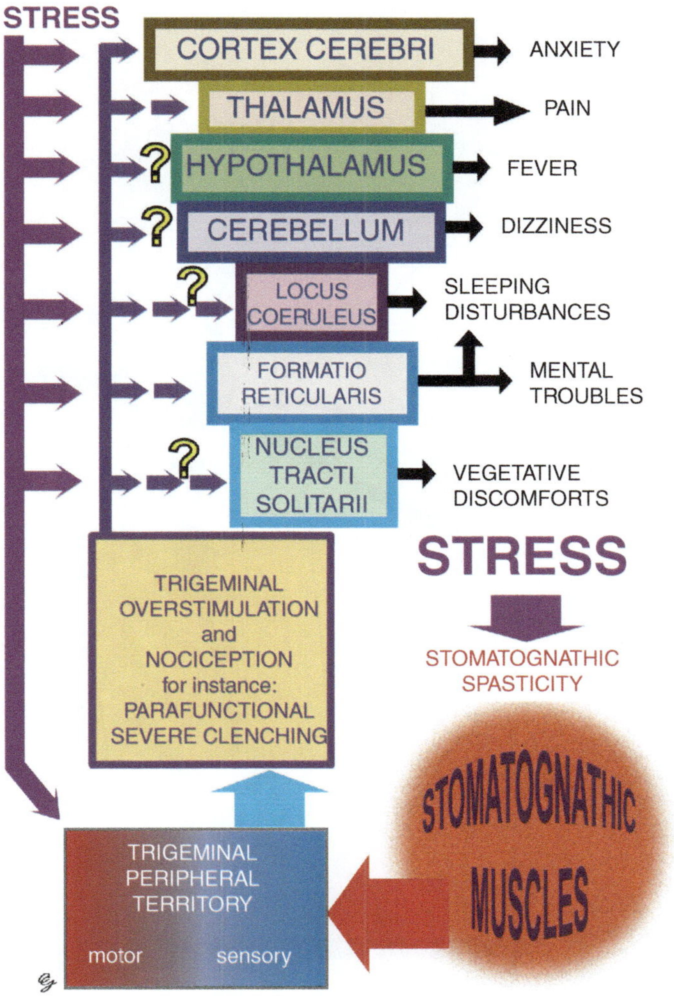

Fig. 2 Stress and possible clinical outcome of severe clenching

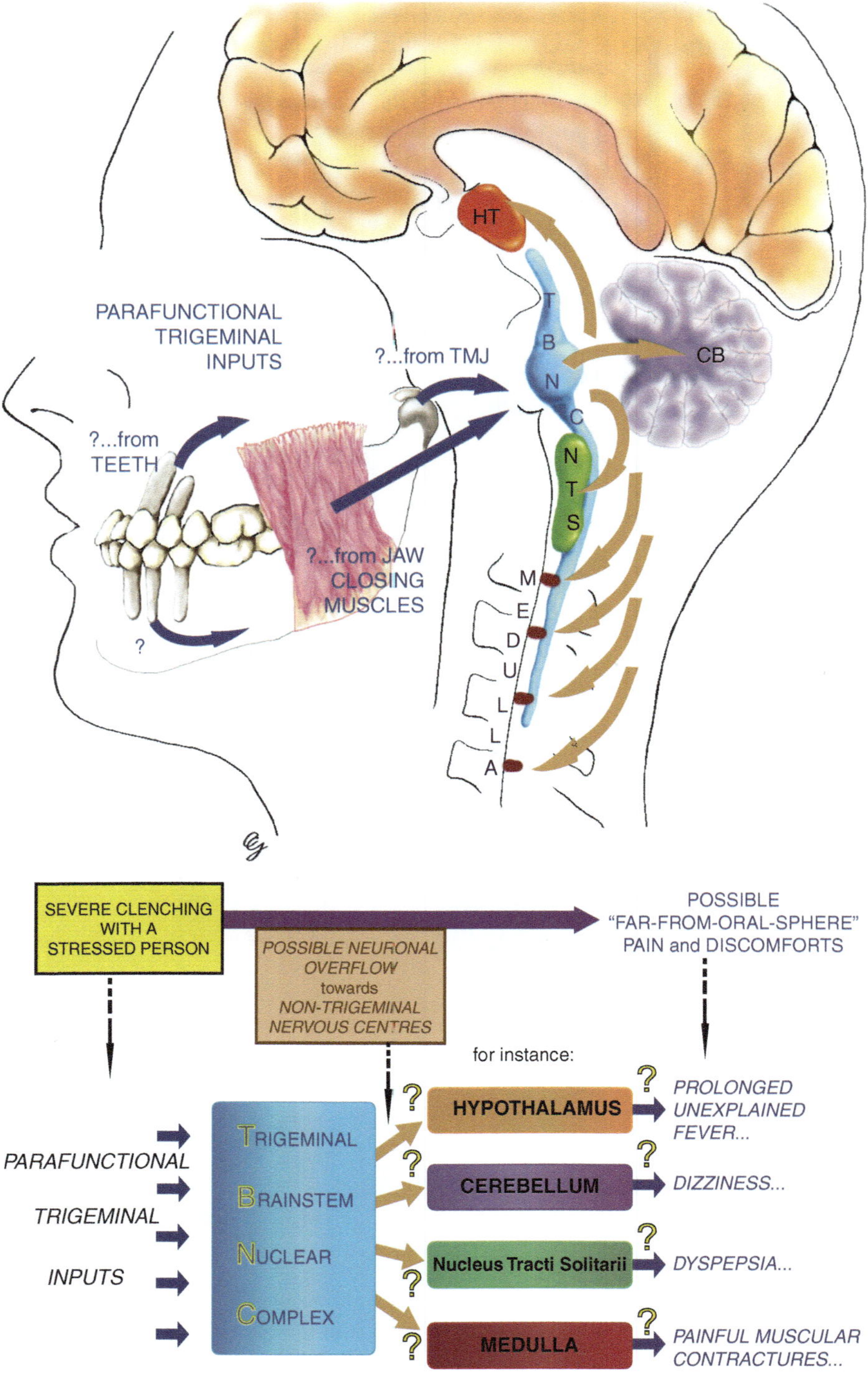

Fig. 3 Projections of parafunctional trigeminal inputs and their possible clinical outcome

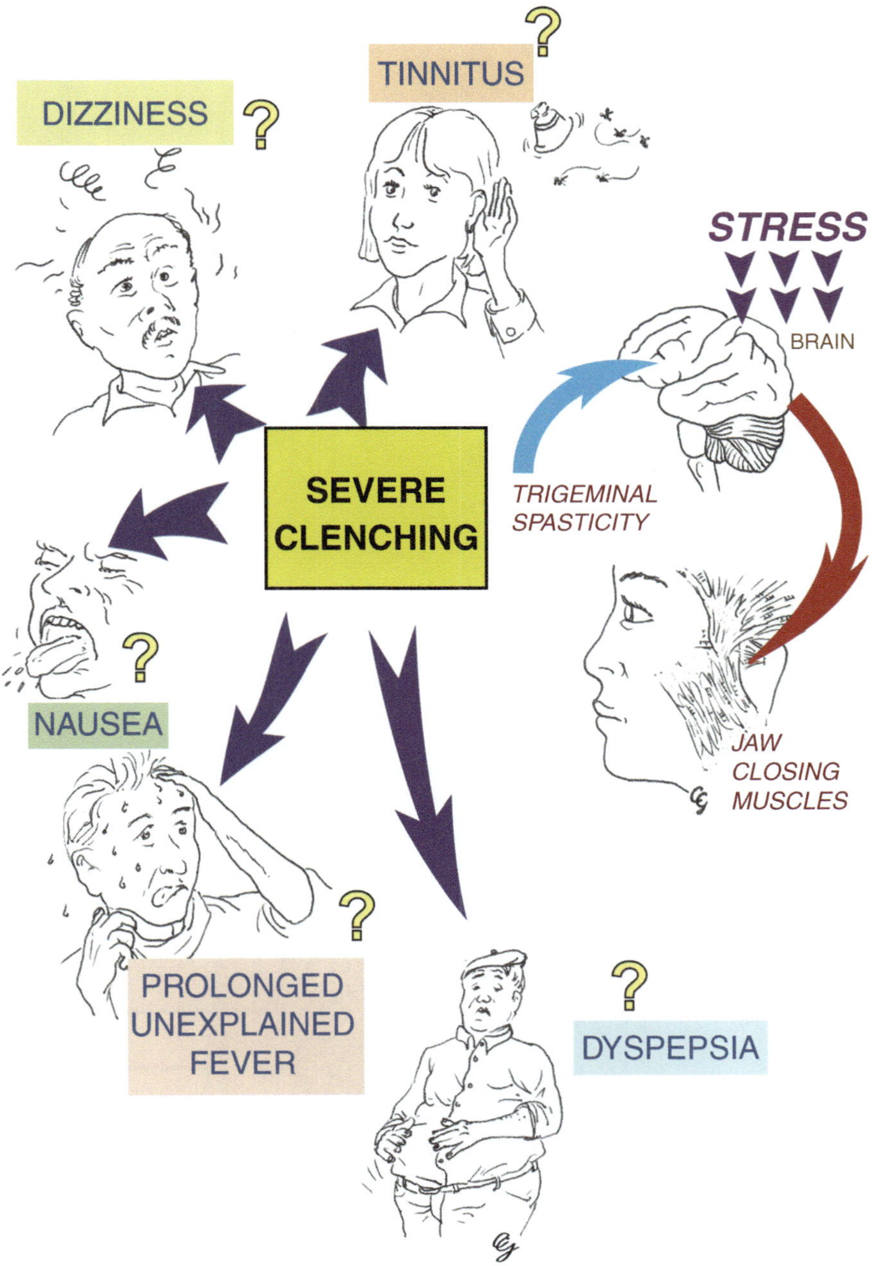

Fig. 4 Several clinical outcomes of severe clenching

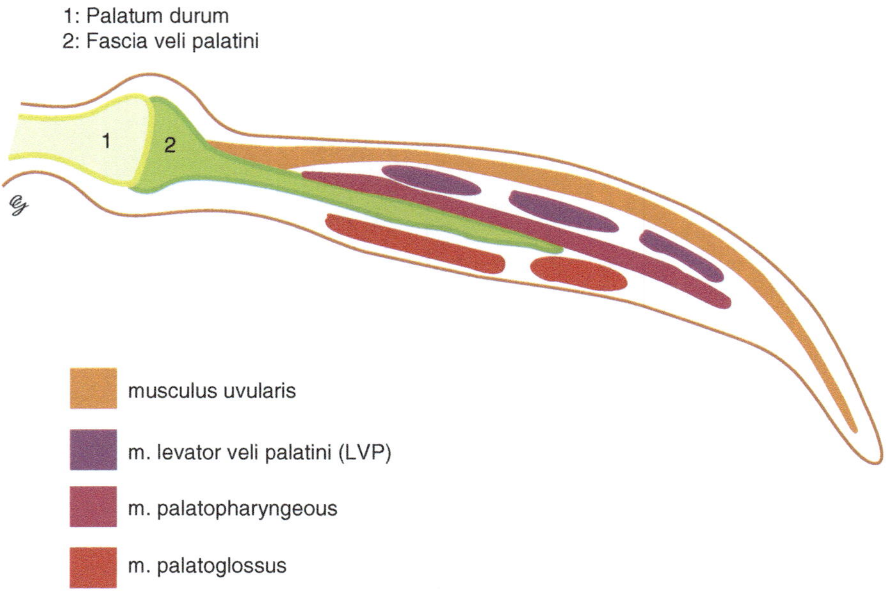

Fig. 5 Musculi palati and faucium (sagittal section) (Modified from Bouchet and Cuilleret [11]). *1* bony palate, *2* fascia veli (terminal tendon of the musculus tensor veli palatini), *3* m. uvulae, *4* m. levator veli palatini, *5* m. palatoglossus, *6* musculus palatopharyngeus

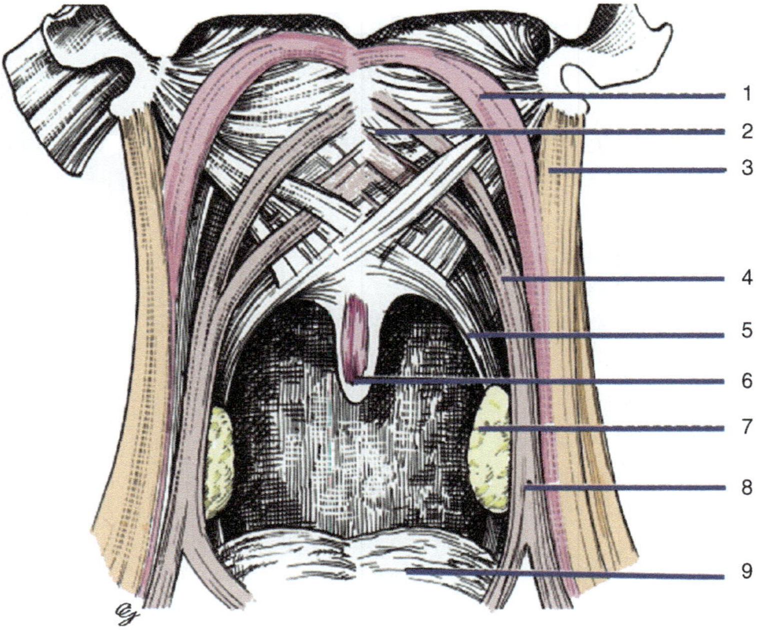

Fig. 6 Soft palate muscles (frontal section) (Modified from Bouchet and Cuilleret [11]). *1* musculus palatopharyngeus (palate fasciculi), *2* fascia veli, *3* musculus palatopharyngeus (fascia pterygoidea), *4* and *8* musculus palatoglossus, *5* musculus palatopharyngeus, *6* musculus uvulae, *7* amygdala, *9* tongue

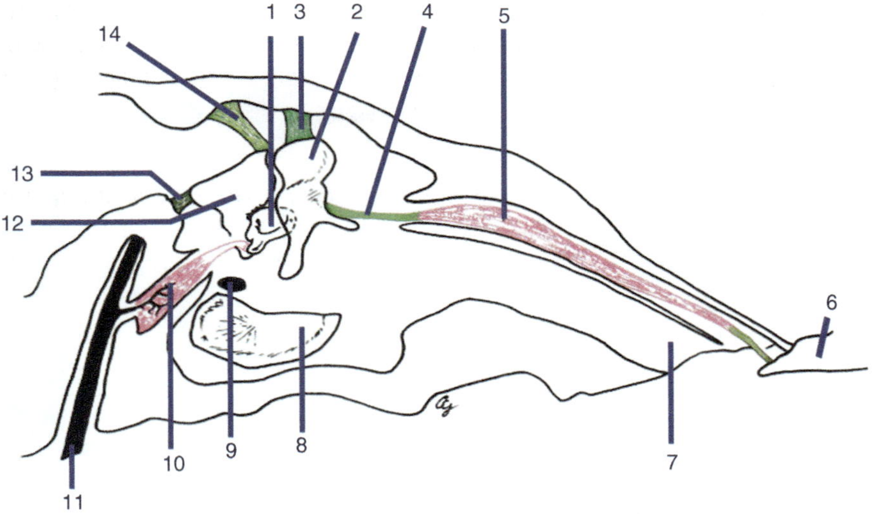

Fig. 7 Anteroposterior vertical section of the middle ear (Modified from Bouchet and Cuilleret [11]). *1* stirrup, *2* malleus, *3* superior ligament of the malleus, *4* tendon of musculus TT, *5* musculus TT, *6* spina ossis sphenoidalis, *7* Eustachian tube, *8* tympanum (partially resected), *9* fenestra cochleae, *10* musculus stapedius, *11* facial nerve(VII), *12* incus, *13* posterior ligament of the incus, *14* superior ligament of the incus

stomatognathic muscle spasticity. Thus increased excitability, especially of the motor neurons of the muscles innervated by the V, could facilitate a dysfunctional phenomenon. Besides the participation of the elevator fibers of the medial pterygoid m. during clenching (Fig. 9), a dysfunction in the regulation of the tension in the tympanic membrane may come from the action of the m. TT (tinnitus). A dysfunction in the opening mechanism of the Eustachian trump [88] may come from the action of the m. TVP (feeling of ear blockage). This muscle spasticity can also originate from dental occlusal disturbances [7, 28, 82] and from traumatisms particularly following motor vehicle accidents [97, 122]. Additionally some experts have identified the loss of the vertical dimension of occlusion (VDO) as a possible factor in the dysfunction of the Eustachian tube. A modification in the tongue position with a global elevation of the glosso-hyoidian set could be the result of a reflex contracting the TVP [2]. Scientific studies [75] have shown that primary trigeminal afferents, especially mandibular afferents (V3), directly project to the trigeminal motor nucleus (MoN). This nucleus is the command center of TT and TVP. Other observations report a projection from the trigeminal ganglion [117] or from a nearby spinal trigeminal tract to the cochlear nuclei [43, 69, 100, 101, 132] which may be involved in the mechanism of tinnitus. Another study shows that a projection from the predominantly somatosensory trigeminal ganglion can influence the activity of central auditory neurons in a manner different from acoustic stimulation, which suggests activation of nonclassical auditory pathways [32].

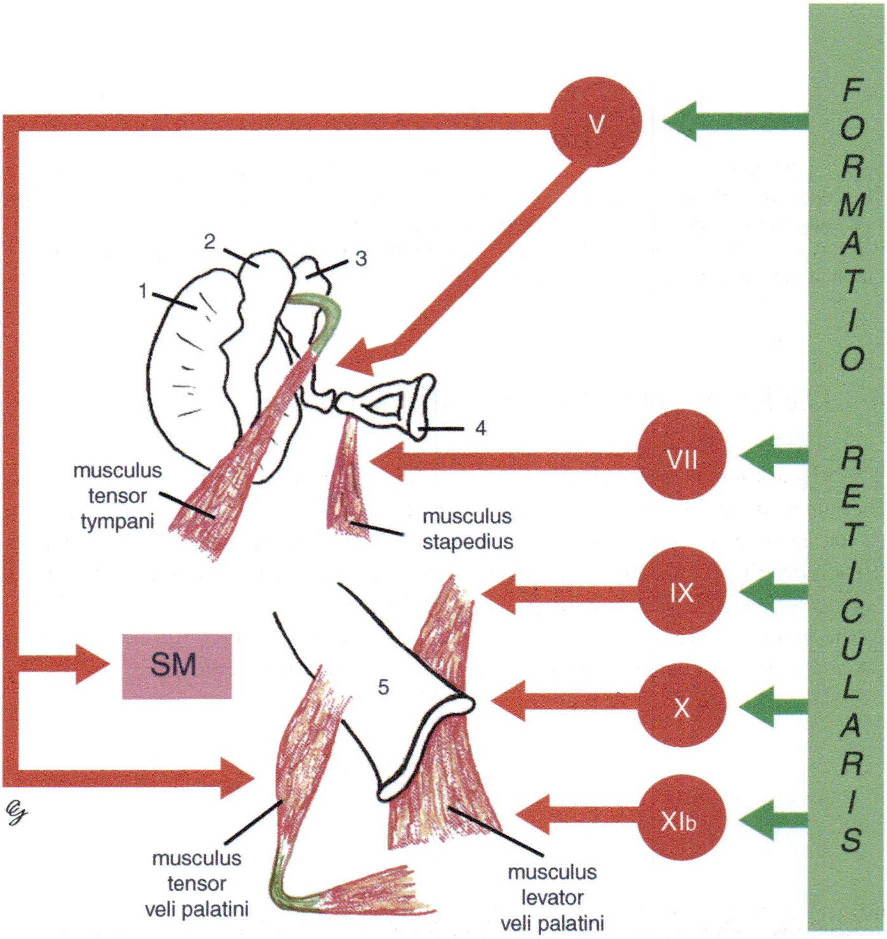

Fig. 8 Reticular influence on the tone of the middle ear and soft palate muscles (Modified from Bossy [10]). *1* tympanum, *2* malleus, *3* incus, *4* stirrup bone, *5* Eustachian tube, *SM* stomatognathic muscles

2 Problems with Swallowing and Phonation

Some scientific studies report the interactions between V and the cranial nerves involved in tongue motor control such as the *hypoglossal nerve* (XII) [131] and motor nerves involved in swallowing such as X and IX [4, 51–53, 64]. Another study shows that only the superior laryngeal nerve afferents (branch of X) have sufficient nervous influence to start the swallowing process [18]. Some studies reveal projections of trigeminal inputs to the motor nuclei of facial (VII) and

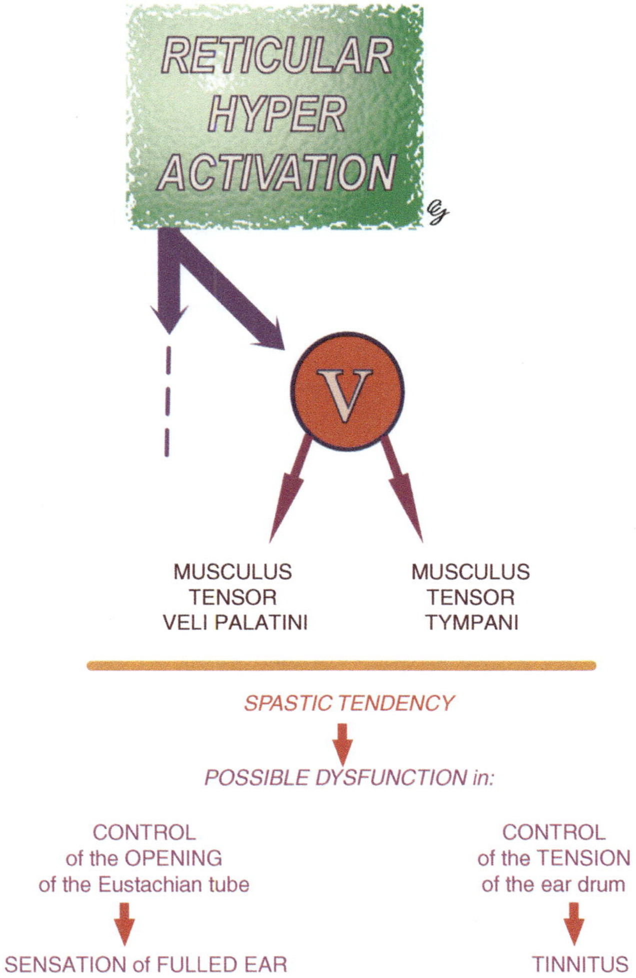

Fig. 9 Reticular influence on the veli palatini and middle ear muscles in spastic conditions

hypoglossal (XII) nerves [89]. In the nucleus of the solitary tract (NST), there is normally a serotoninergic inhibition of the swallowing reflex initiating in the laryngeal nerve during functional acts such as mastication. But in pathophysiological conditions (severe clenching), SP liberated from the SN [116] may respond to overstimulation and nociception and activate a neuroanatomical pathway [106, 123] and be found in the glossopharyngeal and vagal afferents. According to these data, recent EMG studies [41] and clinical results one may suggest that parafunctional trigeminal overstimulation and nociception (severe clenching and major stress conditions) may have aggravating repercussions on a dysfunctional swallowing mechanism. This could explain some pharyngolaryngeal symptoms often attributed by patients to other ailments.

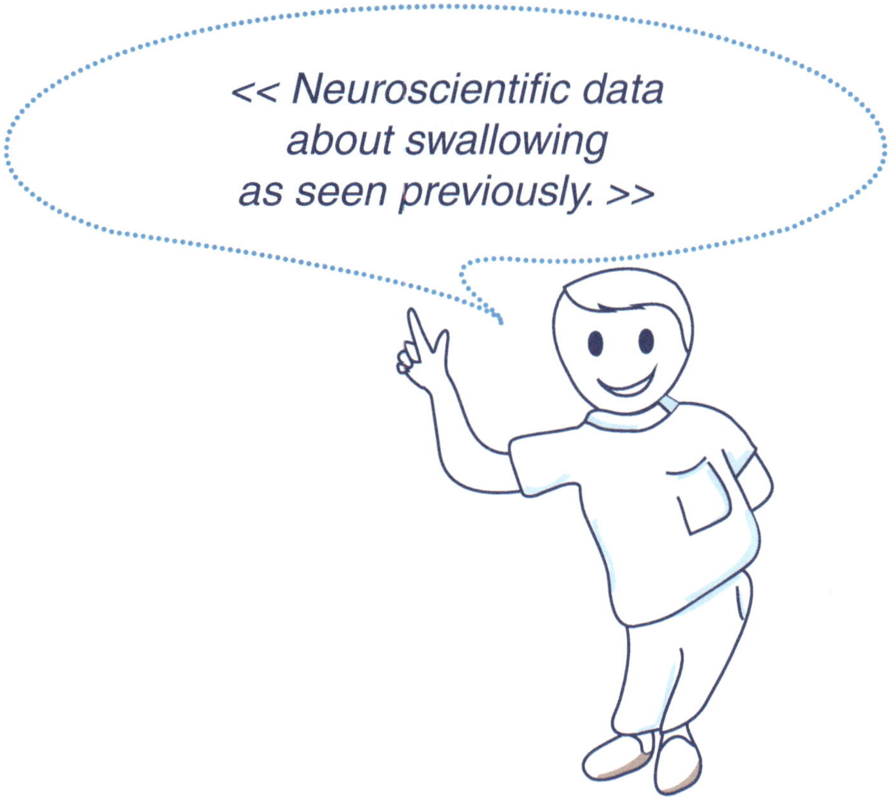

Finally, it must be reminded that some muscles (Fig. 6) are working together to elevate the tongue during a normal swallowing (about 500–1,200 times a day for an adult): m. styloglossi, m. palatoglossi, and m. palatopharyngeuses. As previously described (see Fig. 2 in chapter "Stomatognathic Parafunctions"), in physiological swallowing conditions, that is, when the inferior teeth come to gear with the superior teeth for giving spatial and neural repairs to the brain, the **tongue** must benefit of a sufficient space (large hard palate and superior dental arch). Thus, deficient maxillar and sinusal osteogenesis due to deficient neural inputs in children (too soft food, buccal breathing) mainly appear to be a primum movens of later severe clinical problems in adults especially when parafunction exists.

As for problems with phonation, one should keep in mind the importance of the hyoid bone position in vocal emission. The control of this position relies on supra- and infrahyoid muscles. Trigeminal spasticity or a prosthetic error may cause a dysfunction in these muscles and disrupt the phonation mechanism.

3 Problems with Posture and Vision

Patients complaining of *dizziness* are sometimes diagnosed with Meniere's disease. The classic trio of symptoms includes vertigo, tinnitus, and hearing loss episodes, sometimes with *nausea* and *vomiting*. Some studies have revealed nuchal muscle symptoms such as painful palpation of the attachment of m. trapezius and m. levator scapulae with limited neck mobility [8]. The actual originating factors of Meniere's disease are still unknown. Some questions have been raised about stomatognathic and postural musculoskeletal implications in the etiological mechanism of this disease. Figure 10 reminds the inputs coming from extraocular muscle's proprioception along the n. ophthalmicus (V1). As other trigeminal afferents, they reach the TBNC before projecting to cerebellum. Figures 11 and 12 suggest a possible pattern of neurophysiological connections between the extraocular muscle's proprioceptive afferents and the oculomotor efferents, via the trigeminal system (TBNC), the vestibular nucleus, and the retino-vestibular pathway [91]. Some neuroanatomical data suggest a close link between the trigeminal system and the postural system[3]. For instance, the *periodontal proprioception* usefully completes the visual information and the vestibular inputs. Those come treated by the cerebellum to get a refined balance of the cranio-cervico-facial sphere into postural and motor coordination. Here comes a new concept which inserts the trigeminal component into the oculo-cephalogyrus system. It would actually be more appropriate to speak about the "oculo-trigemino-cephalogyral system". Thus, in spastic conditions the trigeminal sensory overstimulation and nociception could help in tensing head

[3]The ocular motor system is connected to postural muscles by the medial longitudinal fasciculus (MLF); it is a pathway between the motor and sensory nuclei of the cranial nerves and the anterior horn of the spinal cord, connecting the cranial nerves which intervene in head and eye motility [67] and in equilibration based on its important nervous origin in the vestibular nuclei [10, 55]. It has additional connections with the RF, the CC, the cerebellum, and the CGN. Through its ophthalmic branch (V1), V already plays a part in oculomotility, in the development of orientation selectivity, and more largely in the regulation of the oculo-cephalogyrus system. The oculomotor afferents could reach either the trigeminal MeN [23] or the trigeminal SP [74]. Some studies [14, 105] identified the trigeminal afferents pathways (V1) as the external ocular muscles (EOM), trigeminal ganglion, trigeminal SnC, and cervical medulla (C1,C2). Furthermore, fibers from the trigeminal MeN project to the medial vestibular nucleus. A recent study revealed that a monosynaptic pathway exists between vestibular nuclei and masseter motor neurons [24]. Some trigeminal proprioceptive afferents [21, 25, 30, 50, 59, 93, 104, 107] go across the SnI [49, 120] or NP [120] and project to the cerebellum. Some of these trigemino-cerebellar physiological projections come

posture muscles[4]. Some EMG studies [85, 86] have suggested that parafunctional habits and body position are significantly correlated to the clinical symptomatology of the masseter and SCM in TMD patients upon waking up and during moments when they are vigilant. It was noted that imbalance in the stomatognathic muscle activities could disturb postural muscle functions [37]. In fact, inputs coming from the stomatognathic muscles themselves, teeth, tongue, and TMJ affect the motor activities of these muscles as well as muscles responsible for head posture such as SCM. Some observations have revealed that clenching is the only pattern of investigated jaw muscle exercise that results in increased pain in the forehead region [118]. This is indeed one of the principal zones of referred pain from SCM [111]. As for head posture, the jaw-closing muscles (masseter, temporalis, pterygoid) are antigravity muscles. During clenching, these muscles experience an intense con-

---

from PR [31]. Trigeminal afferents (for instance periodontal afferents) have proven that they supplement nicely visual messages to postural stabilization [39]. These are treated by the cerebellum with the purpose of refining the balance of the cranio-cervico-facial sphere in posture and motor coordination. These scientific data confirm previous data about possible trigeminal disturbances in the oculo-cephalogyrus system [79]. The evidence of a relationship between functional neck and trigeminal muscle afferent systems was found in the upper cervical chord and lower medulla where trigeminal afferents activate the m. splenius, m. biventer cervicis, and m. complexus [1]. Studies explain this type of close functional coupling between the trigeminal and cervical systems [12, 13, 33, 47, 126]. Jaw-muscle spindle afferents could reach the spinal cord through relays in the SnO and parvocellular RF [26]. Trigeminal inputs project from the NS to all levels of the cord [76, 94, 119]. Neonative polysynaptic pathways could transmit trigeminal stimulations all the way to the lumbar spinal cord. Electromyographic studies in humans [6, 20, 29, 80, 86, 124, 127] have attempted to prove that the trigeminal afferents could contribute to the regulation and stabilization of head posture during physiological functions such as mastication and swallowing. Let's note that simple changes in the mandibular position have immediate repercussions on the EMG activity of head posture muscles, especially the trapezius [17]. Other EMG studies have also revealed the functional repercussions between the nuchal tonic reflex and the tone of the stomatognathic muscles [36, 38, 63, 71, 96]; trigeminal afferents can modify this reflex [79]. More evidence came from a 7-week-old embryo who responded to a stimulation of trigeminal receptors with a nuchal muscle reflex contraction called the *trigemino-neck reflex* [108]; this reflex is a sign of early nervous connections between the trigeminal system and head posture system. A new variant of trigemino-cervical reflex was observed in swine [62], but it is not yet been demonstrated in humans. A mouth-opening reflex was reported in a 14-week-old human fetus reacting to palmar stimulation [46]; these data confirm the previously noted connections between the V and the superior spinal roots. The activity of the obliquus capitis inferior muscle is EMG recorded during bruxism [124] which could explain some painful cervical symptoms when such stomatognathic parafunctions persist. In the same way the SCM under EMG responds to different masticatory movements and to intense durable voluntary clenching episodes [129]; this is confirmed for the SCM [20] as well as for the m. trapezius [127]. There is a reflex interaction between nociceptive trigeminal afferents and both upper and lower cervical spinal cord motor neurons [98].

[4]These data could help to understand why rifle marksman's results improve after an occlusal equilibration [78].

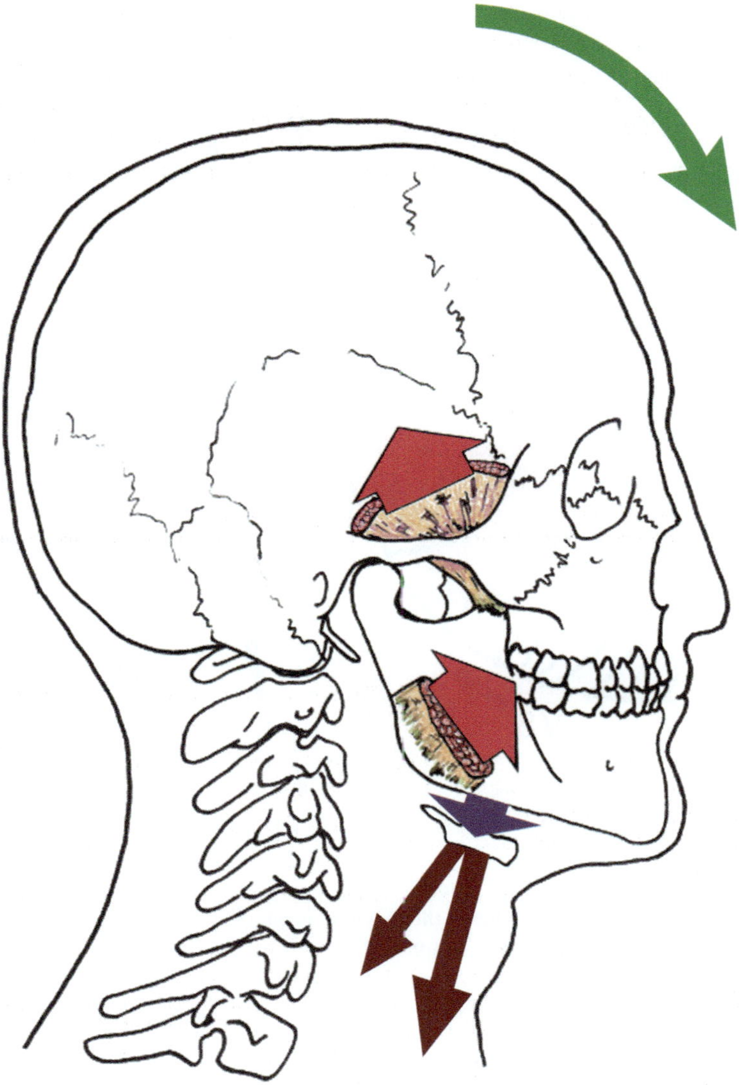

Fig. 10 Role of the stomatognathic muscles on the ventral flexion of the head (Modified from Kapandji [58]). The cervical musculature allows movements of flexion (ventral, dorsal, lateral), movements of rotation, and mixed. Some stomatognathic muscles participate in the physiology of head movements: the mylohyoid m. and the anterior heads of the digastric m. fix the hyoid bone and the jaw; they are innervated by the mandibular nerve (V3). The thyrohyoid m., the sterno-cleidohyoid m., the sternohyoid m., and the omohyoid m. trigger lowering of the jaw. The masseter and the temporalis block the jaw against the superior maxillar. Thus, the isotonic contractions of the suprahyoid (*purple arrow*) and infrahyoid muscles (*brown arrows*), together with an isometric contraction of the masseter and the temporalis (*red arrows*), trigger a ventral flexion of the cervical rachis (*green arrow*), a major factor in head dynamics. We can easily anticipate what dysfunctional occurrences may be generated by severe clenching (i.e., trigeminal spasticity in jaw elevator muscles)

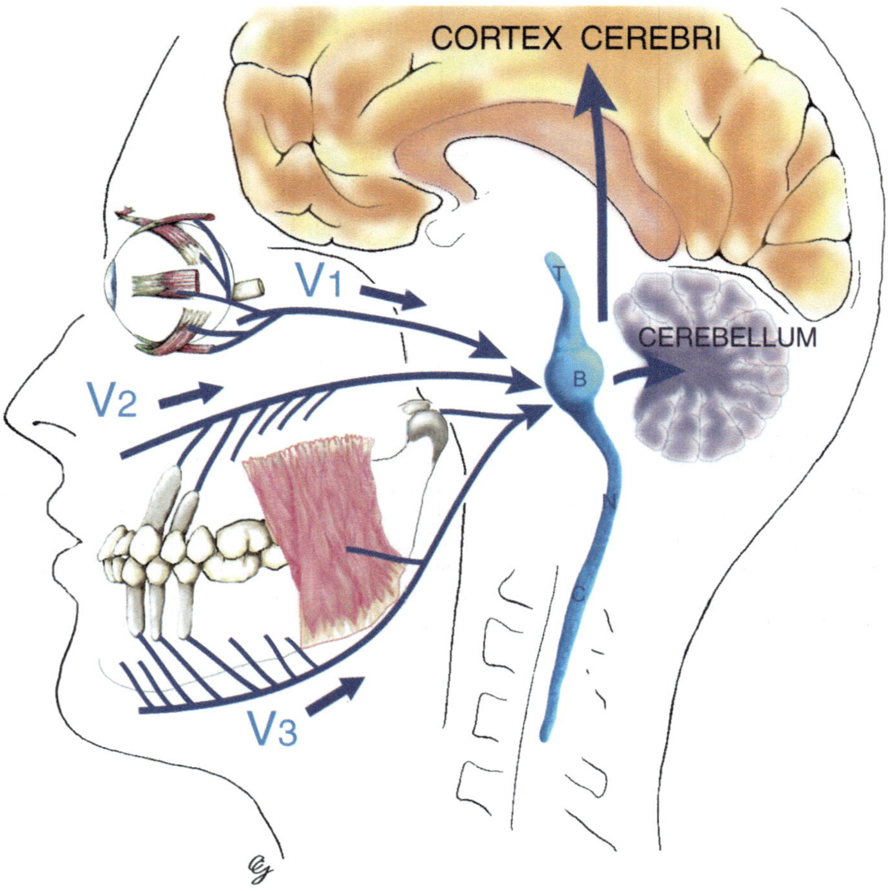

Fig. 11 The three sensory branches of the nervus trigeminus. The first branch (V1) also brings proprioceptive inputs from the extraocular muscles

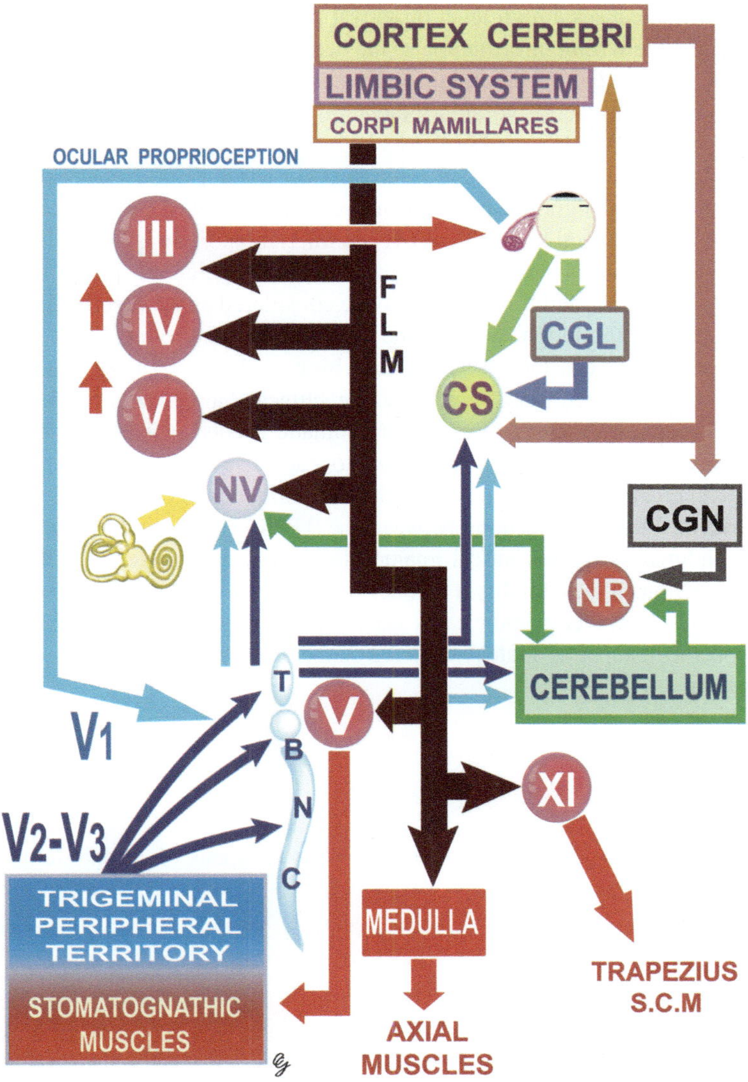

Fig. 12 Central nervous connections between the trigeminal system and the oculocephalogyrus system. *CM* corpus mamillare, *CGE* corpus geniculatum laterale, *CS* colliculus superior, *FPAM* fasciculi propii anterior medullae, *FLM* fasciculus longitudinalis medialis, *NMS* neuromuscular spindle, *FR* formatio reticularis, *CGN* central gray nuclei, *MoN* trigeminal motor nucleus, *NR* nucleus ruber, *NV* nucleus vestibularis, *GTO* Golgi tendon organs, *MP* motor plaque, *in blue* sensory ways, *in red* motor ways

traction which causes a high level of activation of their Golgi tendon organs. This may provide the wrong information on the head position with respect to the vertical axis and thereby disturb the balance. Previously mentioned EMG investigations have shown the impact of voluntary clenching on the forearm [109] and the trunk muscle activity [29, 34]. Another theory suggests that afferents from the dental area may perhaps take part in the head orientation in space [79][5]. Figure 13 presents a pathophysiological hypothesis of the nervous circuits in the oculo-cephalogyrus system and its connections with the *trigeminal system*. Figures 14 and 15 show the connections between trigeminal and vestibular nuclei in physiological and pathophysiological conditions. This may be considered as the mechanism by which trigeminal overstimulation modifies the head posture physiology.

Deleterious repercussions of **severe clenching** on the muscles responsible for posture must be considered when clinical and paraclinical diagnoses fail in identifying the cause of dizziness. In cases of etiologic traumatic events such as *whiplash* injuries, projections of the TMJ receptors are known to reach all areas of the sensory trigeminal nuclei with greater density in the n. sensorius and the subnucleus oralis [16]. Based on the numerous close connections between the TBNC and medullar areas, the tissue trauma endured by the retrodiscal ligaments during *whiplash* (see Fig. 28 in chapter "Objective Signs") may amplify a number of non-oral painful and dysfunctional clinical outcomes. However in some cases stomatognathic spasticity treatment can require more specific therapeutic strategy centered on the postural system and must be referred to a specialist.

4 Fatigue

We shall study this general sign in Part IV when we speak of chronic fatigue.

---

[5]An asymmetrical sensory information originating from that area (e.g., unbalanced occlusion) would affect the head position or its perception and consequently produce a postural asymmetry of other body segments from top to bottom. It has been shown that the loss of occlusal supporting zone has a unilateral and bilateral influence on the weight distribution at the feet during clenching [128]. More recently a potential-evoked-signal investigation revealed that disturbance of the cortical functions regulating visual-motor integration could increase the risk of TMD [99]. Therefore, disorders in head posture regulation – even in body equilibrium – can occur via a *trigemino-ocular dysfunction*; for example, inputs from MOE, via the V1, could be disturbed by excessive V3 afferents elicited by exacerbated clenching. As we know today it is difficult to identify the CNS levels possibly caused by such disturbances: *low pathways* with the TBNC and *high pathways* with the colliculus superior [92], the cerebellum, etc. Regardless, the overstimulated and nociceptive afferent process intensifies reticular influence on motor neurons of stomatognathic [110, 112] and other muscles by creating as much spasticity as the limbic system (emotional factors).

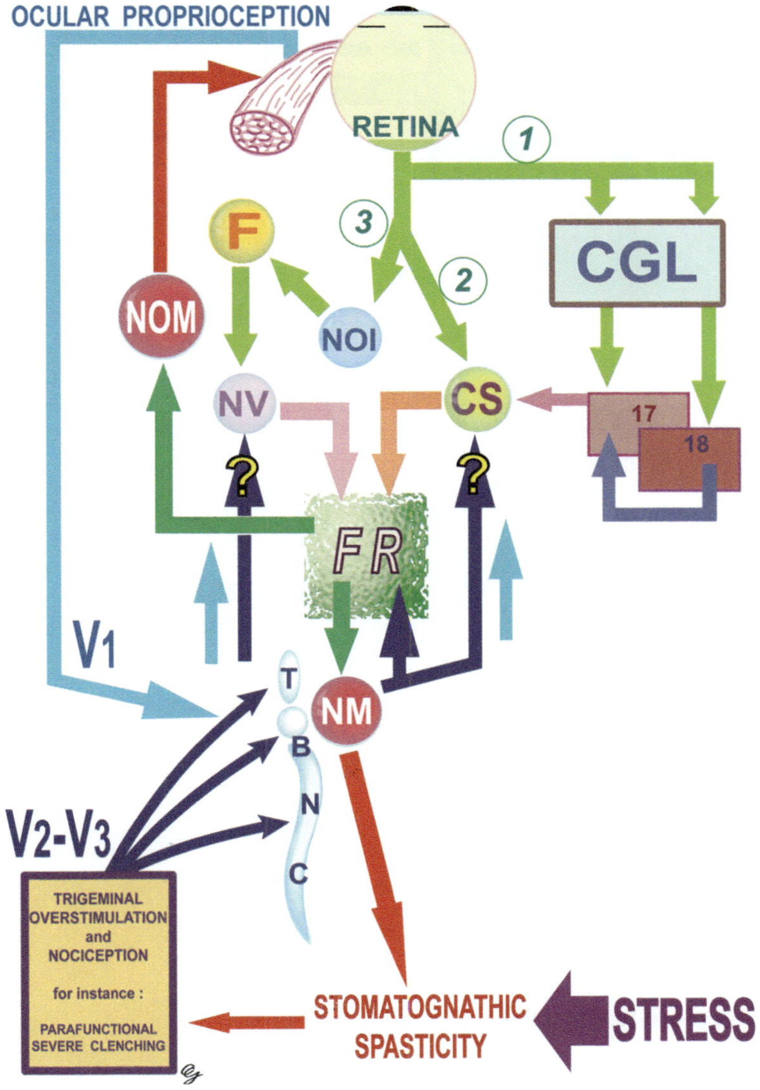

Fig. 13 Impact of trigeminal overstimulation and nociception from stomatognathic spasticity on the dysfunction of the ocular system under stress. A neurophysiological theory. *CGL* corpus geniculatum laterale, *CS* colliculus superior, *NV* nucleus vestibularis, *F* flocculus, *FR* formatio reticularis, *OEM* ocular external muscles, *NO* nucleus n. oculomotorii, *1* retino-geniculo-striated way, *2* retino-collicular way, *3* retino-vestibular way. Some compensations are possible between the different elements responsible for the balance, for example, between a neuro-labyrinthic lack of balance and the craniocervical neuromusculature. Thus when elevator muscles experience spasms and block the jaw (clenching), "the contraction of supra and infra-hyoïd muscles provokes the head flexion on the cervical rachis and the flexion of the cervical rachis on the dorsal rachis, and also a correction of the cervical lordosis" (Kapandji [58]). Inversely the backward head posture would hinder the normal buccal opening and the jaw retropulsive movement. An excessive reflex activity in the jaw protractor and elevator muscles, especially the lateral pterygoid m., could have a noxious repercussion on the breathing mechanism [63]

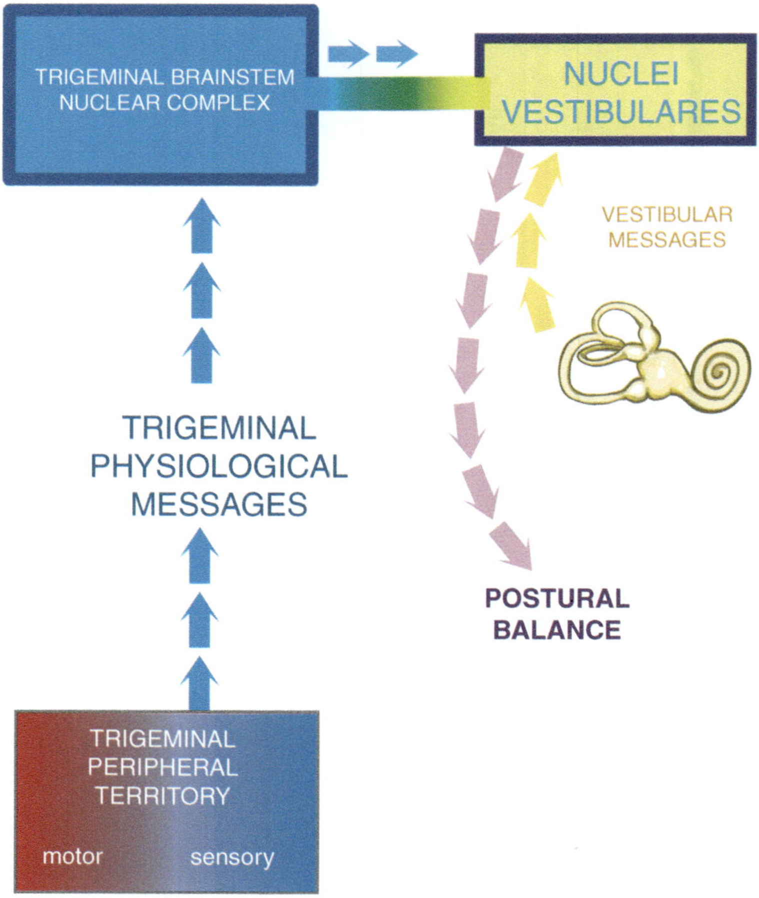

Fig. 14 Physiological trigemino-vestibular connections

5 Sleep Disturbances

If referring to physiological data[6], the 5-HT metabolism disorders could be involved in certain sleep disturbances TMD patients [65]. On the other hand, the dopaminergic system has been implicated at the level of the striatum in nocturnal

[6] During awakening, the serotonin activates some synthesis which is responsible to deferred setting of low sleep and paradoxal sleep (REM) by regulating the biosynthesis of hypnogenic substances. The sleeping would occur by diminution of the 5-HT bulbar neuronal activity and by liberation of these substances. The locus coeruleus is well known to be an important nervous structure in physiology of sleeping. It is rather curious to note that ancient French anatomists have originally given to this locus the name of *trigeminal vegetative nucleus*. Otherwise it has been shown that some hypothalamic 5-HT neurones are activated during awakening particularly during stressful events [54].

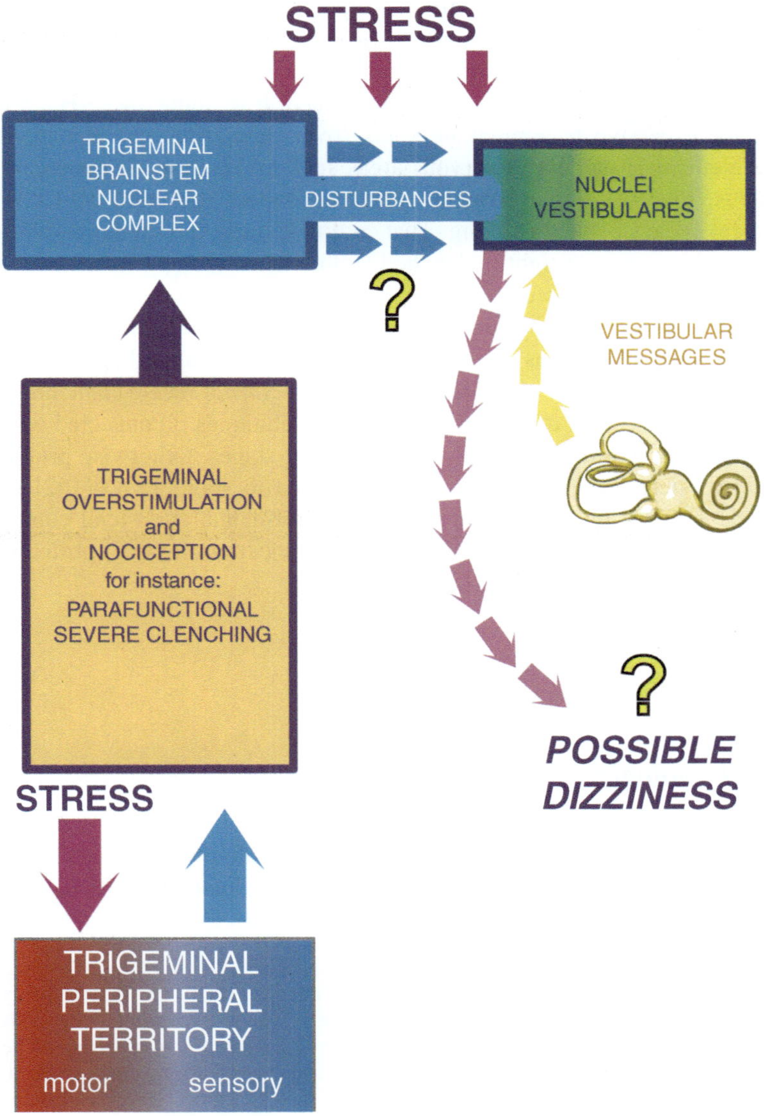

Fig. 15 Pathophysiological trigemino-vestibular connections

bruxism pathophysiology (grinding) [70]. The management of some sleep disturbances which is observed after a trigeminal **Relaxing and Moderating Treatment** (RMT) in TMD patients could allow to more consider the place of these neuromediator disorders. It is particularly true about the 5-HT with the impact of excessive trigeminal afferents (overstimulation and nociception by severe clenching) on central nervous areas such as FR, hypothalamus, or locus coeruleus (Fig. 16). These structures have an important role in controlling the biological cycle sleeping-awaking. That could explicate the sudden awaking during night sleeping with tightly clenched teeth which some patients complain of. About parafunctional nocturnal events, it seems that sleep bruxism may be mainly under the influence of brainstem networks [40, 68]. Should it be desirable to view no longer sleep grinding as a real pathological disorder but perhaps just as a normal variation of behavior [68]? But what about *nocturnal severe clenching*? Great hopes are coming from modern neuroimaging techniques if connected with masticatory EMG recordings during sleep clenching stages. Otherwise problems of obstructive sleep apnea (OSA) have been linked to some TMD [102] with an unfavorable effect on the development of several dental and facial components [130], sometimes treated by a sibilant phoneme registration (SPR) protocol [102] or by orthodontic procedures [44].

6 Prolonged Unexplained Fever

6.1 Physiological Reminders[7]

The rich projection of dental receptors to the hypothalamus can activate or inhibit hypothalamic cells [113, 114]. Various trigeminal craniofacial tissues are known to project their inputs to the hypothalamus [73]. Could they disturb thermoregulation

[7]With the exception of spinal and brainstem detectors, the thermostatic center is primarily represented by the anterior hypothalamus and the preoptic area [10]; more precisely the hypothalamus ventralis posterior fights against cold and the anteromedial supraoptic area fights against heat. The thermosensitive neurons of the region react to blood temperature and to inputs brought by the fibers connected to the cutaneous and muscular thermoreceptors (Ruffini's corpuscles and Krause's corpuscles). In vertebrates fever is a major defensive process; prostaglandins, particularly PGE2, help raise the hypothalamic thermostat. However we know that an experimental destruction of the posterior hypothalamus leads to akinesia and the anterior hypothalamus to hyperkinesia.

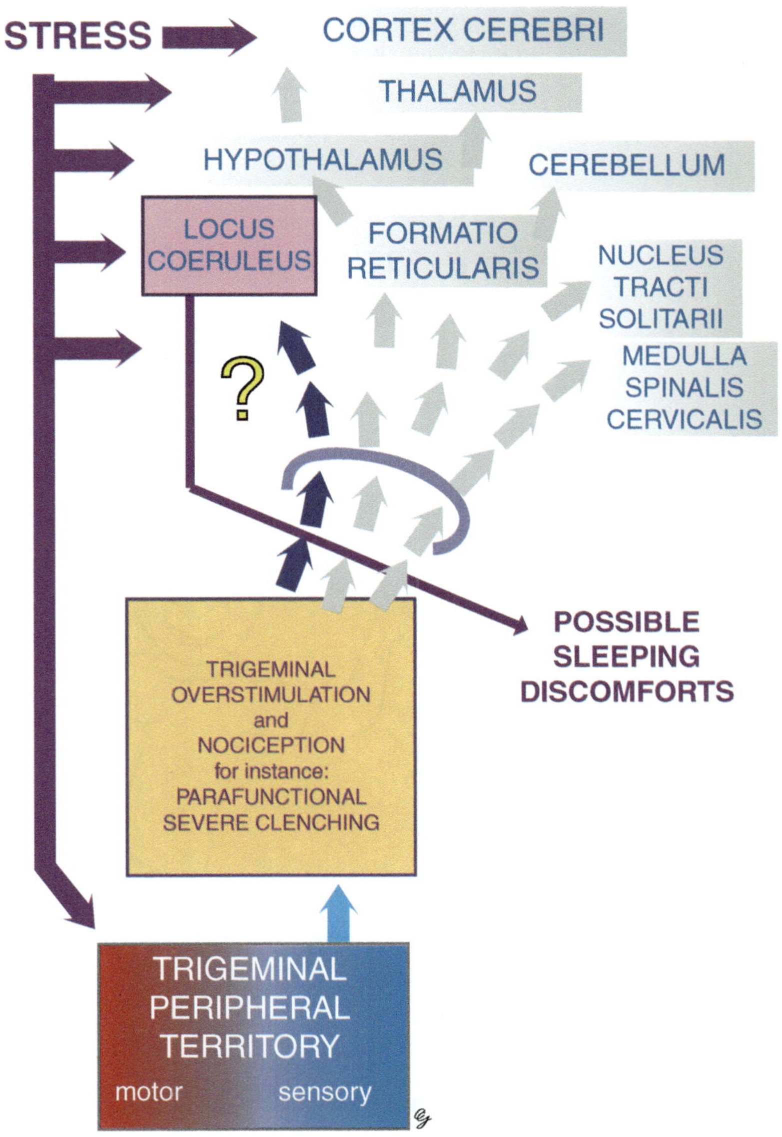

Fig. 16 Supposed impact of severe clenching on sleep disorders as observed in some TMD patients. A pathophysiological theory

in parafunctional conditions, that is, by sensory trigeminal overstimulation from stomatognathic spasticity (Figs. 17 and 18)?

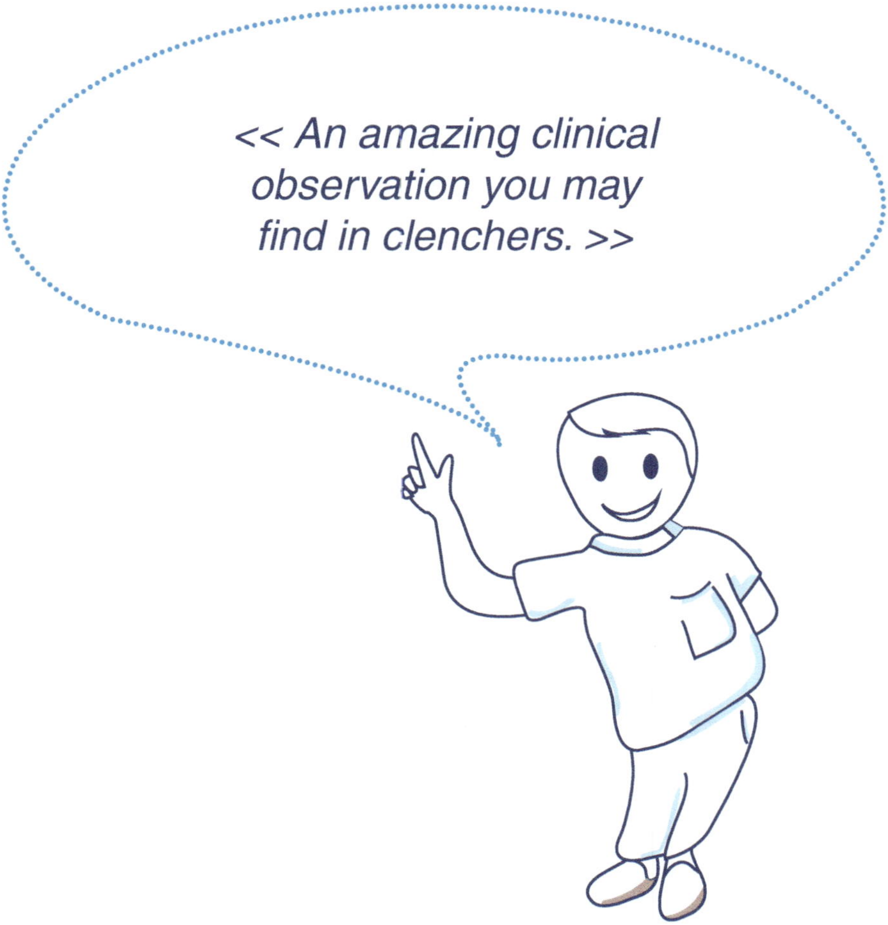

7 Immunodeficiency Problems

A number of authors have reported infectious events associated with chronic orofacial muscle pain [35, 77, 111]; some patients also complain about gastrointestinal, genitourinary, and neurologic symptoms. A psychosomatic approach to TMD may explain this somatization outcome based on the familiar alteration of the hypothalamic-pituitary-adrenal axis function in response to stressful conditions.

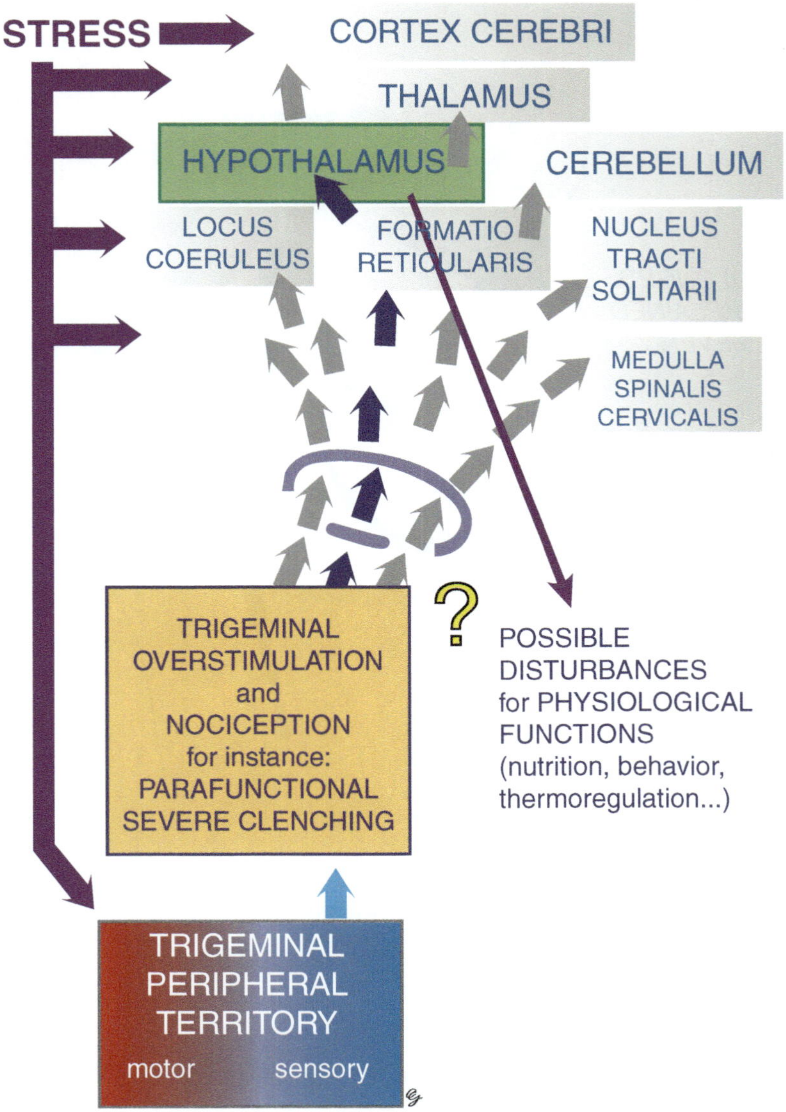

Fig. 17 Clenching and possible hypothalamic dysfunctions. A neurophysiological theory. Clinicians should know that a number of female clenching patients have reported that the amenorrhea they experienced fully disappeared when they stopped clenching. The trigemino-hypothalamic projections may be a possible explanation to such an amazing phenomenon knowing that periodontal inputs may elicite excitative or inhibitive responses at the level of hypothalamic cells [114]

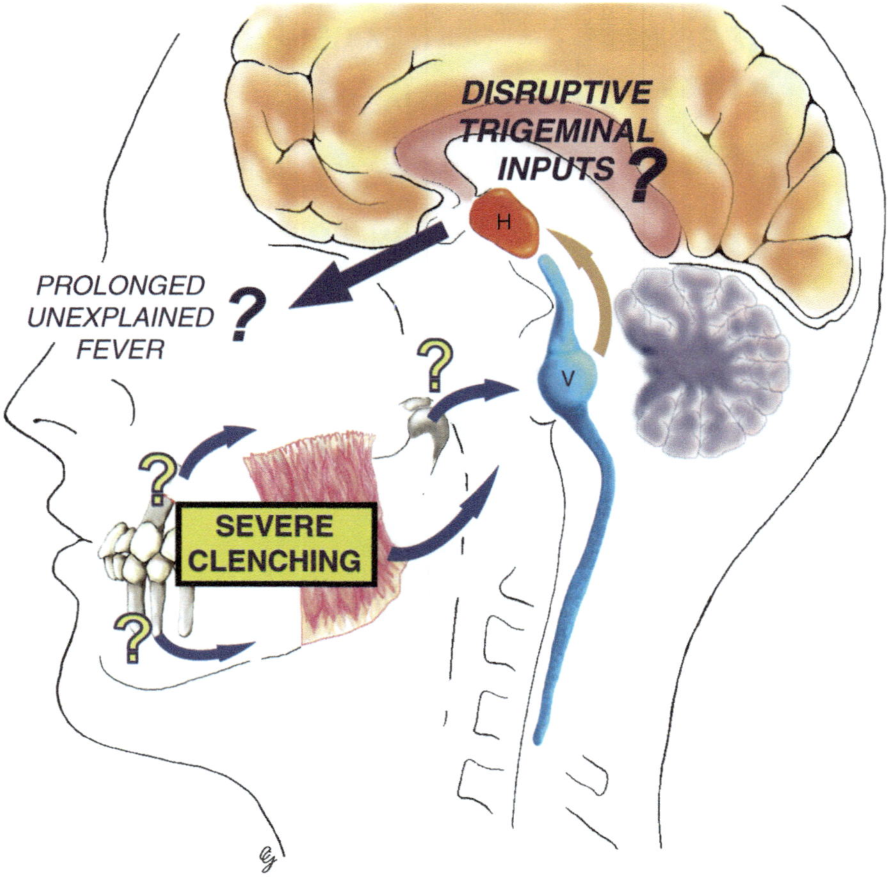

Fig. 18 Parafunctional trigeminal projections and possible thermic dysregulation. Model

8 Autonomic Problems

There is a link between parafunction, dry mouth syndrome, and anxiety [87]. Cardiovascular problems have been noted in TMD patients (see Part I). The area postrema (AP)-nucleus tracti solitarii (NTS) complex, where the vagus nerve inputs converge, is the cardiovascular center of homeostasis [19, 45, 56, 57, 115]. Maixner et al. suggest that "...painful TMD can result, at least in part, from an impairment in central pain regulatory systems that are influenced by resting arterial blood pressure" [72]. Therefore, could trigeminal overstimulation and nociception from *severe clenching* disrupt the integrative function of the NTS and facilitate a *variation in the heart rhythm*? This type of interference might have pathological repercussions in cardiovascular patients [83]. When compared to normal subjects during rhythmic masticatory muscle activity, nocturnal bruxers clearly show a more rapid onset of heart rate increase [61]. For many years we have known that stimulation of the trigeminal ganglion generated

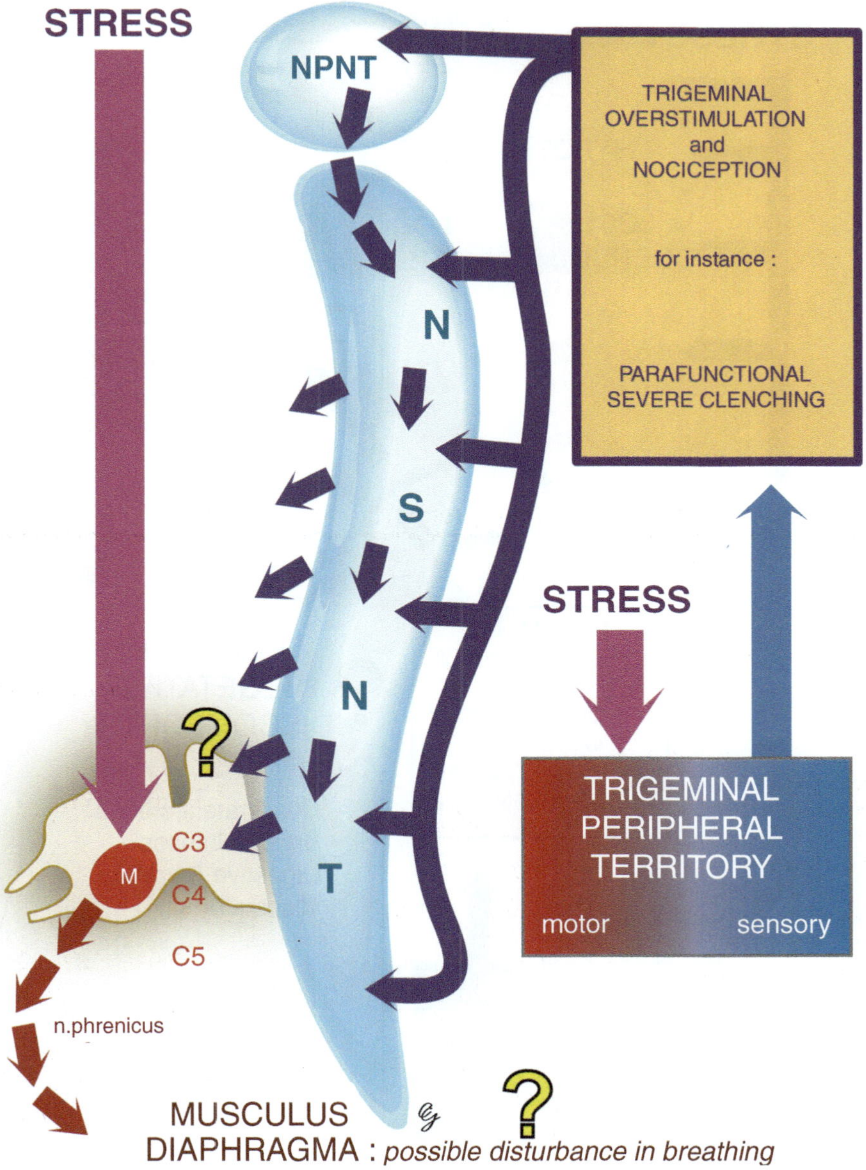

Fig. 19 Trigeminal parafunctional projections to the medullar phrenic nerve motor center which commands the diaphragm muscle

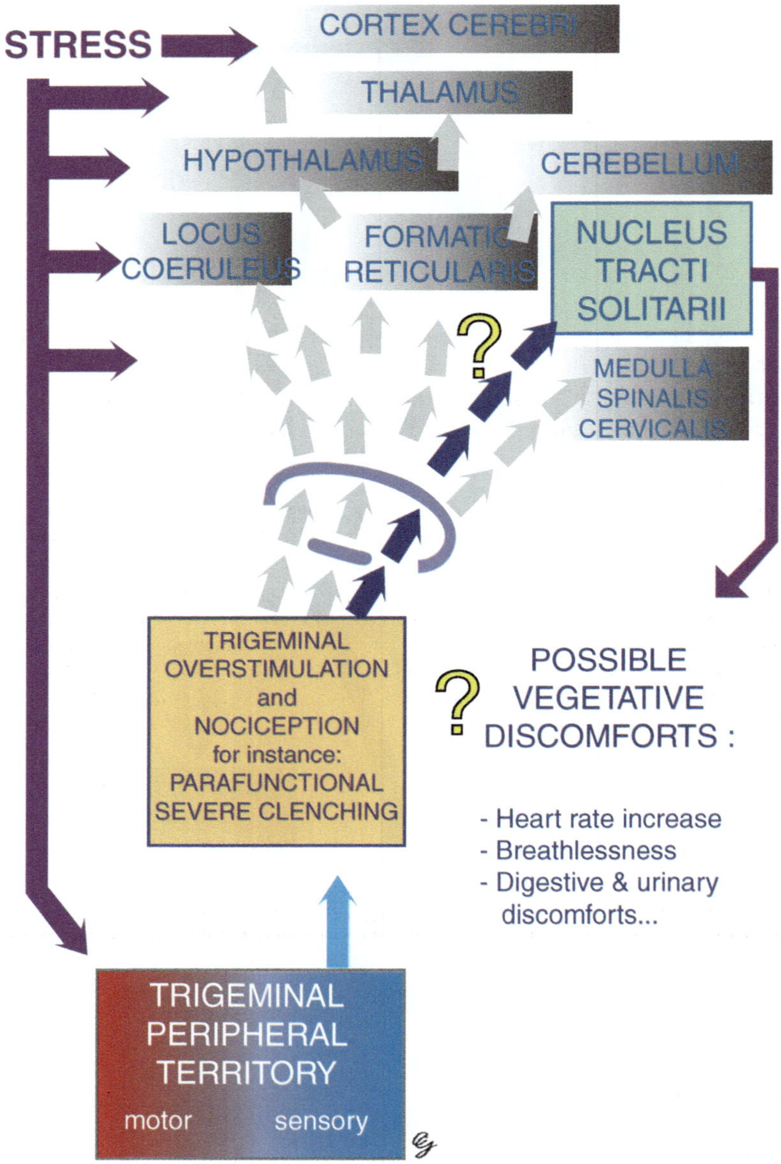

Fig. 20 Trigeminal parafunctional projections to the nucleus tracti solitarii

tachycardia and blood hypertension [27]. This model explains how abnormally intensive and durable trigeminal afferents (creating *overflowing* inputs) could possibly aggravate some autonomic disorders, that is, cardiac, respiratory, digestive, and urinary signs or symptoms (Figs. 19, 20, and 21). In cases of urination among nocturnal bruxing children, the oral parafunction seems to be significantly associated with bed wetting as well as drooling and colic [121].

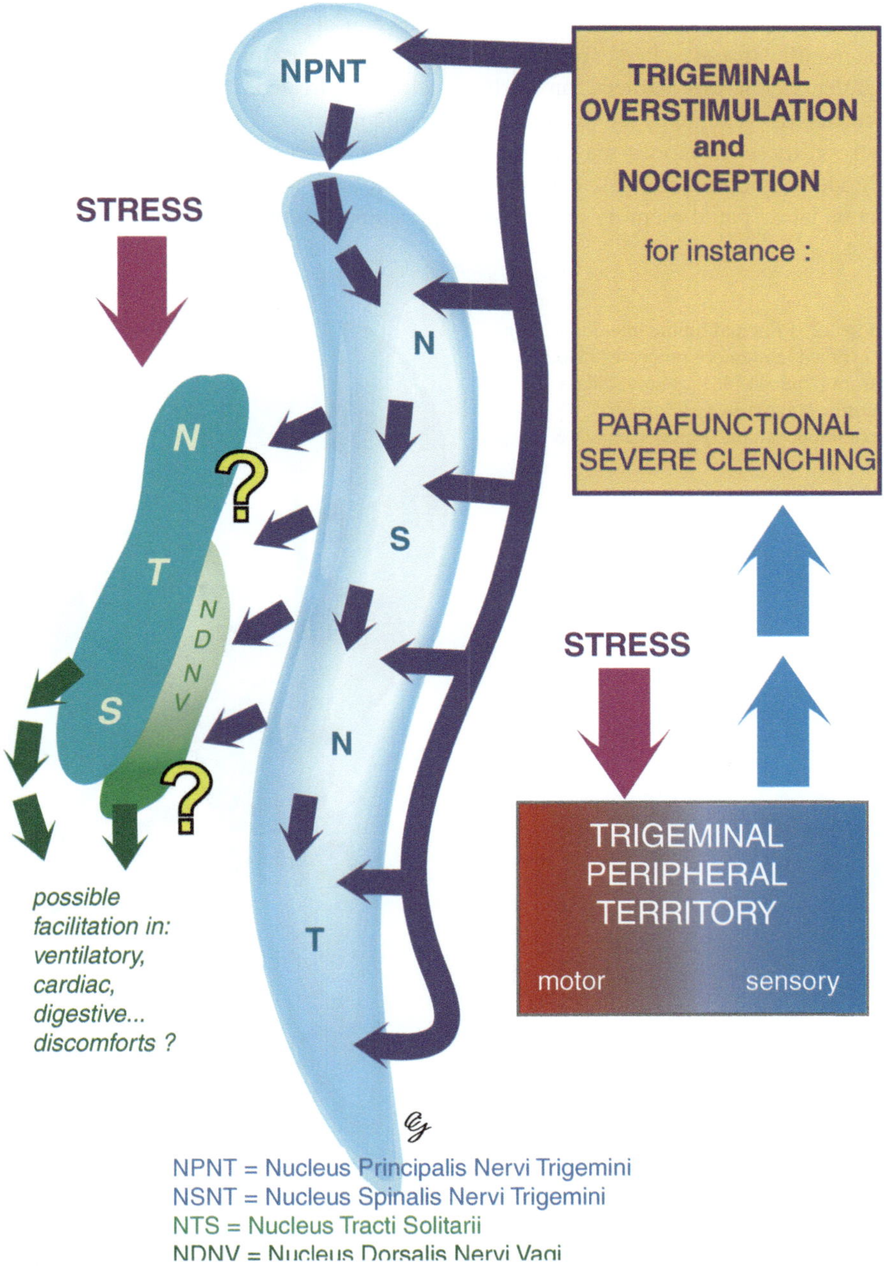

Fig. 21 Trigeminal parafunctional projections from the TBNC to the nucleus tracti solitarii

9 Problems with Memory

Owing to the limbic interconnections (Fig. 22), the richness in (5-HT) receptors in the hippocampus and the disrupted memory acquisition following stimulation of the

(5-HT) neurons of the dorsal raphe nucleus can also explain the role of (5-HT) metabolic troubles in generating anterograde memory problems in some TMD patients. On this subject, an earlier theory implicated the role of endogenic corticoids. When they are released by the corticoadrenal gland as a result of chronic stress, these hormones may cause a functional deficiency, even a destruction of hippocampic neurons [5]. It is very important to know that reduced mastication attenuates spatial memory and causes hippocampal neurons to deteriorate [84]. Is

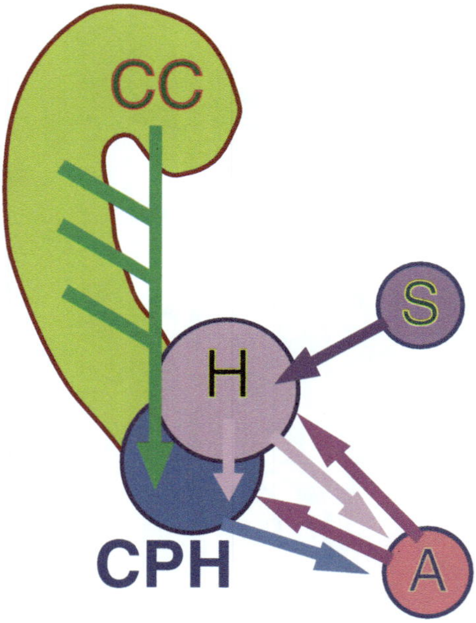

Fig. 22 Principal limbic interconnections involved in memory processes (Modified from Izquiedo [48]). *A* amygdala, *CCi* cortex cingularis, *CPH* cortex parahippocampi, *H* hippocampus, *S* septum

this symptom more obvious in TMD patients than in patients suffering from other diseases (Fig. 23)?

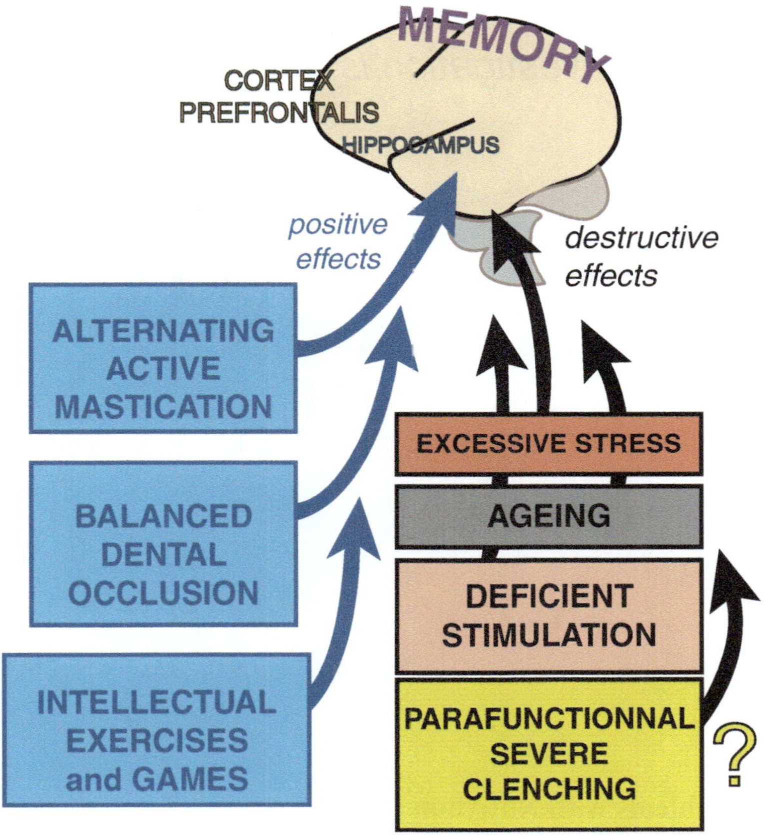

Fig. 23 Stomatognathic activities and memorial impacts. Recent studies enlightened the role of active masticatory inputs to rescue stress-attenuated hippocampal memory process [66, 84]. The question follows: what about the possible aggravating impacts induced by parafunctional oral habits as severe clenching, according to clinical observations about memorial deficiencies with some clenchers?

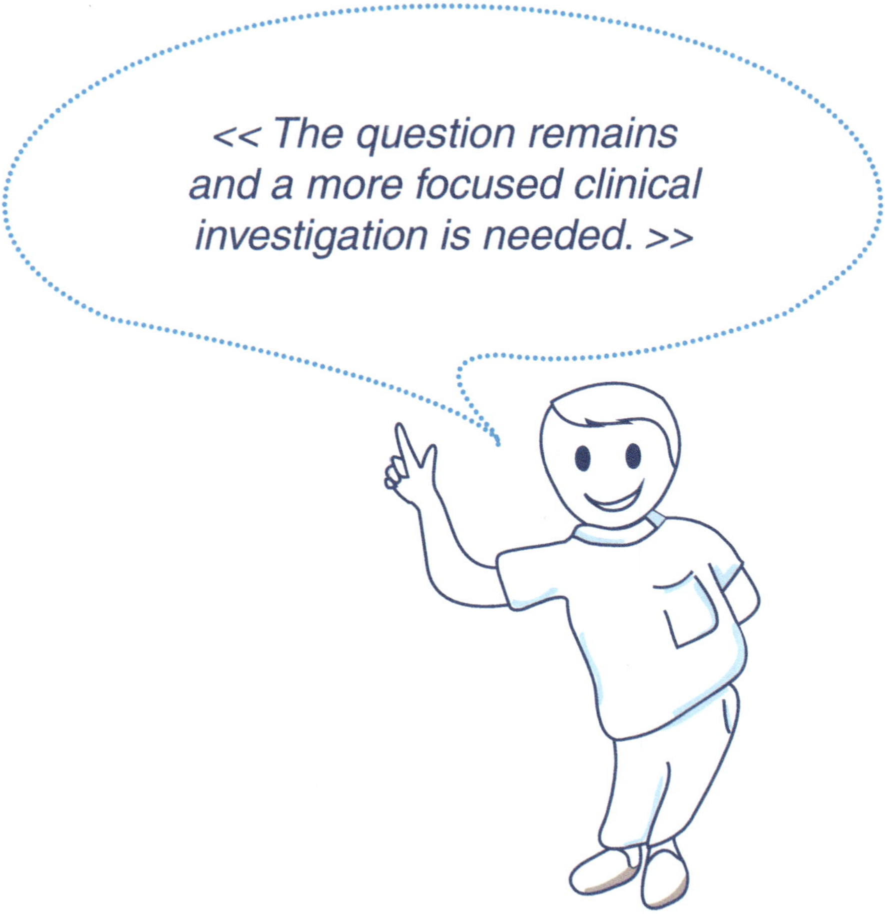

10 Problems with Nutrition

From the oropharyngeal and gastric spheres, a first influence associated with a state of food deprivation may stimulate noradrenergic neurons. These neurons can provoke food intake [42, 60], via the hypothalamus. The same afferents could immediately activate cholinergic neurons that initiate a feeling of satiety, via the hypothalamus. In some TMD patients, a dysfunction with a trigeminal origin or direct action on the ventromedial hypothalamus (VMH) (Figs. 24 and 25) may be considered. The (5-HT) may also contribute to generating some types of nutritive behavior towards carbohydrates particularly in situations of depression possibly linked with photoperiodism [125]. Some studies have also shed light on the role of trigeminal afferents in regulating satiety mechanisms by recruiting histamine neurons in the trigeminal mesencephalic nucleus (MeN) [95]. Therefore, physicians should not be surprised to notice weight problems in TMD clenching patients and some positive changes when using the RMT protocol.

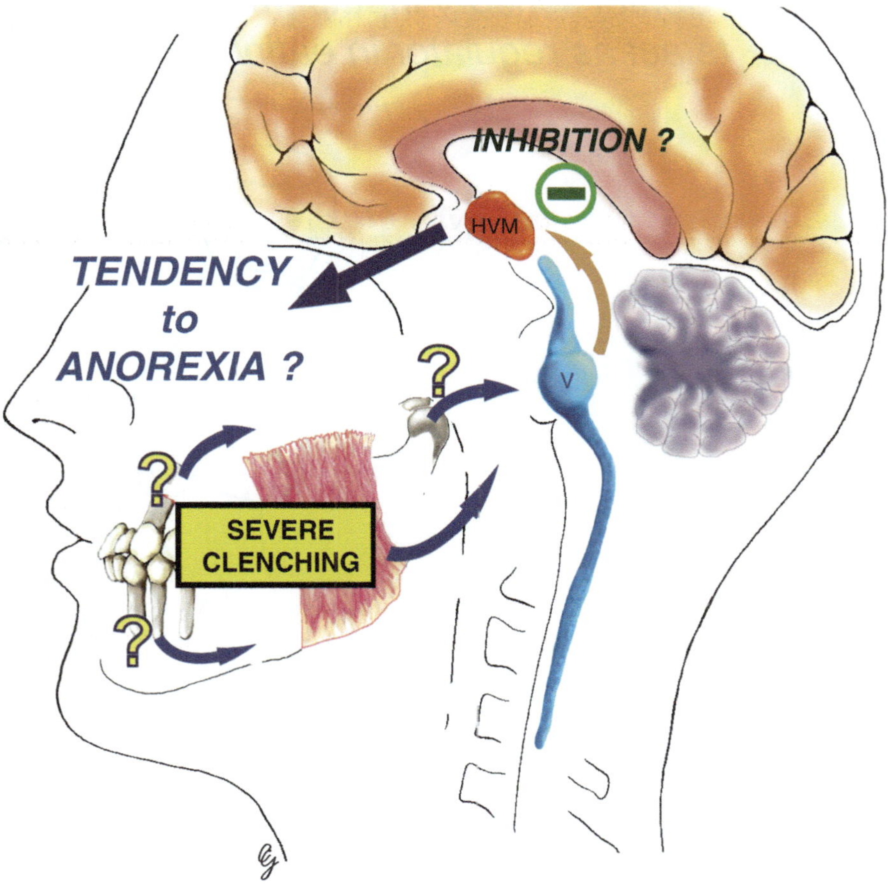

Fig. 24 Trigeminal parafunctional inputs and tendency to anorexia. Model

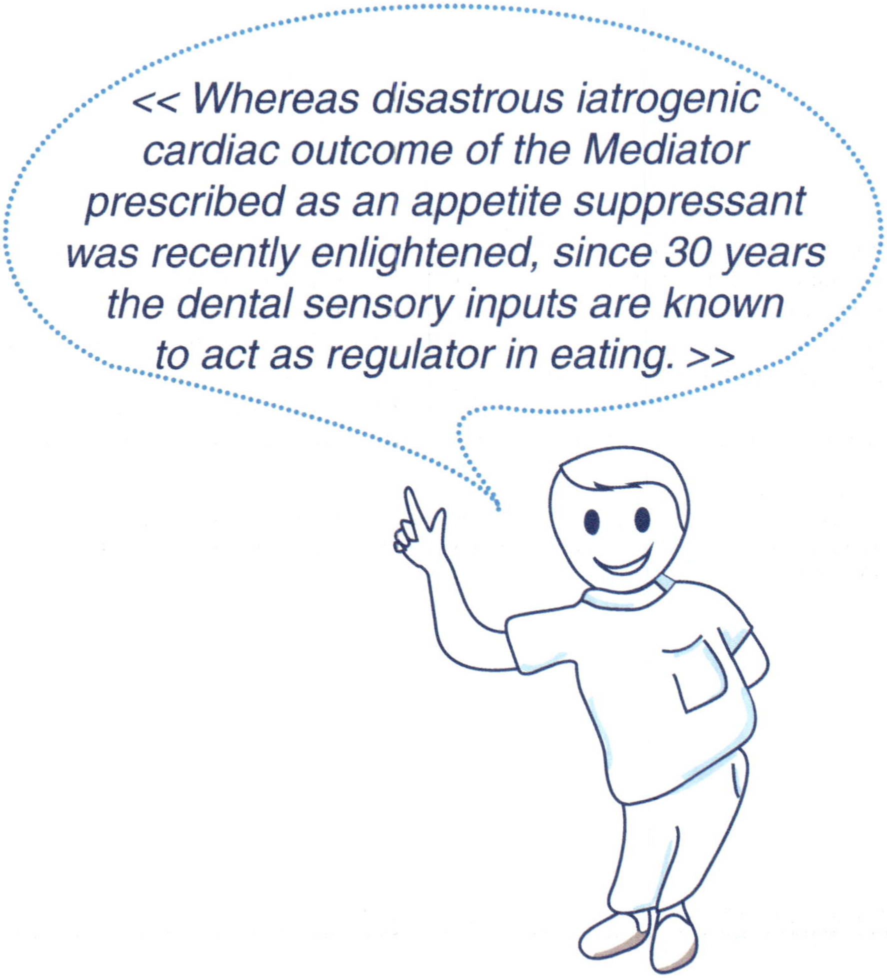
<< Whereas disastrous iatrogenic cardiac outcome of the Mediator prescribed as an appetite suppressant was recently enlightened, since 30 years the dental sensory inputs are known to act as regulator in eating. >>

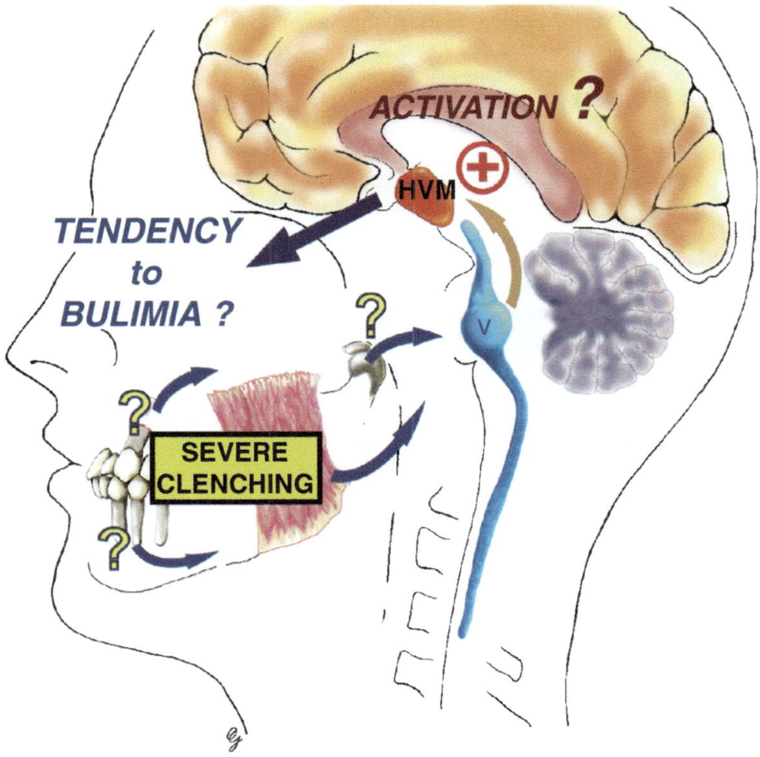

Fig. 25 Trigeminal parafunctional inputs and tendency to bulimia. Model

References

1. Abrahams VC, Anstee G, Richmond FJ, Rose PK (1979) Neck muscle and trigeminal input to the upper cervical cord and lower medulla of the cat. Can J Physiol Pharmacol 57(6):642–651
2. Ackermann F (1964) Occlusodontologie et occlusodontie. Rev Franç Odont Stomatol 1053–1054
3. Alkofide EA, Clark E, El Bermani W et al (1997) The incidence and nature of fibrous continuity between the sphenomandibular ligament and the anterior malleolar ligament of the middle ear. J Orofac Pain 11(1):7–14
4. Amri M, Car A, Jean A (1984) Medullary control of the pontine swallowing neurons in sheep. Exp Brain Res 55:105–110
5. Bader JM (1991) Le stress met les neurones à mort. Sci Vie 889:52–59
6. Bazzotti L (1998) Mandible position and head posture: electromyography of sternocleidomastoids. Cranio 16:100–108
7. Berstein JM, Mohl ND, Spiller H (1969) Temporomandibular joint dysfunction masquerading as disease of the ear, nose and throat. Trans Am Acad Ophthalmol Otolaryngol 73:1208
8. Bjorne A, Berven A, Agerberg G (1998) Cervical signs and symptoms in patients with Meniere's disease: a controlled study. Cranio 16(3):194–202

9. Block SL (1976) Possible etiology of ear stuffiness (barohypoacousis) in MPD syndrome TMJ and facial pain. J Dent Abstract 55, 752:B250
10. Bossy J (1990) Anatomie clinique: neuro-anatomie. Springer Verlag (éd), Paris
11. Bouchet A, Cuilleret J (1980) Anatomie topographique, descriptive et fonctionnelle. La face, la tête et les organes des sens. Simep ed, Paris
12. Browne PA, Clark GT, Yang Q, Nakano M (1993) Sternocleidomastoid muscle inhibition induced by trigeminal stimulation. J Dent Res 72(11):1503–1508
13. Browne PA, Clark GT, Kuboki T, Adachi NY (1998) Concurrent cervical and craniofacial pain. A review of empiric and basic science evidence. Oral Surg Oral Med Oral Pathol Oral Radiol Endod 86(6):633–640
14. Buisseret P, Buisseret-Delmas C, Epelbaum M, Lepercq H (1991) Projections proprioceptives primaires des muscles oculaires extrinsèques sur les noyaux vestibulaires et la région cervicale haute. Résultats anatomiques. Rev Oto Neuro Ophalmol 14:13–17
15. Burch JG (1966) The cranial attachment of the sphenomandibular ligament. Anat Rec 156:433
16. Capra NF (1987) Localization and central projections of primary afferent neurons that innervate the temporomandibular joint in cats. Somatosens Mot Res 4(3):201–213
17. Ceneviz C, Mehta NR, Forgione A et al (2006) The immediate effect of changing mandibular position on the EMG activity of the masseter, temporalis, sternocleidomastoid and trapezius muscles. Cranio 24(4):237–244
18. Ciampini G, Jean A (1980) Rôle des afférences glosso-pharyngiennes et trigéminales dans le déclenchement et le déroulement de la déglutition. J Physiol 76:49–66
19. Ciriello J, Caverson MM (1986) Bidirectional cardiovascular connections between ventrolateral medulla and nucleus of the solitary tract. Brain Res 367:273–281
20. Clark GT, Browne PA, Nakano M, Yang Q (1993) Co-activation of sternocleidomastoid muscles during jaw clenching. J Dent Res 72(11):1499–1502
21. Cody FW, Richardson HC (1978) Mossy and climbing fibre projections of trigeminal inputs to cerebellar cortex in the cat. Brain Res 53:352–356
22. Coleman RD (1970) Temporomandibular joint: relation to the retrodiscal zone to Meckel's cartilage and lateral pterygoid muscle. J Dent Res 49:626
23. Cooper S, Daniel P, Whitteridge D (1951) Afferent impulses in the oculomotor nerve, from extrinsic eye muscle. J Physiol 113:363–374
24. Cuccurazzu B, Deriu F, Tolu E (2007) A monosynaptic pathway links the vestibular nuclei and masseter muscle motoneurons in rats. Exp Brain Res 176(4):665–671
25. Darian-Smith I, Philipps G (1984) Secondary neurones within a trigemino-cerebellar projection to the anterior lob of the cerebellum in the cat. J Physiol Lond 353:42
26. Dessem D, Iyadurai OD, Taylor A (1988) The role of periodontal receptors in the jaw-opening reflex in the cat. J Physiol 406:315–330
27. Dominguez J, Lobato RD, Rivas JJ (1994) Changes in systemic blood pressure and cardiac rhythm induced by therapeutic compression of the trigeminal ganglion. Neurosurgery 34(3):422–428
28. Draft DW, Klocker D, Theissing J (1971) Costen syndrom und Schallperzeptions Schwerhörigkeit. H N O 19:179
29. Ehrlich R, Garlick D, Ninio M (1999) The effect of jaw clenching on the electromyographic activities of 2 neck and 2 trunk muscles. J Orofac Pain 13(2):115–120
30. Elias SA, Taylor A (1984) Direct projections of jaw proprioceptor first-order afferents to the cerebellar cortex in the ferret. J Physiol 353:42
31. Elias SA, Taylor A, Somjen G (1987) Direct and relayed projection of periodontal receptor afferents to the cerebellum in the ferret. Proc R Soc Lond B Biol Sci 231:199–216
32. El-Kashlan HK, Shore SE (2004) Effects of trigeminal ganglion stimulation on the central auditory system. Hear Res 189(1–2):25–30
33. Eriksson PO, Haggman-Henrikson B, Nordh E, Zafar H (2000) Co-ordinated mandibular and head-neck movements during rhythmic jaw activities in man. J Dent Res 79:1378–1384
34. Fink M, Wähling K, Stiesch-Scholtz M, Tschernitschek H (2003) The functional relationship between the craniomandibular system, cervical spine, and the sacroiliac joint: a preliminary investigation. Cranio 21(3):202–208

35. Fonder AC (1988) The dental distress syndrome (quantified). Quant Med 1:1
36. Forsberg CM, Hellsing E, Linder-Aronson S, Sheikholeslam A (1989) EMG activity in neck and masticatory muscles in relation to extension and flexion of the head. Eur J Orthod 7:177–184
37. Frumker SC, Kyle MA (1985) The dentist's contribution to rehabilitation of cervical posture and function: orthopedic and neurological considerations in the treatment of craniomandibular disorders. Basal Facts 9(3):105–109
38. Funakoshi A, Amano NO (1974) Periodontal jaw reflexes in the albino rat. J Dent Res 53:598–605
39. Gangloff P, Perrin PP (2002) Unilateral trigeminal anaesthesia modifies postural control in human subjects. Neurosci Lett 330(2):179–182
40. Gastaldo E, Quatrale R, Graziani A et al (2006) The excitability of the trigeminal motor system in sleep bruxism: a transcranial magnetic stimulation and brainstem reflex study. J Orofac Pain 20(2):145–155
41. German RZ, Crompton AW, Thexton AJ (2009) Integration of the reflex pharyngeal swallow into rhythmic oral activity in a neurologically intact pig model. J Neurophysiol 102:1017–1025
42. Grossman SP (1968) Hypothalamic and limbic influences on food intake. Fed Proc 27:1349–1360
43. Haenggeli CA, Pongstaporn T, Doucet JR, Ryugo DK (2005) Projections from the spinal trigeminal nucleus to the cochlear nucleus in the rat. J Comp Neurol 484(2):191–205
44. Hamada T, Ono T, Otsuka R et al (2007) Mandibular distraction osteogenesis in a skeletal Class II patient with obstructive sleep apnea. Am J Orthod Dentofacial Orthop 131(3):415–425
45. Higgins GA, Hoffman GE, Wray S, Schwaber JS (1984) Distribution of neurotensin-immunoreactivity within baroreceptive portions of the nucleus of the tractus solitarius and the dorsal vagal nucleus of the rat. J Comp Neurol 226:155–164
46. Humphrey T (1969) The prenatal development of mouth opening and mouth closure reflexes. Pediatr Dig 11:28–40
47. Igarashi N, Yamamura K, Yamada Y, Kohno S (2000) Head movements and neck muscle activities associated with the jaw movement during mastication in the rabbit. Brain Res 871:151–155
48. Izquiedo I (1992) Trends in pharmacological. Sciences 13:7
49. Jacquart G, Mahler P, Kachani-Mansour R (1986) Growth of trigemino-cerebellar areas in infant rat studied by micrometric and cytophometric methods. Arch Oral Biol 31(9):573–576
50. Jacquin MF, Semba K, Rhoades RW, Egger MD (1982) Trigeminal primary afferents project bilaterally to dorsal horn and ipsilaterally to cerebellum reticular formation and cuneate, solitary, supratrigeminal and vagal nuclei. Brain Res 246:285–291
51. Jean A (1984) Brainstem organization of the swallowing network. Brain Behav Evol 25:109–116
52. Jean A (1990) Brainstem control of swallowing localization and organization of the central pattern generator for swallowing. In: Taylor A (ed) Neurophysiology of the jaw and teeth. McMillan (eds), Basingstoke, pp 294–321
53. Jean A, Amri M, Calas A (1983) Connections between the ventral medullary swallowing area and the trigeminal motor nucleus of the sheep studied by tracing techniques. J Auton Nerv Syst 7:87–96
54. Jouvet M (1984) Le comportement onirique. In: Le Cerveau. Pour la Science (éd), Berlin/Paris, p 146
55. Kahle W, Leonhardt H, Platzer W (1981) Anatomie. Tome 3: système nerveux et organes des sens. Flammarion (éd), Paris
56. Kalia M, Melusam MM (1980) Brain stem projections of sensory and motor components of the vagus complex in the cat: I – the cervical vagus and nodose ganglion. J Comp Neurol 193:435–465
57. Kalia M, Sullivan JM (1982) Brainstem projection of sensory and motor components of the vagus nerve in the rat. J Comp Neurol 211:248–264
58. Kapandji AI (1982) Physiologie articulaire. Tome 3: Tronc et rachis. Maloine (éd), Paris

59. Karamandilis A (1968) Trigemino-cerebellar connections in the goat studied by means of the retrograde cell degeneration method. J Comp Neurol 133:71–88
60. Karli P (1976) Neurophysiologie du comportment. In: Kayser C (ed) Physiologie. Flammarion (ed), Paris, pp 1331–1454
61. Kato T, Rompré PH, Montplaisir JY et al (2001) Sleep bruxism: an oromotor activity secondary to microarousal. J Dent Res 80:1940–1944
62. Kato S, Papuashvili N, Okada YC (2003) Identification and functional characterization of the trigeminal ventral cervical reflex pathway in the swine. Clin Neurophysiol 114(2):263–271
63. Kawamura Y (1974) Physiology of mastication. Kawamura (ed), Basel
64. Kessler J-P, Jean A (1985) Identification of the medullary swallowing regions in the rat. Exp Brain Res 57:256–263
65. Kreisberg MK (1986) Headache as a symptom of craniomandibular disorders I: pathophysiology. Cranio 4(2):135–142
66. Kubo KY, Ichihashi Y, Kurata C et al (2010) Masticatory function and cognitive function. Okajimas Folia Anat Jpn 87(3):135–140
67. Larmande P, Larmande A (1989) Neuro-ophtalmologie. Masson (éd), Paris, pp 147–148
68. Lavigne GJ, Kato T, Kolta A, Sessle BJ (2003) Neurobiological mechanisms involved in sleep bruxism. Crit Rev Oral Biol Med 14(1):30–46
69. Levine RA (1999) Somatic (craniocervical) tinnitus and the dorsal cochlear nucleus hypothesis. Am J Otolaryngol 20(6):351–362
70. Lobbezoo E, Souly JP, Montplaisir JY, Lavigne GJ (1996) Striatal D2 receptor binding in sleep bruxism: a controlled study with iodine-123-iodobenzamide and single-photon-emission computed tomography. J Dent Res 75:1804–1810
71. Lund JP, Nishiyama T, Möller E (1970) Postural activity of the muscles of mastication with the subject upright, inclined and supine. Scand J Dent Res 78:417–424
72. Maixner W, Fillingim R, Kincaid S (1997) Relationship between pain sensitivity and resting arterial blood pressure in patients with painful temporomandibular disorders. Psychosom Med 59(5):503–511
73. Malick A, Burstein R (1998) Cells of origin of the trigeminohypothalamic tract in the rat. J Comp Neurol 400:125–144
74. Manni E, Palmieri G, Marini R (1971) Extra-ocular muscle proprioception and the descending trigeminal nucleus. Exp Neurol 33:195–204
75. Marfurt CF, Rajchert DM (1991) Trigeminal primary afferent projections to "non-trigeminal" areas of the rat central nervous system. J Comp Neurol 303:489–511
76. Matsushita M, Okado N, Ikeda M, Hosoya Y (1981) Descending projections from the spinal and mesencephalic nuclei or the trigeminal nerve to the spinal cord in the cat. A study with the horseradish peroxidase technique. J Comp Neurol 196:173–187
77. Mc Gregor NR, Butt HL, Zerbes M et al (1996) Assessment of pain (distribution and onset), symptoms, SCL-90-R inventory responses, and the association with infectious events in patients with chronic orofacial pain. J Orofac Pain 10(4):339–350
78. Meyer J (1977) Participation des afférences trigéminales dans la régulation tonique posturale orthostatique. Intérêt de l'examen systématique du système manducateur chez les sportifs de haut niveau. Thèse 3ème cycle Sci Odontol Paris
79. Meyer J, Baron JB (1976) Participation des afférences trigéminales à la régulation tonique posturale. Aspects statique et dynamique. Agressiologie 17(A):33–40
80. Miyahara T, Haglya N, Ohyama T, Nakamuna Y (1996) Modulations of human soleus H-reflexes in association with voluntary clenching of the teeth. J Neurophysiol 76:2033–2041
81. Morgan DH, Gooder RL, Christiansen RL, Tiner LW (1995) The TMJ-ear connection. Cranio 13(1):42–43
82. Myrhaug H (1984) The incidence of ear symptoms in cases of malocclusion and temporomandibular joint disturbances. Br J Oral Surg 2:28
83. Okeson JP, Philips BA, Berry DTR, Baldwin RM (1994) Nocturnal bruxing events: a report for normative data and cardiovascular response. J Oral Rehabil 2(1):623–630
84. Ono Y, Yamamoto T, Kubo KY, Onozuka M (2010) Occlusion and brain function: mastication as a prevention of cognitive dysfunction. J Oral Rehabil 37(8):624–640

85. Ormeno G, Miralles R, Santander H et al (1997) Body position effects on sternocleidomastoid and masseter EMG pattern activity in patients undergoing occlusal splint therapy. Cranio 15(4):300–309
86. Palazzi C, Miralles R, Soto MA et al (1996) Body position effect on EMG activity of sternocleidomastoid and masseter muscles in patients with myogenic cranio-cervical-mandibular dysfunction. Cranio 14(3):200–209
87. Paterson AJ, Lamb AB, Clifford TJ, Lamey PJ (1995) Burning mouth syndrome: the relationship between the HAD scale and parafunctional habits. J Oral Pathol Med 24(7):289–292
88. Philipp U, Munker G, Komposh G (1972) Die funktion der Tube Eustachii bei Patienten mit Kiefergelenkerkrangungen. Dtsch Zanhärztl Z 27:806
89. Pinganaud G, Bernat I, Buisseret P, Buisseret-Delmas C (1999) Trigeminal projections to hypoglossal and facial motor nuclei in the rat. J Comp Neurol 415:91–104
90. Pinto OF (1962) A new structure related to the temporomandibular joint and middle ear. J Prosthet Dent 12:95
91. Reydy R, Hartmann F (1992) Le role du nerf trijumeau dans l'oculomotricité. Arqu Portug Oftalmol 3:7–23
92. Rhoades RW, Fish SE, Chiaia NL et al (1989) Organization of the projections from the trigeminal brainstem complex to the superior colliculus in the rat and hamster: anterograde tracing with Phaseolus vulgaris leucoagglutinin and intra-axonal injection. J Comp Neurol 289(4):641–656
93. Richardson HC, Cody FWJ, Paul VE, Thomas AG (1978) Convergence of trigeminal and limb inputs onto cerebellar interpositus nuclear neurones in the cat. Brain Res 156: 355–359
94. Ruggiero DA, Ross CA, Reis DJ (1981) Projections from the spinal trigeminal nucleus to the entire length of the spinal cord in the rat. Brain Res 225:225–233
95. Sakata T, Yoshimatsu H, Masaki T, Tsuda K (2003) Anti-obesity actions of mastication driven by histamine neurons in rats. Exp Biol Med 228:1106–1110
96. Sasaki K, Watanabe M, Inai T, Kanuma A (1984) Change of mandibular position elicited by tonic reflex under EMG biofeedback. J Dent Res 63(4):556
97. Schwartz HC, Kendrick RW (1984) Internal derangements of the temporomandibular joint: description of clinical syndromes. Oral Surg Oral Med Oral Pathol 58(1):24–29
98. Serrao M, Rossi P, Parisi L et al (2003) Trigemino-cervical-spinal reflexes in humans. Clin Neurophysiol 114(9):1697–1703
99. Shibukawa Y, Ishikawa T, Kato Y et al (2007) Cerebral cortical dysfunction in patients with temporomandibular disorders in association with jaw movement observation. Pain 128(1–2):180–188
100. Shore SE, Vass Z, Wys NL, Altschuler RA (2000) Trigeminal ganglion innervates the auditory brainstem. J Comp Neurol 419(3):271–285
101. Shore SE, El Kashlan H, Lu J (2003) Effects of trigeminal ganglion stimulation on unit activity of ventral cochlear nucleus neurons. Neuroscience 119(4):1085–1101
102. Singh GD, Olmos S (2007) Use of a sibilant phoneme registration protocol to prevent upper airway collapse in patients with TMD. Sleep Breath 11(4):209–216
103. Smelee LE (1988) Odontogeny of relationship of human middle ear and temporomandibular joint. Acta Anat 131:338–341
104. Somana R, Kotchabakdhi N, Walberg F (1980) Cerebellar afferents from the trigeminal sensory nuclei in the cat. Exp Brain Res 38:57–64
105. Steinbach MJ (1987) Proprioceptive knowledge of eye position. Vision Res 27(10):1737–1744
106. Strand FL, Kenneth JR, Zuccarelli LA et al (1991) Neuropeptides hormones as neurotrophic factors. Physiol Rev 71(4):1034–1035
107. Strazielle C, Mahler P, Jacquart G (1987) Localisation des afférences primaires trigémino-cérébelleuses chez le rat. Wistar Symp Int Physiol Oro Fac Nancy 57–65
108. Sumino R, Nozaki S, Kato M (1980) Trigemino-neck reflex. In: Oral-facial sensory and motor functions. International oral physiology symposium, Rappongi, pp 28–29
109. Takahashi T, Ueno T, Ohyama T (2003) Modulation of H reflexes in the forearm during voluntary teeth clenching in humans. Eur J Appl Physiol 90(5–6):651–653

110. Takamatsu T, Inoue T, Tsuruoka M (2005) Involvement of reticular neurons located dorsal to the facial nucleus in activation of the jaw-closing muscle in rats. Brain Res 1055(1–2):93–102
111. Travell JG, Simons DG (1983) Myofascial pain and dysfunction. The trigger-point manual. Williams & Wilkins (ed), Baltimore, 713p
112. Travers JB, Yoo JE, Chandran R et al (2005) Neurotransmitter phenotypes of intermediate zone reticular formation projections to the motor trigeminal and hypoglossal nuclei in the rat. J Comp Neurol 488(1):28–47
113. Trub M, Mei N, Orsini JC (1991) Macro and micro-electrode study of hypothalamic projections of periodontal afferents in the rat and cat. Brain Res Bull 27:29–34
114. Trub M, Mei N (1991) Effects on periodontal stimulation on VMH neurones in anesthetized rats. Brain Res Bull 27(1):29–34
115. Van Giersbergen PL, Palkovits M, De Jong W (1992) Involvement of neurotransmitters in the nucleus tractus solitarii in cardiovascular regulation. Physiol Rev 72(3):789–824
116. Van Willingen JD (1983) Motoriek van het trigeminussystem. In: Van Willigen JD (ed) Morfologie en functie van het orofaciale systeem. Bohn, Scheltema & Holkema (ed), Utrecht
117. Vass Z, Shore SE, Nuttall AL, Miller JM (1998) Direct evidence of trigeminal innervation of the cochlear blood vessels. Neuroscience 84(2):559–567
118. Villarosa GA, Moss RA (1995) Oral behavior patterns as factors contributing to the development of head and facial pain. J Prosthet Dent 54(3):427–430
119. Vinay L, Cazalets JR, Clarac F (1995) Evidence for the existence of a functional polysynaptic pathway from trigeminal afferents to lumbar motoneurons in the neonatal rat. Eur J Neurosci 7:143–151
120. Watson CRR, Switzer RL (1978) Trigeminal projections to cerebellar tactile areas in the rat origin mainly from noyau interpolaris and noyau principalis. Neurosci Lett 10:77–82
121. Weideman CL, Bush DL, Yan-Go FL et al (1996) The incidence of parasomnias in child bruxers versus nonbruxers. Pediatr Dent 18(7):456–460
122. Weinberg S, Lapointe H (1987) Cervical extension-flexion injury (whiplash) and internal derangement of the temporomandibular joint. J Oral Maxillofac Surg 45(8):653–656
123. Wen-Bin Z, Ji-Shud L, Hui-Li L (1991) SP-like immunoreactivity in the primary trigeminal neurons projecting to the nucleus tractus solitarii. Brain Res 558:87–89
124. Widmalm SE (1984) Electromyographic activity in neck muscles at tooth grinding. J Dent Res 63(289):1066
125. Wurtman R, Wurtman J (1989) Glucides et dépression. Pour la Science 137:44–51
126. Yamabe Y, Yamashita R, Fujii H (1999) Head, neck and trunk movements accompanying jaw tapping. J Oral Rehabil 26:900–905
127. Yoshimatsu T, Namikoshi T, Koyama Z et al (1989) Changes of muscles activities in neck and shoulder region during sustained isometric contractions of jaw muscles. Nippon Hotetsu Shika Gakkai Zasshi 33(5):1044–1049
128. Yoshino G, Higashi K, Nakamura T (2003) Changes in head position due to occlusal supporting zone loss during clenching. Cranio 21(4):89–98
129. Young S, Jordan JC (1982) EMG activity of the sternomastoid muscles in relation to mouth movement. J Dent Res Abstract 61, 4:158
130. Zettergren-Wijk L, Forsberg C-M, Linder-Aronson S (2006) Changes in dentofacial morphology after adeno-/tonsillectomy in young children with obstructive sleep apnoea – a 5-year follow-up study. Eur J Orthod 28(4):319–326
131. Zhang J, Luo P, Pendlebury WW (2001) Light and electron microscopic observations of a direct projection from mesencephalic trigeminal nucleus neurons to hypoglossal motoneurons in the rat. Brain Res 917(1):67–80
132. Zhou J, Shore S (2004) Projections from the trigeminal nuclear complex to the cochlear nuclei: a retrograde and anterograde tracing study in the guinea pig. J Neurosci Res 78(6):901–907

Part II
In Conclusion

In the stomatognathic system, neuromuscular hyperactivity principally involves the paired V. Trigeminal spasticity under the influence of central factors, particularly reticular and limbic factors, affects primarily the extensor muscles called *jaw-closing muscles*. At this level, a disorder of the jaw posture occurs with a reduction or even a loss of the physiological free way space at rest. Though masticating, speaking, and even teeth grinding are movement activities, parafunctional clenching is motionless that indicates a deleterious mood for trigeminal and postural muscular tissues. Moreover the misunderstood oral habit generates an overstimulation and nociception from the trigeminal territory. These are high-potential disruptive factors for trigeminal and non-trigeminal nervous pathways through a supposed *neuronal overflowing* mechanism. In stressed patients the projection of these trigeminal afferents to the brain could explain some amazing clinical manifestations: TMD as well as some atypical forms of migraine, fibromyalgia, and chronic fatigue. Patients often call on the clinician's sagacity by asking the key question: *Why do I clench my teeth*? Clenching may be a behavioral response comparable to *action inhibition* predominantly obvious at the level of orality, that is, of the major sphere of human expression. From this point of view, it would be appropriate to give value to the great role of the paired V in a number of pathophysiological implications. The theory about behavioral problems helps to better consider the importance of psychological and emotional factors. We hope that (1) it encourages clinicians to rely more on the experience of experts in human behavior, on the one hand and (2) it encourages experts to acknowledge the oral manifestations of these disorders, on the other hand. This would indeed help understand the reasons why, instead of *rather flight than fight*, those patients often unconsciously seem to prefer to abide by *neither fight, nor flight nor speak but fright...so clench.*

Part III
Therapeutics

Introduction

Among the various pathologies due to uncompensated stress, TMD are a very serious and costly health problem for patients and society [48]. To respond to complaints about constant pain or discomfort, a large variety of ongoing treatments are used (Fig. 1). They still include different clinical approaches often based on signs and symptoms, on statistical data, and more rarely on various causal factors that are difficult to evaluate. It is difficult to identify etiological factors; it is even more difficult to classify their role. As the same factors can generate different problems depending on the patient's specific response, different symptoms may appear and lead to different diagnoses and treatment strategies. So, all appropriate treatments must be enlarged to include various elements specific to each patient [53]. Anyhow, invasive or irreversible tools require clinicians to exercise maximum caution. One must keep in mind an old medical principle: *Medicus curat, Natura sanat.* In most cases lending a listening ear to a patient's complaint and noting the right information about his or her behavioral habits is enough for the clinician to manage recent symptoms. In order to handle long-standing painful symptoms and discomforts, a multidisciplinary approach is required. According to Fonder, "It is impossible to divide a patient into neat little areas to be treated in dichotomized fashion without consideration of the resultant affect upon the total person, psyche and soma" [20]. For many years a number of experts have used *splints* (Fig. 2) on dental arches[1] to get an immediate effect on muscular tension [18, 44] by possibly canceling periodontal inputs. It may contribute to reduce some parafunctional activities [21, 23, 31] particularly nocturnal bruxism [35, 38, 45, 56]. The use of a splint is logically preferable to any kind of long drug treatment (anti-inflammatory, analgesic, psychotropic) [28] even though it may have a placebo effect [10]. But unfortunately this

[1]We are referring to the *occlusion splint* aiming at reducing [6, 12, 15–17, 21, 25, 32, 33, 36, 37, 41, 42, 47, 50]. Please note that the stabilization splint to recapture the TMJ disc is not mentioned here. The *occlusion splint* covers the entire occlusal area [2] or the incisor-canine part [43] with a nonpermanent device to avoid risks in posterior teeth regression. The retro-incisor biting plan is a particular system that brings immediate interesting sedating results on painful muscular contractures and contributes to reeducate the lingual function specially during swallowing [27].

F. Hartmann, G. Cucchi, *Stress and Orality*,
DOI 10.1007/978-2-8178-0271-8_13, © Springer-Verlag France 2014

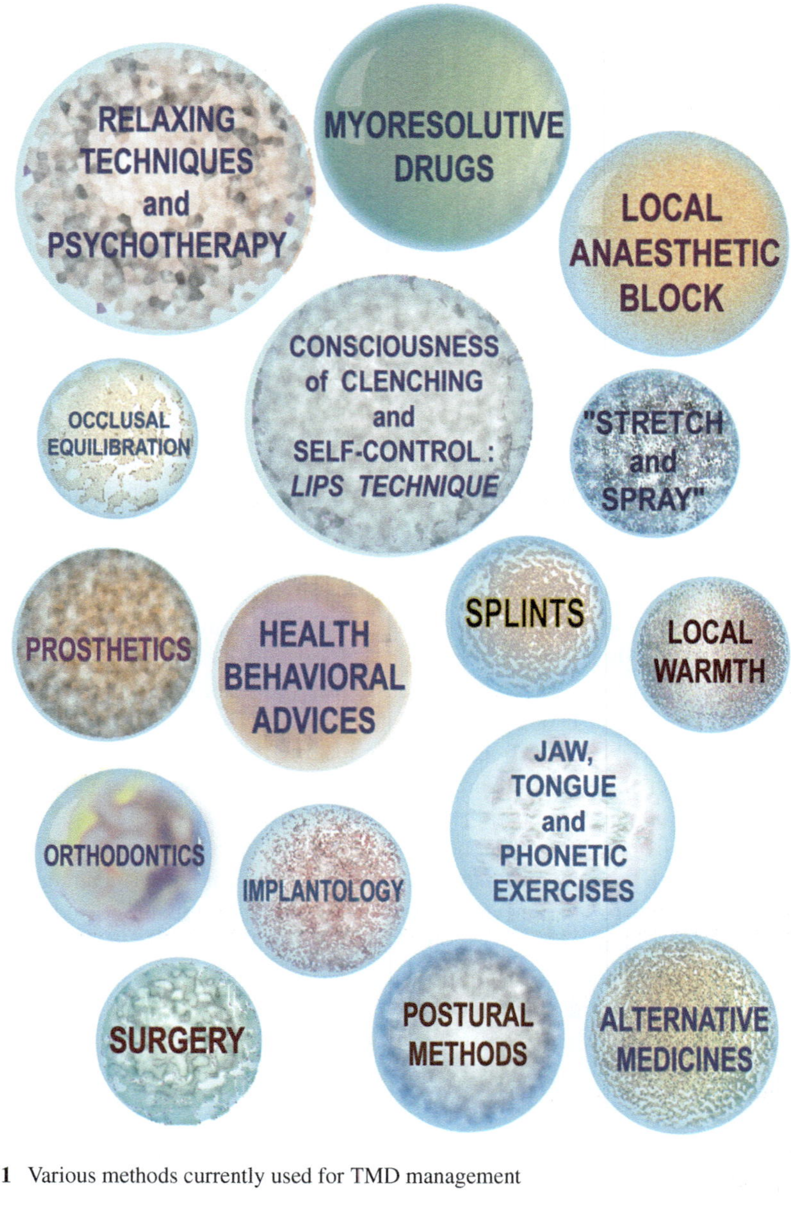

Fig. 1 Various methods currently used for TMD management

method is not always durable [26, 39]. Moreover, its efficiency in the medium and long term becomes uncertain for the treatment of severe clenching, especially when it is early set [34]. When a splint is used in an isolated mode [1], it cannot compete with the instantaneous relaxing action of local anesthetics on myospasm (see below). What's more, some patients become *splint dependant* [52, 55] and use it quasi permanently which can be uncomfortable for those relying on verbal skills for professional activities. Treatments frequently require more complex methods [49], and a

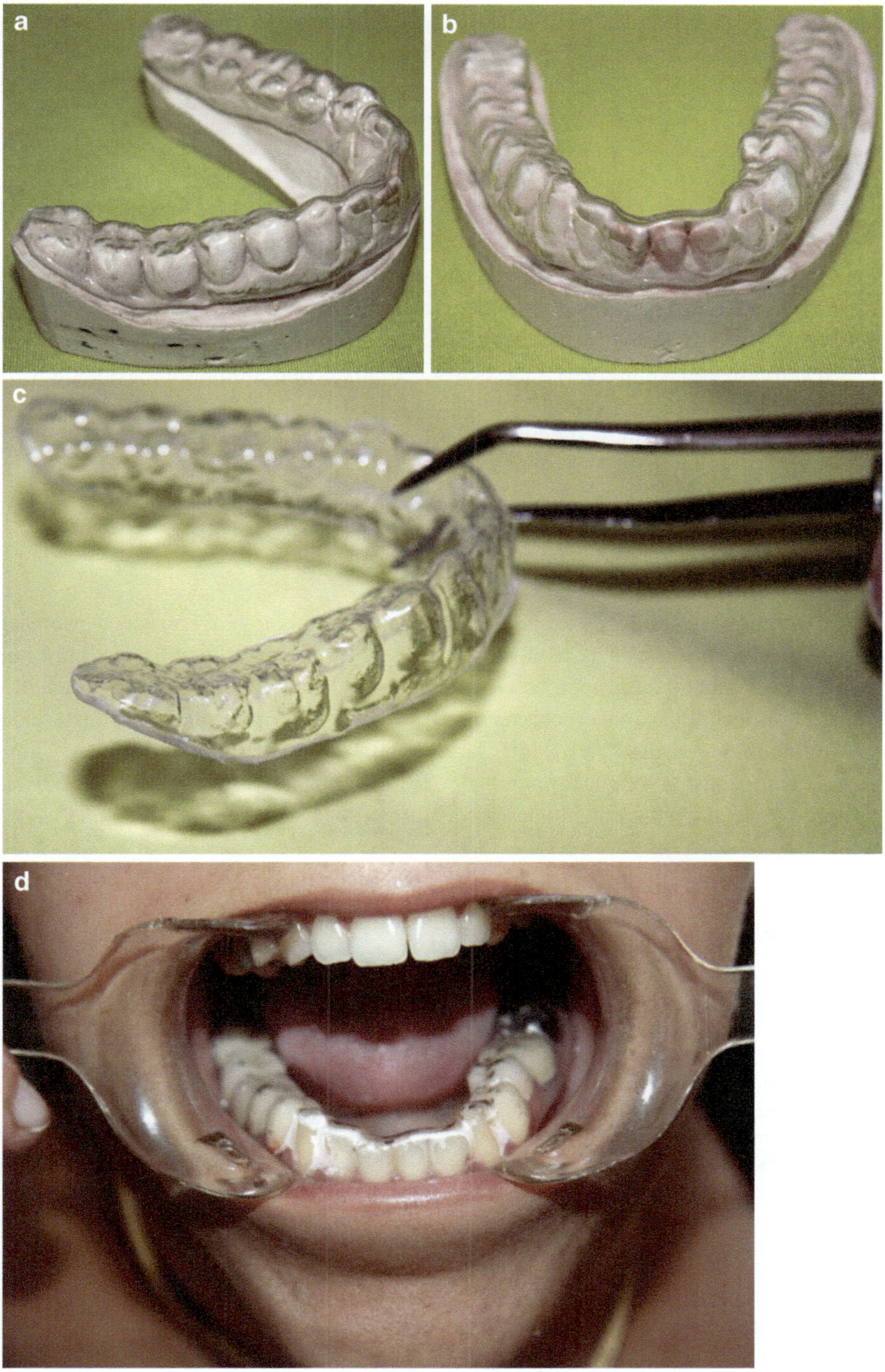

Fig. 2 (**a**–**d**) Occlusal mandibular soft splint

simple occlusal splint is not sufficient [58]. Certain experts consider splints as possible aggravating factors [27]. Negative effects on the cervical spine [54] and functional ventilation [9] have been observed. Some authors even referred to splints as *crutches* [11]. Splints have long been a major means of providing priceless helps to clinicians and patients, whereas many neuromuscular elements were still unknown. Nevertheless, in spite of their drawbacks, their use can be perfected. Splints could reach optimal effect when fitted after some weeks of Relaxing and Moderating Treatment (RMT) (see below). For instance, based on our personal experience, an interesting protocol may be used for better efficiency of splints without *splint dependence*. We advise to have the patient fitted after the fourth session of local anesthetic block (see below). Great results are also obtained if the patient has performed the *lips technique* conscientiously (see below). Dentists and stomatologists used to fit patients with occlusal splints only out of empiricism. Now they should really benefit when focusing on misjudged neurophysiologic laws.

Alternative Methods

Other techniques as biofeedback [14, 22], neuroreflexotherapy [4] have been evaluated to reduce myospasm and its outcomes. One method is to combine biofeedback and relaxation as a therapeutic approach to bruxism management [40]. Electroacupuncture stimulation techniques have been recommended to limit current use of nonsteroidal anti-inflammatory drugs (NSAI) [30], laser therapy [5, 7, 19], ultralow-frequency transcutaneous electrical neural stimulation [8, 29], and acupuncture [3, 13, 24, 51, 57] can successfully expand a number of combined protocols [46].

References

1. Agerberg G, Carlsson GE (1974) Late results of treatment of functional disorders of the masticatory system. J Oral Rehabil 1:309–316
2. Alajbeg IZ, Valentic-Peruzovic M, Alajbeg I, Illes D (2003) Influence of occlusal stabilization splint on the asymmetric activity of masticatory muscles in patients with temporomandibular dysfunction. Coll Antropol 27(1):361–371
3. Bergström I, List T, Magnusson T (2008) A follow-up study of subjective symptoms of temporomandibular disorders in patients who received acupuncture and/or interocclusal appliance therapy 18–20 years earlier. Acta Odontol Scand 66(2):88–92
4. Berguer A, Kovacs F, Abraira V et al (2007) Neuro-reflexotherapy for the management of myofascial temporomandibular joint pain: a double-blind, placebo-controlled, randomized clinical trial. J Oral Maxillofac Surg 66(8):1664–1677
5. Cetiner S, Kahraman SA, Yucetas S (2006) Evaluation of low-level laser therapy in the treatment of temporomandibular disorders. Photomed Laser Surg 24(5):637–641
6. Clark GT, Seligman DA, Solberg WK, Pullinger AG (1990) Guidelines for the treatment of temporomandibular disorders. J Craniomandib Disord 4:80–88
7. Conti PC (1997) Low level laser therapy in the treatment of temporomandibular disorders (TMD): a double-blind pilot study. Cranio 15(2):144–149

8. Cooper BC, Kleinberg I (2008) Establishment of a temporomandibular physiological state with neuromuscular orthosis treatment affects reduction of TMD symptoms in 313 patients. Cranio 26(2):104–117
9. Daly P, Preston CB, Evans WG (1982) Postural response of the head to bite opening in adult males. Am J Orthod 82:157–160
10. Dao TT, Lavigne GJ, Charbonneau A et al (1994) The efficacy of oral splints in the treatment of myofascial pain of the jaw muscles: a controlled clinical trial. Pain 56:85–94
11. Dao TT, Lavigne GJ (1998) Oral splints: the crutches for temporomandibular disorders and bruxism? Crit Rev Oral Biol Med 9(3):345–361
12. Dawson PE (1977) Les problèmes de l'occlusion. Evaluation diagnostique et traitement. In: Traduction de Perelmuter S, Liger F. J Prélat (éd), Paris
13. DeBar LL, Vuckovic N, Schneider J, Ritenbaugh C (2003) Use of complementary and alternative medicine for temporomandibular disorders. J Orofac Pain 217(3):224–236
14. Dohrmann RJ, Laskin DM (1978) An evaluation of electromyographic feedback in the treatment of myofascial pain-dysfunction syndrome. J Am Dent Assoc 96:656–662
15. Ekberg E, Vallon D, Nilner M (2003) The efficacy of appliance therapy in patients with temporomandibular disorders of mainly myogenous origin. A randomized, controlled, short-term trial. J Orofac Pain 17(2):133–139
16. Ekberg E, Nilner M (2004) Treatment outcome of appliance therapy in temporomandibular disorder patients with myofascial pain after 6 and 12 months. Acta Odontol Scand 62(6):343–349
17. Ekberg E, Nilner M (2006) Treatment outcome of short-and long-term appliance therapy in patients with TMD of myogenous origin and tension-type headache. J Oral Rehabil 33(10):713–721
18. Ferrario VF, Sforza C, Tartaglia GM, Dellavia C (2002) Immediate effect of a stabilization splint on masticatory muscle activity in temporomandibular disorder patients. J Oral Rehabil 29(9):810–815
19. Fikackova H, Dostalova T, Navratil L, Klaschka J (2007) Effectiveness of low-level laser therapy in temporomandibular joint disorders: a placebo-controlled study. Photomed Laser Surg 25(4):297–303
20. Fonder AC (1988) The dental distress syndrome (quantified). Quant Med 1:1
21. Gelb H (1977) Clinical management of head, neck and TMJ pain and dysfunction: a multi-disciplinary approach to diagnosis and treatment. WB Saunders Co (ed), Philadelphia/London/Toronto
22. Gessel AH (1975) Electromyographic biofeedback and tricyclic antidepressants in myofascial pain-dysfunction syndrome: psychological predictors outcome. J Am Dent Assoc 91:1048–1052
23. Glaros AG, Owais Z, Lausten L (2007) Reduction in parafunctional activity: a potential mechanism for the effectiveness of splint therapy. J Oral Rehabil 34(2):97–104
24. Goddard G (2005) Short term pain reduction with acupuncture treatment for chronic orofacial pain patients. Med Sci Monit 11(2):71–74
25. Green CS, Laskin DM (1972) Splint therapy for the myofascial pain dysfunction (MPSyndrome): a comparative study. J Am Dent Assoc 84:624–628
26. Holmgren K, Sheikholeslam A, Riise C (1993) Effect of a full-arch maxillary occlusal splint on parafunctional activity during sleep in patients with nocturnal bruxism and signs and symptoms of craniomandibular disorders. J Prosthet Dent 69:293–297
27. Jeanmonod A (1988) Occlusodontie. Applications cliniques. Cah Proth (éd), Paris
28. Johansson-Cahlin B, Samuelsson N, Dahlstrom L (2006) Utilization of pharmaceuticals among patients with temporomandibular disorders: a controlled study. Acta Odontol Scand 64(3):187–192
29. Kamyszek G, Ketcham R, Garcia R Jr, Radke J (2001) Electromyographic evidence of reduced muscle activity when ULF-TENS is applied to the Vth and VIIth cranial nerves. Cranio 19(3):162–168
30. Kim K, Lee KY, Kim KS (2000) A comparative study of muscle relaxation appliance therapy, electroacupuncture stimulation therapy, and pharmacological therapy for masticatory muscle disorders. J Orofac Pain Abstract 14, 3:11

31. Kobayashi Y, Ishikawa T, Itoh Y (1986) The influence of psychosomatic aspects on the E.M.G. silent period. J Dent Res Abstract 65, 143:741
32. Kuttila M, Le Bell Y, Savolainen-Niemi E et al (2002) Efficiency of occlusal appliance therapy in secondary otalgia and temporomandibular disorders. Acta Odontol Scand 260(4):248–254
33. Lerman MD (1987) The hydrostatic splint: new muscle-directed TMJ-PDS treatment technique. CDS Rev 80(4):31–34
34. Mc Carroll RS, Naeije M, Kim YK, Hansson TL (1989) Short-term effect of a stabilization splint on the asymmetry of submaximal masticatory muscle activity. J Oral Rehabil 16(2):171–176
35. Mohl ND, Zarb GA, Carlsson GE, Rugh JD (1988) A textbook of occlusion. Quintes Pub Co Inc, Chicago
36. Morgan DH, Hall WP, Vanwas SJ (1977) Diseases of the temporomandibular apparatus. CV Mosby Co (ed), St Louis
37. Ogus HD, Toller PA (1981) Common disorders of temporomandibular joint. J Wright & Sons Limited (ed), Bristol
38. Okesson JP (1989) Management of temporomandibular disorders and occlusion. CV Mosby Co (ed), St Louis
39. Pierce CJ, Gale EN (1988) A comparison of different treatments for nocturnal bruxism. J Dent Res 67:597–601
40. Pourre F, Lubespere A, Albaret JM, Lubespere R (1986) Intérêt d'une approche comportementale du bruxisme: aspects théoriques et perspectives thérapeutiques. Cah Proth 53:109–131
41. Quayle AA, Gray RJ, Metcalfe RJ et al (1990) Soft occlusal splint therapy in the treatment of migraine and other headaches. J Dent 18(3):123–129
42. Raphael KG, Marbach JJ, Klausner JJ et al (2003) Is bruxism severity a predictor of oral splint efficacy in patients with myofascial face pain? J Oral Rehabil 30(1):17–29
43. Rugh JD, Johnson RW (1984) Vertical dimension discrepancies and masticatory pain-dysfunction. In: Solberg WK, Clark GT (eds) Abnormal jaw mechanics: diagnosis and treatment. Quintes Pub Co Inc, Chicago, p 117
44. Santander H, Miralles R, Jimenez A et al (1994) Influence of stabilization occlusal splint on cranio-cervical relationship. Part II: electromyographic analysis. Cranio 12:227–233
45. Satoh T, Hadara Y (1973) Electrophysiological study on tooth-grinding during sleep. Electroencephalogr Clin Neurophysiol 35:267–275
46. Schneider J, Vuckovic N, DeBar L (2003) Willingness to participate in complementary and alternative medicine clinical trials among patients with craniofacial disorders. J Altern Complement Med 9(3):389–401
47. Schokker RP, Hanson TL, Ansink Ben JJ (1990) The result of treatment of the masticatory system of chronic headache patients. J Craniomandib Disord 4:126–130
48. Shimshak DG, Kent RL, DeFuria M (1997) Medical claims profiles of subjects with temporomandibular joint disorders. Cranio 15:150–158
49. Shimshak DG, De Furia MC (1998) Health care utilization by patients with temporomandibular joint disorders. Cranio 16(3):185–193
50. Slavicek R (1983) Les principes de l'occlusion. Rev Orthop Dent Fac 17:449–490
51. Smith P, Mosscrop D, Davies S et al (2007) The efficacy of acupuncture in the treatment of temporomandibular joint myofascial pain: a randomised controlled trial. J Dent 35(3):259–267
52. Taddey JJ (1990) Rationale for sequential use of both maxillary and mandibular orthopedic appliances in the treatment of TMJ disorders. J Craniomandib Disord 4:273–275
53. Turk DC, Rudy TE, Kubinski A, Zaki HS, Greco CM (1996) Dysfunctional patients with temporomandibular disorders: evaluating the efficacy of a tailored treatment protocol. J Consult Clin Psychol 64(1):139–146
54. Urbanowicz M (1987) Alteration of vertical dimension and its effect on head and neck posture. Cranio 5:51–53
55. Whinery J (1990) Anomalie de la posture mandibulaire. Clin Odont 4:281–286

56. Wilkinson T, Hansson TL, Mc Neil C (1992) A comparison of the success of 24-hour occlusal splint therapy versus nocturnal occlusal splint therapy in reducing craniomandibular disorders. J Craniomandib Disord 6:64–70
57. Wong YK, Cheng J (2003) A case series of temporomandibular disorders treated with acupuncture, occlusal splint and point injection therapy. Acupunct Med 21(4):138–149
58. Yatani H, Minakuchi H, Matsuka Y et al (1998) The long-term effect of occlusal therapy on self-administered treatment outcomes of TMD. J Orofac Pain 12:75–88

Objectives

The therapeutic objectives defined in this book remain centered on *counteracting spastic conditions in stomatognathic muscles*. This means both excessive central inputs from the brain and excessive afferents from trigeminal receptors. Hence, an interceptive, specific, and early therapeutic objective is to reach both myorelaxation and moderation of these abnormal inputs. Early diagnosis and basic treatments evidently decrease the risks of aggravating TMD chronic conditions [4, 13] even though those often need active long-lasting management in some patients. Many different factors – central and/or peripheral – can combine to trigger the disease. But an accurate evaluation remains very difficult. What should be treated first? What signs are secondary – even insignificant enough to be neglected? Yet, in this confused clinical picture, an oral parafunctional habit is still too often misunderstood: **severe teeth clenching**. While it is expressed through complex harmful behavior, it can be diagnosed early and eliminated rapidly and successfully by treatment. It seems as a *Gordian knot* to be mainly sliced through (Fig. 1). In some clinical cases, the interruption of this parafunctional habit alone decreased, even stopped several painful symptoms. Therefore, the primary objective of an appropriate treatment must be global relaxation of the stomatognathic muscles involved in clenching, that is, the jaw-closing muscles. This helps break up the spastic circle between muscles and CNS [1, 6].

Spastic conditions always make exact diagnoses about possible peripheral factors more difficult. Dental malocclusion or postural problems are harder to evaluate accurately. Moreover spasticity still upsets physical, osteopathic, or chiropractic treatments[1]. Sedative treatments, if successful at first, often lead to relapse. So *breaking off the stomatognathic β–γ loop is the first step* in therapeutic procedures[2].

[1]Dental surgeons are advised that early myorelaxation combined with exercise contributes to restoring the harmonious function of stomatognathic muscles, which is essential to allow occlusal recording and rehabilitation [12]. A study in rats showed that occlusal disharmony was a factor for chronic stress. So dentist surgeons have to be aware that an overocclusion could elicite severe central neurobiological perturbances (high rate of stress neuromediators) to delay even for a long time.

[2]This should be followed by a useful intermediate step before occlusal or prosthetic rehabilitation, consisting in a retro-incisor occlusal plan used as an individual pattern [5].

F. Hartmann, G. Cucchi, *Stress and Orality*,
DOI 10.1007/978-2-8178-0271-8_14, © Springer-Verlag France 2014

In a second phase, the *causal factors* (peripheral and/or central) will be easily evaluated and eliminated by adapted methodical responses (Fig. 2). Ancient Romans used to teach *Causa oblata, tollitur effectus*[3]. This helps decrease the risks of relapse. Another positive factor is that the patient's spirits are raised as treatment quickly reduces and even eliminates some symptoms. We decided to call our method as **Relaxing and Moderating Treatment** (RMT). Figure 3 presents the RMT three combined therapeutic actions: towards sensory inputs, motor inputs, and central spastic factors. In some clinical cases, stomatognathic spasticity management can be complemented by a procedure based on appropriate postural methods.[4]

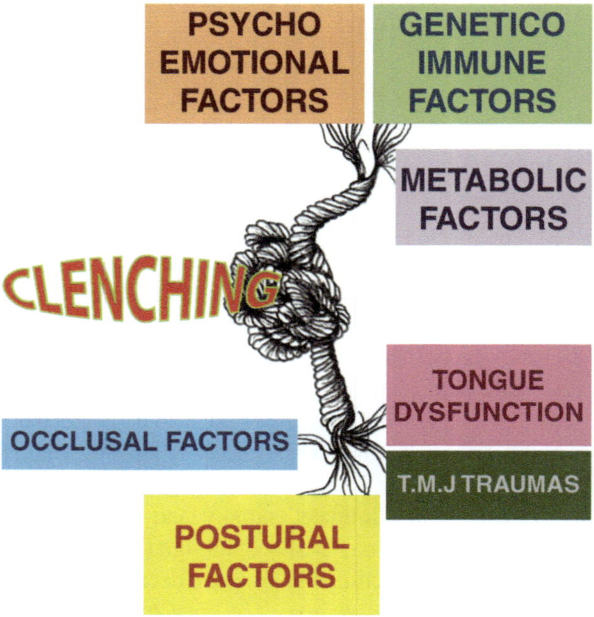

Fig. 1 Clenching as a *Gordian knot*

[3]"As the cause is removed, the effect disappears."

[4]This issue is not dealt with here. The reader can refer to specialized publications [2, 3, 7–11].

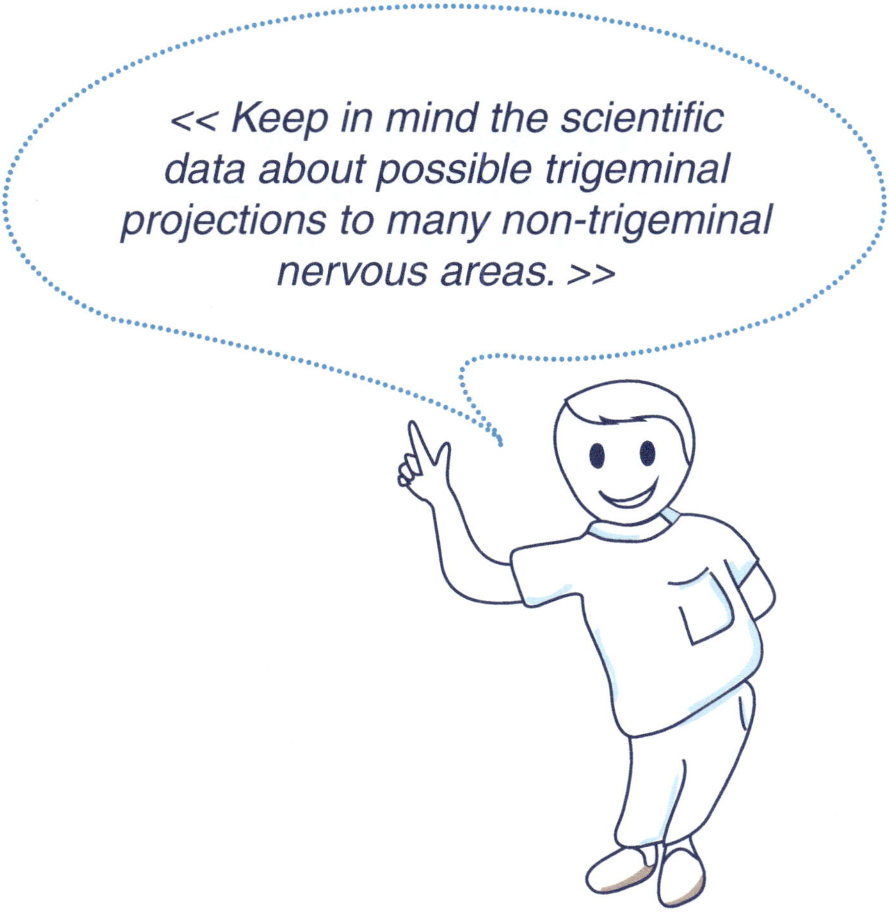
<< Keep in mind the scientific
data about possible trigeminal
projections to many non-trigeminal
nervous areas. >>

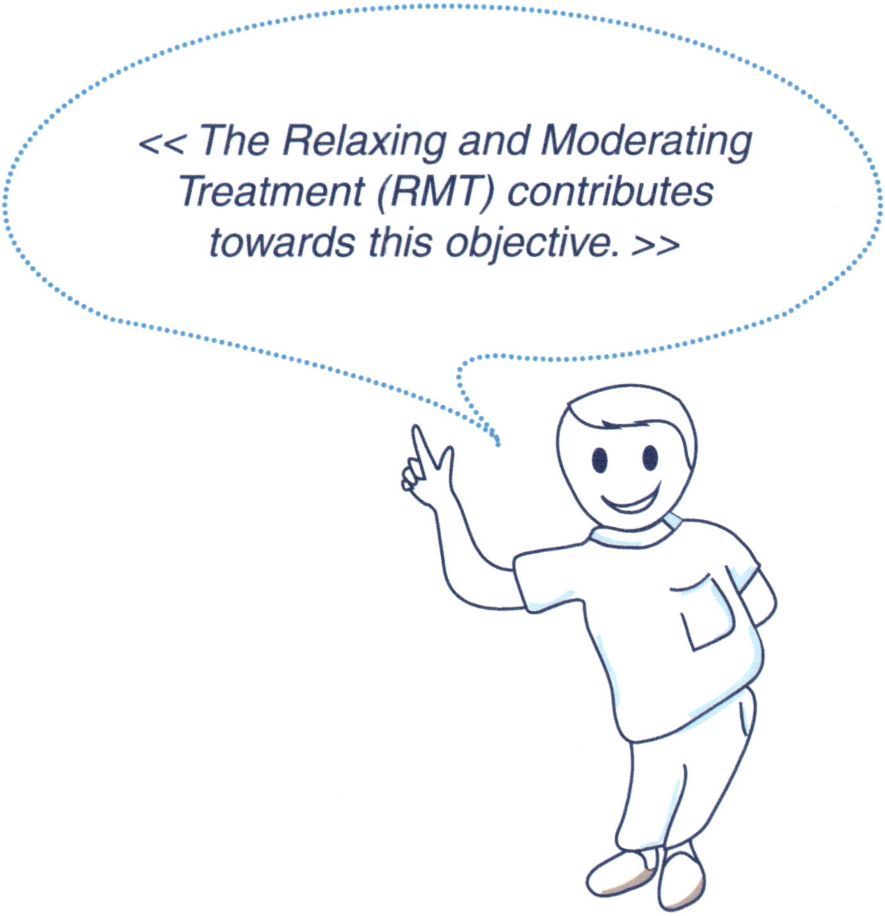
<< The Relaxing and Moderating Treatment (RMT) contributes towards this objective. >>

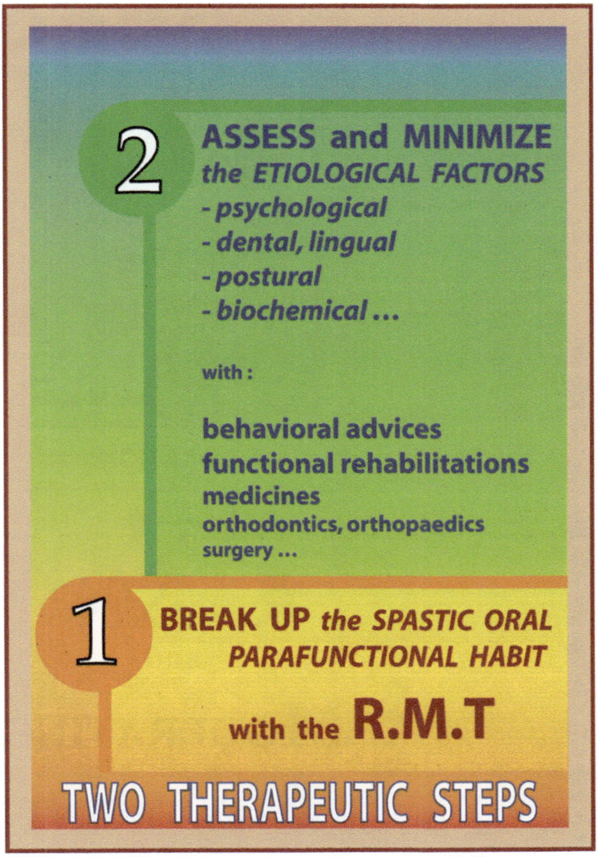

Fig. 2 The *two-step* therapeutic procedure

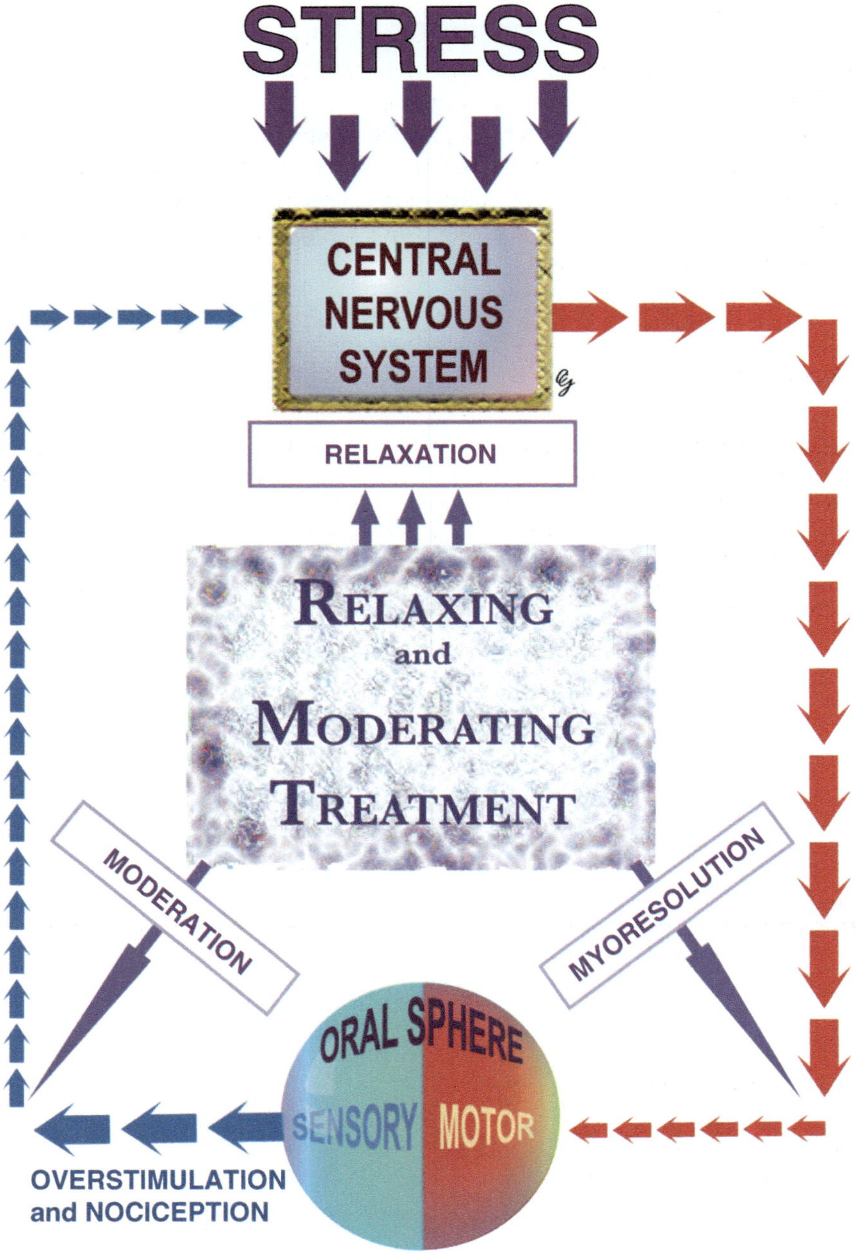

Fig. 3 The Relaxing and Moderating Treatment. The RMT has a triple action: on the central nervous system and psycho-emotional factors (through general relaxation), on the peripheral motor side and its spastic conditions (through local myoresolution), on the peripheral sensory side and its overstimulation and nociception (through moderating influence)

References

1. Beard CC, Clayton JA (1980) Effects of occlusal splint therapy on TMJ dysfunction. J Prosthet Dent 44:324–335
2. Clauzade M, Darraillans B (1992) L'homme, le crâne, les dents. SEOO (éd), Perpignan, 163p
3. Clauzade M, Marty J-P (1998) Orthoposturodontie. SEOO (éd), Perpignan, 214p
4. Epker J, Gatchel RJ, Ellis E (1999) A model for predicting chronic TMD: practical application in clinical settings. J Am Dent Assoc 10:1470–1475
5. Jeanmonod A (1988) Occlusodontie. Applications cliniques. Cah Proth (éd), Paris
6. Krogh-Poulsen WG (1979) Examen et diagnostic des troubles du système manducateur. Encycl Médic Chir, Paris, Stomato 22030 G10
7. Makofsky H, August B, Ekkis J (1989) A multidisciplinary approach to the evaluation and treatment of temporomandibular joint and cervical spine dysfunction. Cranio 7(3):205–213
8. Mohl ND (1976) Head posture and its role in occlusion. N Y State Dent J 42:17–23
9. Nahmani L, Amiel M, Casteyde JP et al (1990) Kinésiologie, Théorie et Pratique. Comedent (éd), Paris
10. Nahmani L, Zarrinpour A, Lumbroso C (1995) La mise en articulateur selon le concept posturo-kinésiologique. Orthod Franç 66:605–626
11. Servière F (1989) L'examen postural en exodontie quotidienne. Cah Proth 65:36–42
12. Steed PA (2004) The longevity of temporomandibular disorder improvements after active treatment modalities. Cranio 22(2):110–114
13. Syrop SB (2002) Initial management of temporomandibular disorders. Dent Today 21(8):52–57

The Relaxing and Moderating Treatment (RMT)

Classic anti-inflammatory drugs treat muscle tissue inflammation locally but often prove ineffective against muscular spasticity and its tenacious outcomes, that is, **referred pain** [3]. To the contrary, through the use of local anesthetics and myorelaxant drugs [14, 46, 47, 50, 98], the RMT directly regulates the important β–γ-loop. Stomatognathic muscular spasticity imposes repeated traumatic forces on articular tissues, under a central factor [78, 91]. The RMT facilitates diagnosis and management of peripheral factors which contribute to myo-articular disorders. What's more, the outcome of pain to the brain (central sensitization) stimulates the interception of these nociceptive inputs while blocking the periphery repeatedly with anesthetics [87]. Figure 1 is a schematic view of the different therapeutic tools according to many levels that are implicated in TMD. The work of the RMT affects both the peripheral side (sensory and motor) and the central side (relaxation to eliminate stressing psycho-emotional factors) (Fig. 2).

1 Local Procedures

Travell [104] was probably the first clinician to bring medical attention to anesthetic[1] procedures (procaine)[2] for local treatment of spasmed muscles [105]. The value of repeated local anesthetic injections is supported by some studies with significant continual decrement in muscle sensitivity to pressure testing (algometer) [69]. Such

[1]Long mistrusted, anesthetics began to attract a number of clinicians [1, 7, 37, 41, 46, 47, 65, 74, 79, 81, 92]. Injection of bupivacaine 0.5 % or etidocaine 2 % in painful muscles [41, 43] has a long-lasting sedative effect on craniofacial pain, while the physiological serum has only a transitory effect.

[2]Today a molecule with amine function is preferred for its minor allergic risk: 2 or 3 % lidocaine (or lignocaine) and 3 % mepivacaine. However, whatever the molecule, an associated vasoconstrictor remains absolutely contraindicated. In effect, any vasoconstrictor interferes with a relaxation objective because muscular tissue is injured by an ischemic and anoxic phenomenon [26, 64, 73, 100].

F. Hartmann, G. Cucchi, *Stress and Orality*,
DOI 10.1007/978-2-8178-0271-8_15, © Springer-Verlag France 2014

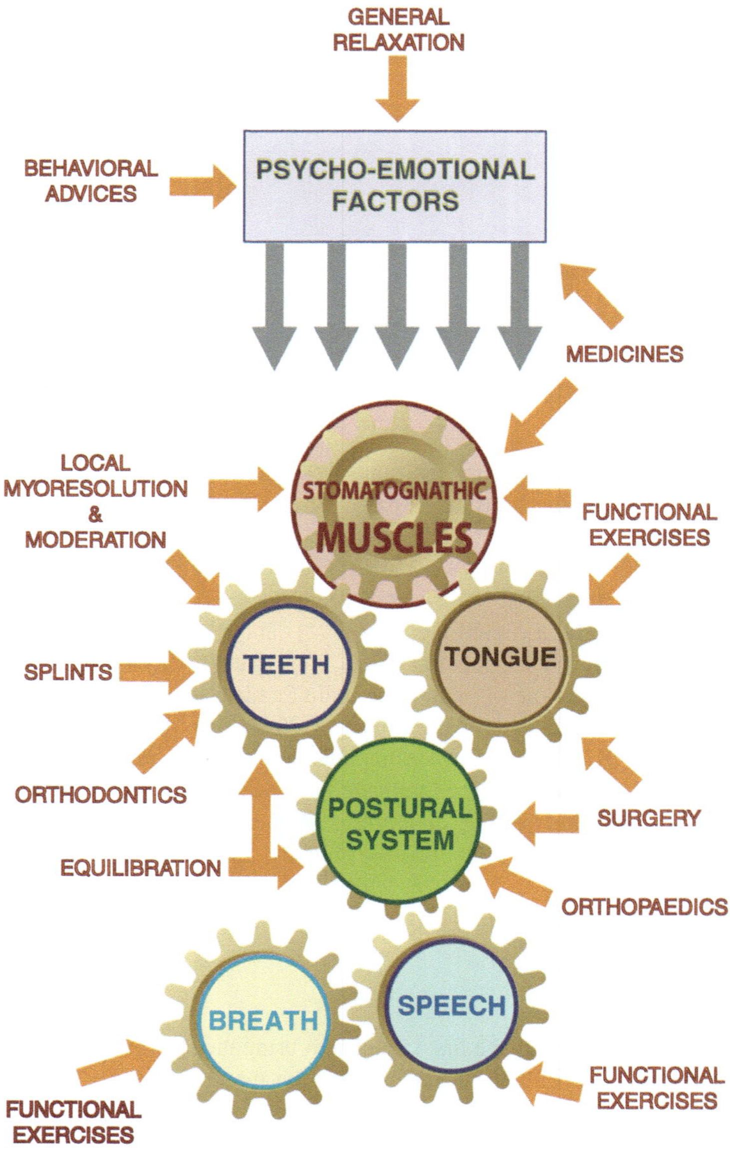

Fig. 1 Different tools for treating several implicated levels in TMD

principle can also constitute a diagnostic evaluation method of the neuromuscular origin of pain [3, 7]. Local block can directly affect the TMJ [99] with a sedative action on head and neck pain [21, 58]. However, this kind of injection must be reserved to extremely acute pain for which classic procedures have failed [110]. Previous studies have discussed results of sphenopalatine ganglion blocks [27, 54, 56, 84] or cervical sympathetic gg. blocks (such as the stellate gg.) [61] to manage orofacial pain.

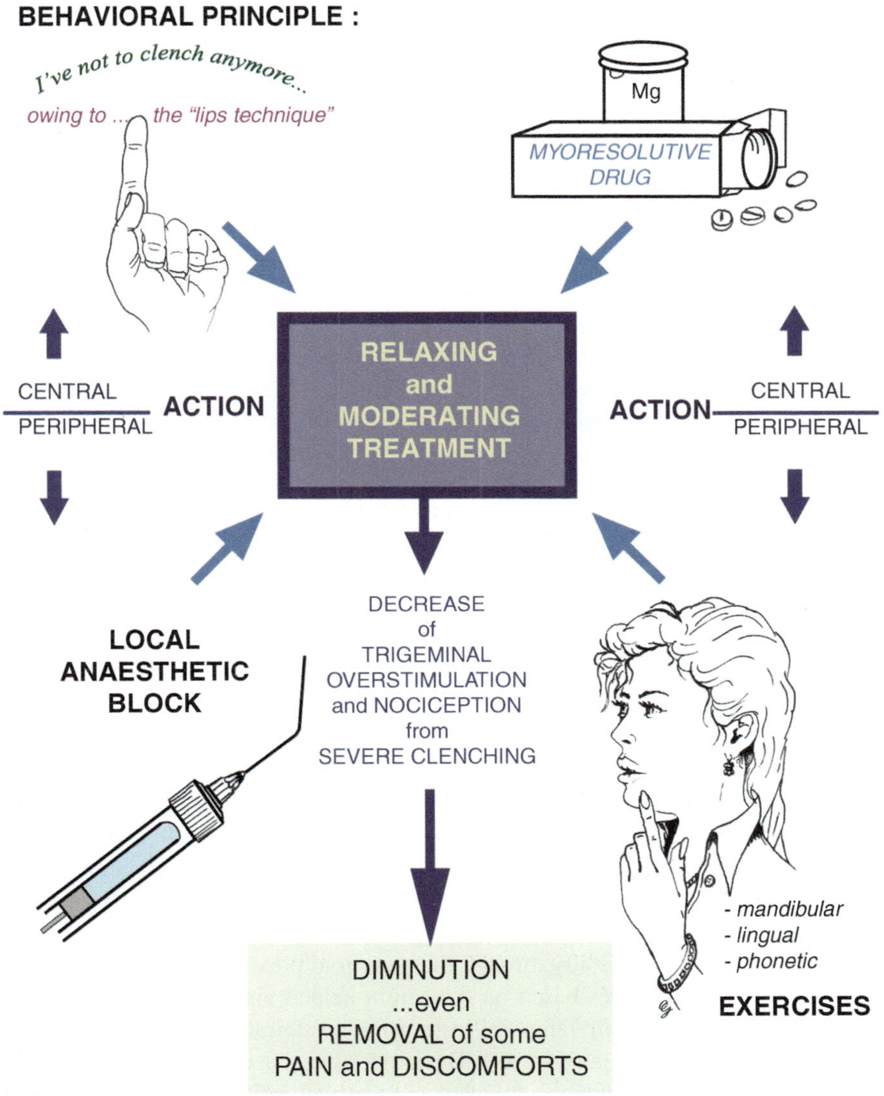

Fig. 2 Therapeutic tools of the RMT

There may also be similar anesthetic improvements in the otic gg. when are injected in the fossa infratemporalis. Thus, positive results on cases of migraines may be explained by this protocol. As the major nerve in the oral sphere, the V is largely involved in TMD with some repercussions to other nervous territories. The classic Slüder syndrome could be updated. In these conditions, clinicians should no longer be surprised to observe the *impact of local blocks on areas distant from the oral sphere* such as the neck, shoulder, arm, and loins. That is true also of certain symptoms such as chronic hiccup, bronchospasm, and dysmenorrhea. One must keep in mind some obvious precautions in using local anesthetics. A questionnaire must investigate about previous allergic events and current drug prescription which might interfere with anesthetics[3]. Furthermore, the individual's receptivity to any chemical substance requires a great deal of vigilance from clinicians. One patient's reaction may be stronger than another's, no matter how low the dose of local anesthetics without vasoconstrictor, that is, one regular dose on each side. In most cases, the use of only two doses during a clinical session at the rate of one session a week protects against neurological toxicity by chemical overdosing. As for the risk of infection, it is nonexistent as long as bad oral hygiene is totally avoided. Finally, it is a fact that once opened, anesthetic vials can never be reused in other sessions, even on the same patient.

Since 1980s, neurologic experts have used botulinum toxin to treat some ailments such as orofacial dystonia or spasms or chronic [4, 8, 13, 28, 52, 53, 55, 93, 94, 97, 102, 108, 109]. The hypotonic results following local injection prompted some ENT specialists and dentists to use this toxin in TMD therapeutic procedures [55]. It is also recommended to stop bruxism following anoxic brain injury [52]; a case of a patient who received this therapy in both the right and left lower heads of the LPMs was reported [106]. This approach to research should be envisaged because any myorelaxant tool is much appreciated.

1.1 Technical Methods

First and foremost, all clinicians must be aware of one peculiarity: the following technique is not similar to the classic external way used by specialists for alcohol destruction of V3 fibers in the treatment of trigeminal neuralgia. In that case, the spindle must enter into the foramen ovale to ensure the perforation of the V3 going across. Of course, the RMT objectives are totally different. The fossa infratemporalis would be a very important zone with regard to cranio-maxillomandibular morphogenesis [24, 51], especially through the pterygoid plexus which covers the top of this fossa. Some studies based on dissection helped visualize the long needle orientation for reaching infratemporal fossa using this intraoral way[4], that is, a rear lateral line towards the tragus [48, 49]. The major objective remains the injection of anesthetics into the *infratemporal fossa* which is hermetically closed [62]. One must approach the inferior belly of LPMs on its lateral lower side to avoid injury to the internal maxillary artery or the nearby deep pterygoid venous plexus. This plexus has close connections with the medial carotid plexus and cavernous sinus. Any block in this zone can diffuse anesthetics into the brain vascular circulation through

[3]For instance, there is danger in associating anesthetics with a β-blocking treatment. There is fundamental incompatibility with antiarrhythmics (tocainide, β-lytic, digitalin, etc.). Other interactions with antimyasthenics can cancel their therapeutic effects.

[4]At any rate, clinicians must keep in mind that disparities do exist between patients in morphology and size.

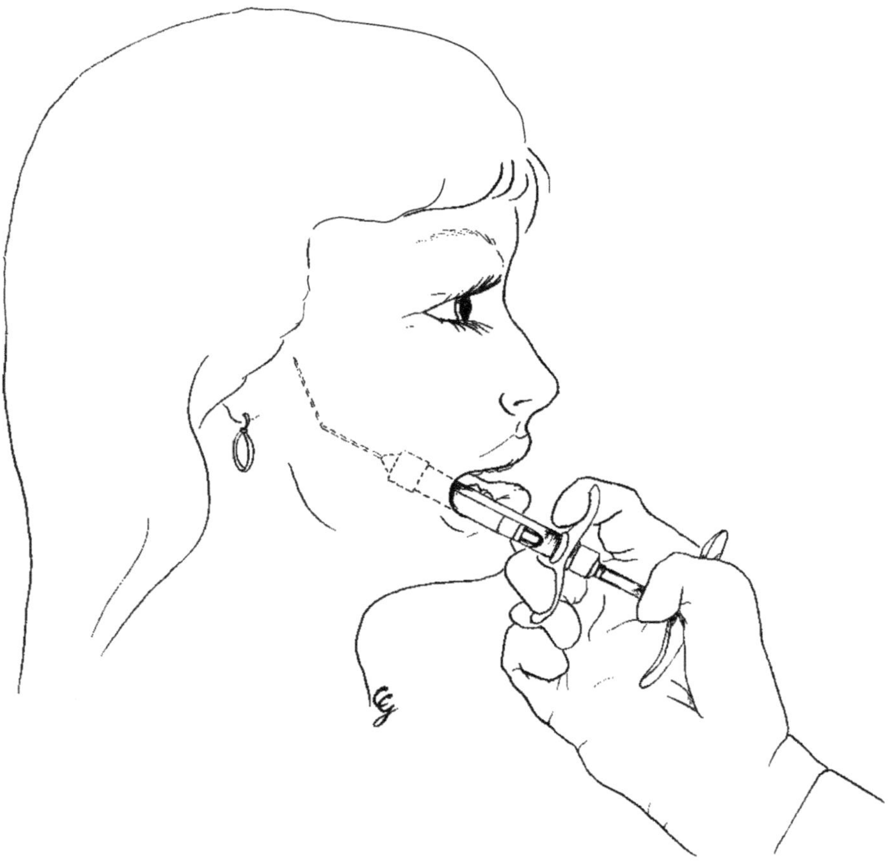

Fig. 3 Anesthetic block inserted into the fossa infratemporalis when using an intraoral way (lateral view). To facilitate the placing of the syringe and needle into the fossa infratemporalis, the clinician may ask the patient to close his mouth halfway and slightly lower his mandible on the side to be injected

the skull's base holes and cause strange feelings or light dizziness to the patient. Furthermore, if the needle's penetration is too high or too medial, close to the base of the skull, the risk of injury to the trunk of V3 with dilacerations of nervous fibers is very high (see the inappropriate ways as red draws in Figs. 3 and 4). Such an event could bring on incoercible iatrogenic neuralgia. Finally, if a needle's direction is too anterior and medial (towards the retrotuberositar zone), it can be painful and ineffective. Three technical points must be underscored. Prior to the injection, practitioners must disinfect the retrotuberositar zone where the needle will penetrate into the mucosa[5]. The anesthetic liquid must be warmed and slowly injected. The needle must progress without resistance which would be a sign of wrong modality. If these

[5]Disinfectant containing heavy metal must be eliminated due to local risks of irritation and edema.

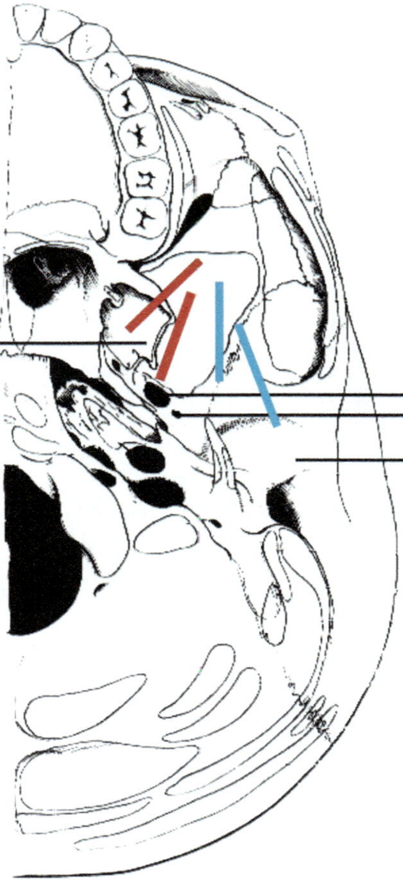

Fig. 4 Anesthetic block inserted into the fossa infratemporalis when using an intraoral way (inferior view). Needle directions: *blue draws* correct ways, *red draw* inaccurate way

instructions are followed, the technique proves painless. The intraoral technique is illustrated in Figs. 3, 4, 5, 6, 7, 8, 9, 10, and 11. Therapeutic results are conditioned by two constraints. The first one is the bilateral injection relating to the physiology of the *stomatognathic muscles-TMJ* functional set. For instance the two LPMs and the contiguous articular structures work simultaneously on the right and left sides during all jaw movements. The block minimizes the clenching tendency, inasmuch as this action involves both right and left muscles (bilateral injections). The second constraint is the need for a minimum **8 weeks of sessions**. In these conditions repeated local infiltrations (1 session a week) significantly help the symptoms attenuate and reduce the frequency and intensity of pain. In some rare cases where patients experience severe pain, a treatment with 2 sessions a week may be necessary to manage painful symptoms.

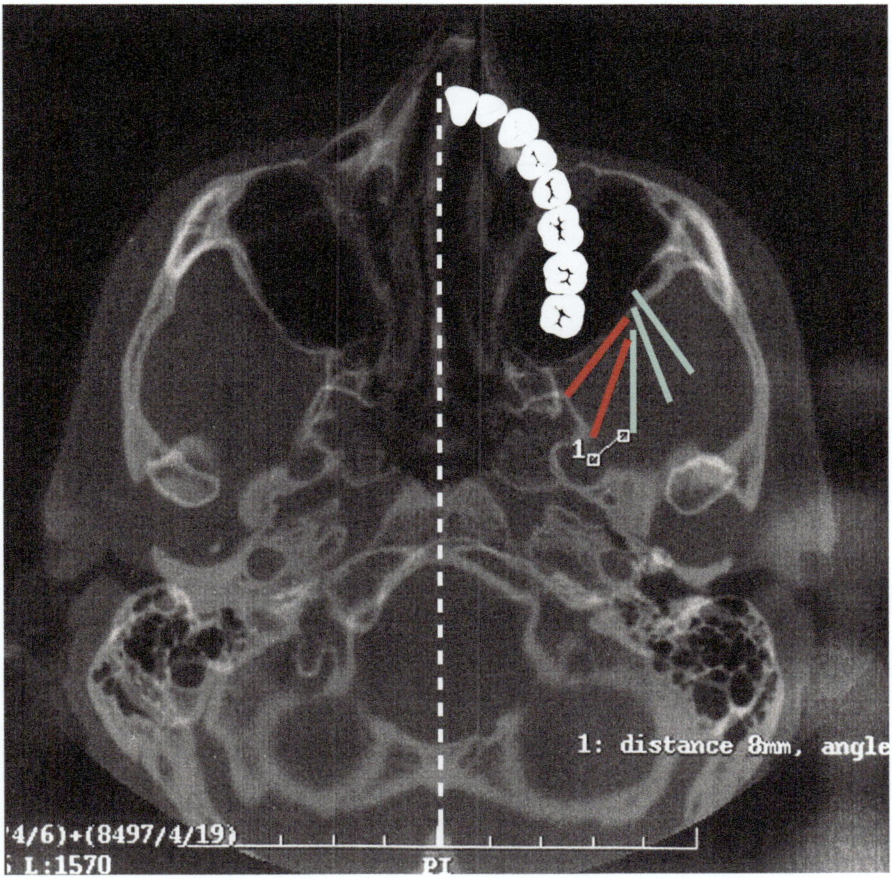

Fig. 5 Correct ways (*blue draws*) and inaccurate ways (*red draws*) of the needle as shown on a scanner view. *1* foramen ovale. On this shot the tip of the needle comes within 8 mm of the foramen ovale: this is the furthest point the needle can reach for a safe injection. For easier view, the upper dental arch was drawn in projection in an approximate position

1.2 *Possible Actions*

One must keep in mind that the V3 is the only branch of V with both sensitive and motor inputs. Anatomical and physiological data can explain how the LPMs retain a strategic role in jaw dynamic actions. Therefore, in pathophysiological conditions, this muscle is perhaps a weak element in the stomatognathic system. Now the exact action mode of the liquid still remains unknown[6]. Close functional relationships

[6]One may imagine combining the anesthetic liquid with a radio-opaque substance to identify it precisely in the radiological status. Inversely this protocol may not be appropriate to track the anesthetic liquid for the next hours or days, because of possible variation in the mixture viscosity.

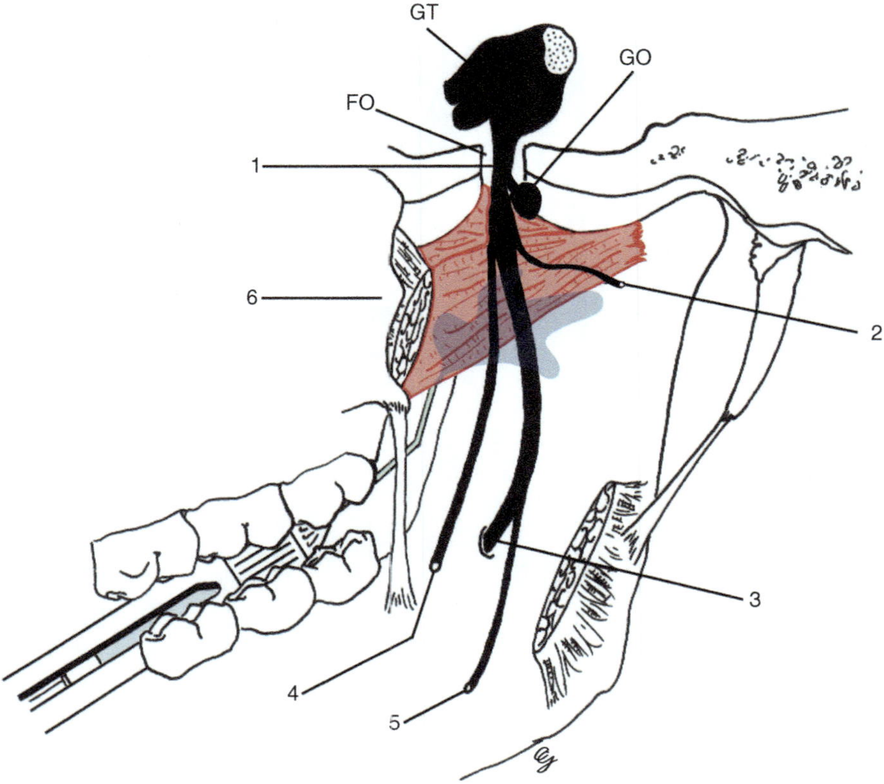

Fig. 6 Anesthetic block inserted into the fossa infratemporalis when using an intraoral way (internal view). *FO* foramen ovale, *GT* ganglion trigeminale, *GO* ganglion oticus. *1* nervus mandibularis, *2* nervus auriculo-temporalis, *3* nervus alveolaris inferior, *4* nervus lingualis, *5* nervus musculi mylohyoidei, 6 apophysa pterygoidea

between LPMs and TMJ are well known [15, 36]. But a dual diffusion towards LPM and V3 is perfectly conceivable. Apart from a direct myorelaxant effect on LPM, we may theorize that the blocking action also works at moderating *both the afferent and efferent inputs of the stomatognathic muscles*. It may affect those innervated by V3 which goes across the infratemporal fossa, particularly jaw-closing muscles (masseter, temporal, lateral, and medial pterygoid m.) but also the TT, TVP, mylohyoidean and digastric muscles. As regards some of these muscles, we may reflect on possible therapeutic actions against symptoms such as craniofacial and suprahyoid pain, nausea, vomiting, and tinnitus[7]. Progressive relaxation of jaw-closing muscles comes with the patient's awareness of the deleterious dimension of

[7]About tinnitus, both Relaxing and Moderating Treatment (RMT) and awareness of clenching give good results in managing some cases of tinnitus such as buzzing caused by trigeminal dysfunction; but patients who complain about whistling must be informed that this treatment is noneffective for this particular symptom.

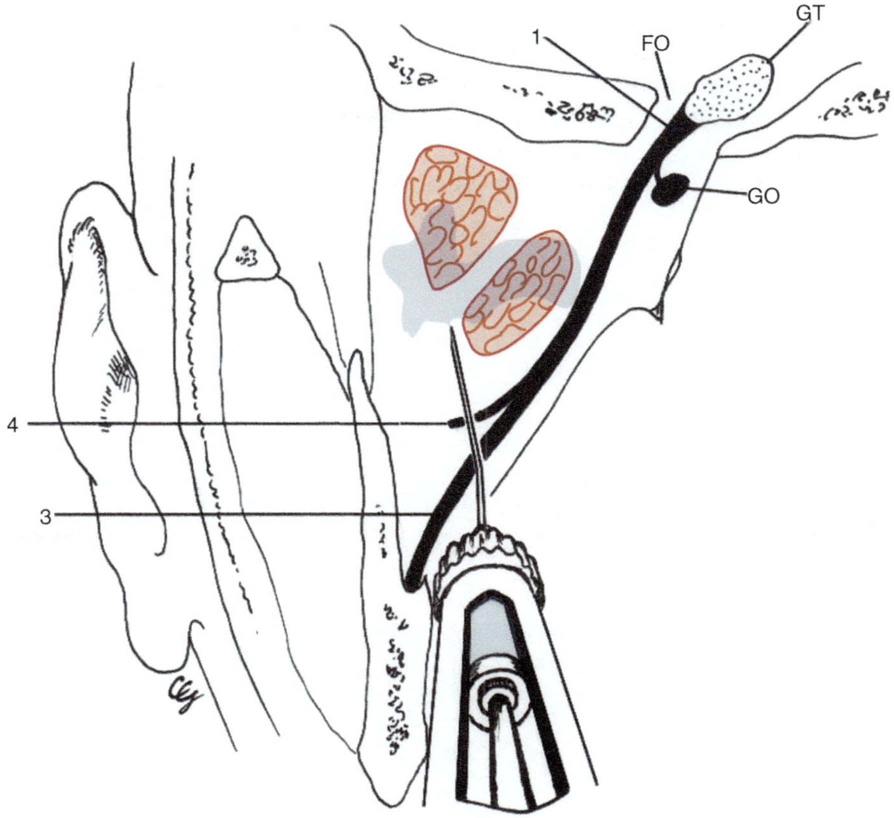

Fig. 7 Anesthetic block inserted into the fossa infratemporalis when using an intraoral way (frontal view). Position of a curved needle for injecting into the infratemporal fossa. The needle should be directed vertically or towards the outside so as not to reach the neurovascular plexus pterygoideus or arteria pterygoidea. *FO* foramen ovale, *GT* ganglion trigeminale, *GO* ganglion oticus. *1* nervus mandibularis, *3* nervus alveolaris inferior, *4* nervus lingualis

parafunctional clenching. The diffusion of the anesthetic molecule can benefit two therapeutic components. The first one is the *immediate relaxing effect* on V3 afferent and efferent inputs. The second one is a *residual effect* which goes far beyond the first effect. It may come from a myorelaxant and moderating action on neuromuscular circuits. This second effect should be reinforced by functional lingual, mandibular, and phonetic exercises. What's more, if other mandibular inputs (periodontal, articular, mucosal, etc.) are involved in trigeminal overstimulation, the block may also involve them in its moderating action. However, it seems that there is no immediate intensive block of sensitivity such as the earlier occurrence in a regional block because sensitive perception remains in the V3 areas. Some patients just complain about impaired mastication when the injection is given less than 2 h before a meal. This tends to confirm the blocking action on PLMs which are largely implicated in all masticatory movements. Moreover injections do not fully interrupt motor activity. To complete the myorelaxant effect of the block, we recommend

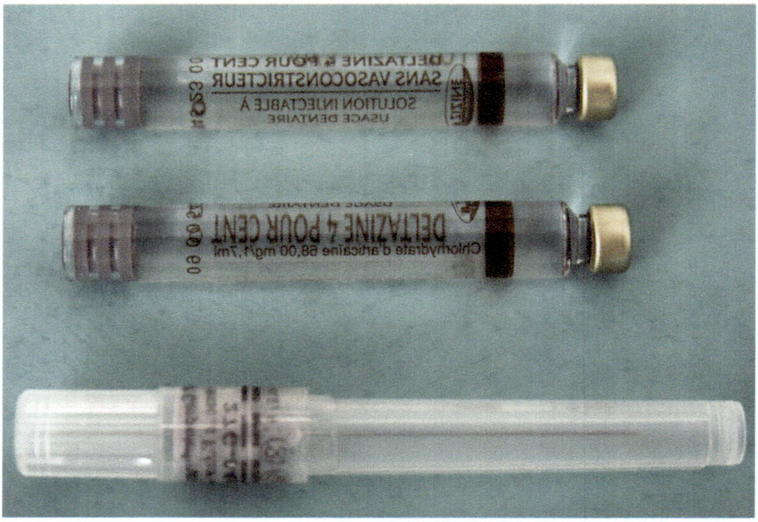

Fig. 8 Needle (long model) and anesthetic doses without vasoconstrictor

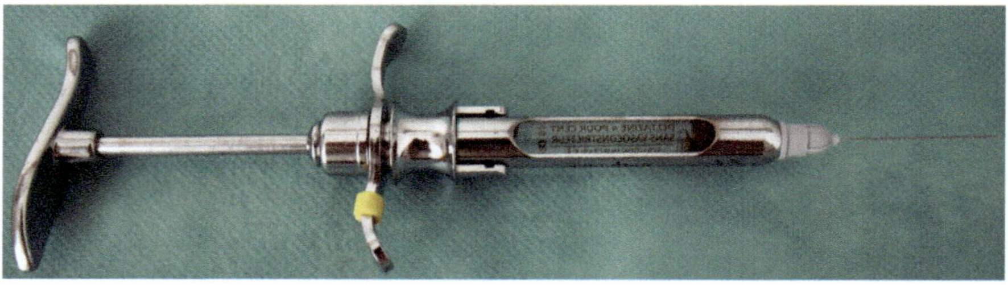

Fig. 9 A long needle when set on its syringe

using the Cyriax technique, that is, *short intraoral massages of the LPMs* [20][8]. Several beneficial effects have been reported [6] particularly on TMJ cracking and pain. Some questions remain unanswered: does the anesthetic liquid stay in the fossa after the injection and how long? How does it work to reduce or release some symptoms, especially those which are linked to non-trigeminal structures? Generally speaking, how long does this local procedure contribute to a therapeutic action against TMD in terms of awareness of parafunctional oral habits and behavioral suggestions to stop clenching habits? Since the 1950s Travell has been recommending an external technique referred to as *stretch and spray* [105]. The value of this technique as a complement of intraoral block seems to be supported by thermographic studies [85]. While this *stretch and spray* technique must be performed by

[8] As written in the Part I (chapter "Objective Signs"), the direct digital contact with the PLMs is real [6].

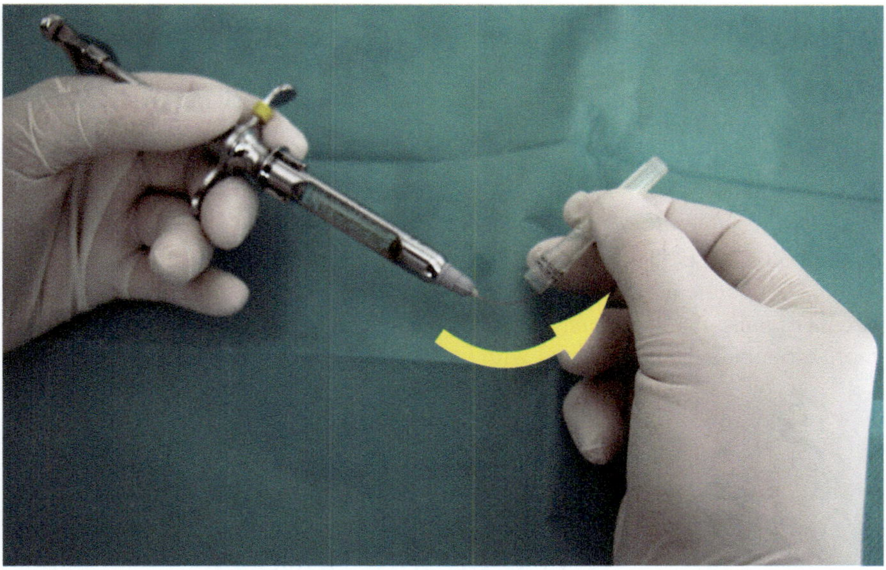

Fig. 10 How to curve the long needle with its own sterile cap

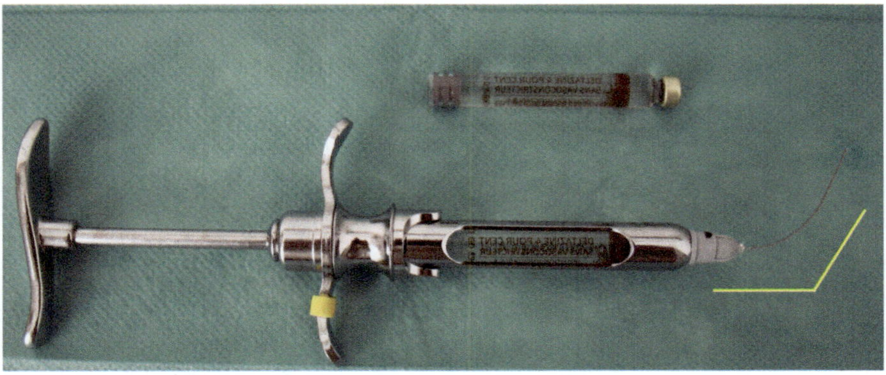

Fig. 11 The final result: about a 45° angle

a clinician, another local myorelaxant technique can be used at home by patients: long application of hot cloth pads on superficial muscles such as the masseteris, SCM, and trapezius several times a day. More recently clinicians have been advised to use locally a topical cream for TMJ and afflicted stomatognathic muscles. It contains zinc and copper, whose anti-inflammatory and myorelaxant properties are well known [60]. Massages and IR rays performed locally also relax spasmed muscles. All these easy techniques should really be considered by clinicians before they engage in more complex procedures [88].

2 Functional Exercises

A myorelaxant prescription can never go without functional exercise [14, 18, 29, 37, 42, 57, 63, 68, 70, 74, 77, 78, 80, 86, 113] since regular exercise has a great value in reducing the inflammatory process [83]. Therefore, patients must engage in daily jaw exercises to help their stomatognathic muscles regain their physiological tone. We recommend two sessions a day with dental brushing (after breakfast and upon bedtime). They include closing, opening, lateral, and propulsion movements with gentle manual resistance [18] (Figs. 12, 13, 14, 15, and 16). Moreover in case of muscular disorders, TMD self-management instructions are significantly more effective when associated with posture stretching exercises [112].

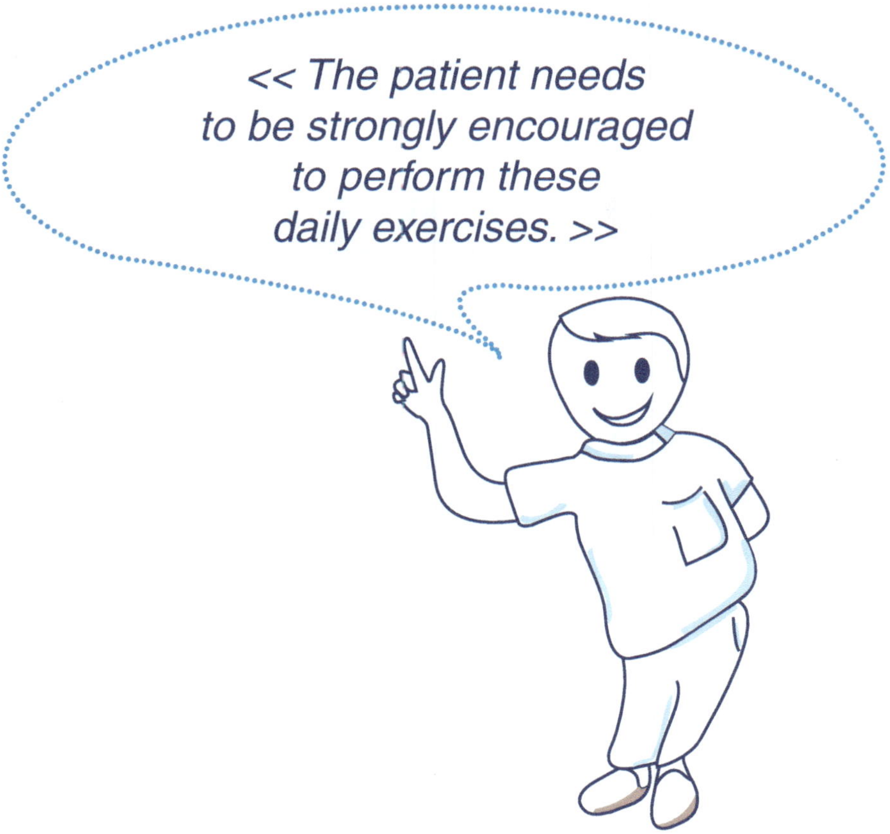

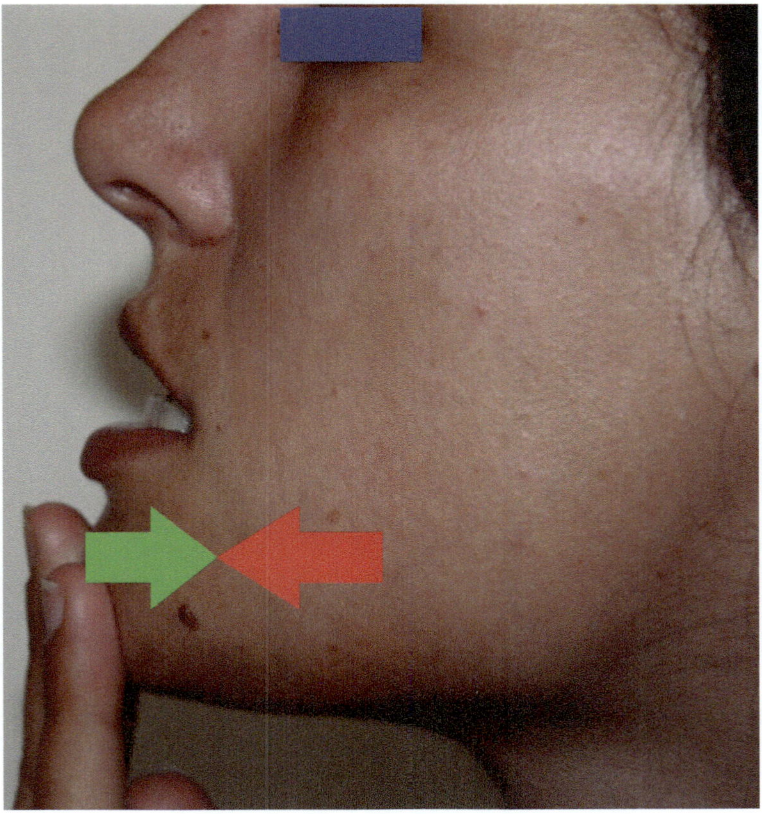

Fig. 12 Propulsion: the patient stands his or her jaw in a normal rest position. He or she makes a propulsion movement (*red arrow*) against a soft manual resistance (*green arrow*). Then he or she lets the spontaneous natural retropulsion of the jaw going. This exercise draws the pterygoid complex (lateral and medial pterygoid m.). It must be performed ten times

Also, in cases of atypical swallowing (infantile deglutition) often associated with wide anterior opening, it is possible to awaken the patient's stereognosis by touching lightly the retro-incisor papilla with an oral mirror. The patient must then apply the tip of his tongue on the area while he proceeds to swallow. The patient must perform this exercise ten times. He should keep his fingers on the thyroid zone to be more aware of the physiological swallowing mechanism. Here are some useful daily exercises to reeducate lingual and some stomatognathic functions:

Lingual exercises

Muscular reinforcement, (4 × 10 *exercises/day*) (*keep* 6–10 s):

- Piston: the tongue pushes upwards the palate with a countereffort under the throat.
- Clacking: keep laid on upwards the tongue and make a clacking with a rounded and then smiling mouth.

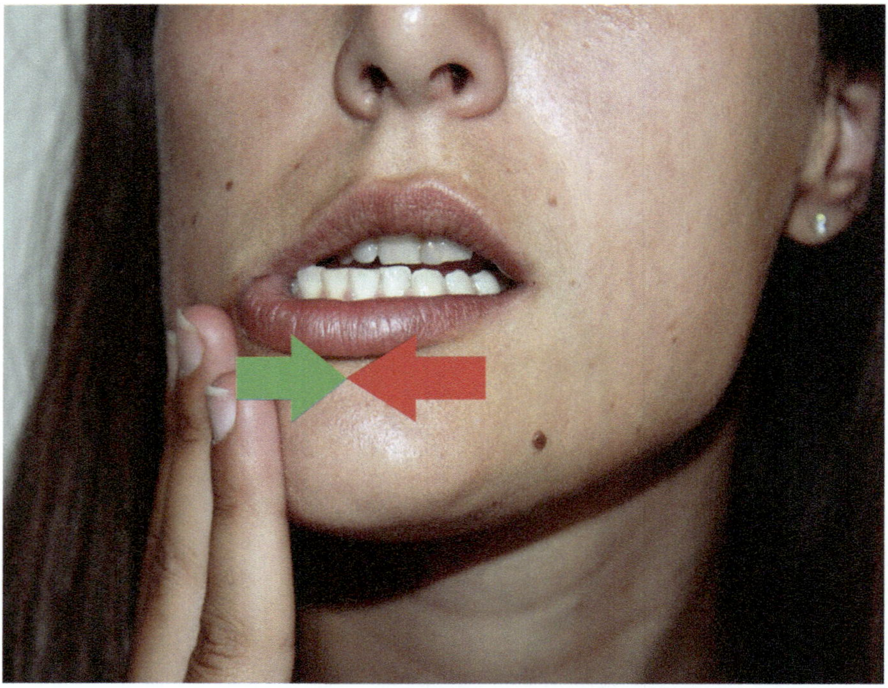

Fig. 13 Lateral movements on the right: with a right head in front of a mirror, coming from a medial jaw rest position, the patient slides laterally the jaw (*red arrow*) as the fingers hold a soft resistance (*green arrow*) in an inverse. The patient must perform ten go and return

- Yawning: laid on the tongue far backwards and down into the mouth.
- Pointed tongue: pull out the tongue then contract it (making a pointed form).

Correction of the resting function: while jaw is resting, be aware to keep uncontacted teeth with the tongue upwards laid on the front part of the palate.

Correction of the swallowing function (6×6 *exercises/day*): take a water sip, lightly contact the teeth, tongue upwards laid on the front part of the palate, and then swallow.

Correction of the phonating function (1×2 *exercises/day*): pronounce (as in duck) la la la, na na na, da da da, ta ta ta, etc. while upwards contacting the tongue on the front part of the palate (in any way between the teeth).

Stomatognathic exercises

Relaxing (3×10 *exercises/day*): inspire by the nose, and then dynamically expire by the mouth with the tongue between the teeth (without pressure).

Stretching (4×5 *exercises/day*) (*keep* 6–10 s).

Each exercise must be preceded by an expiration while keeping the mouth opened:

- Monkey: strongly push with the tongue against the upper lip.
- Pan: progressively push ahead the jaw as far as possible.

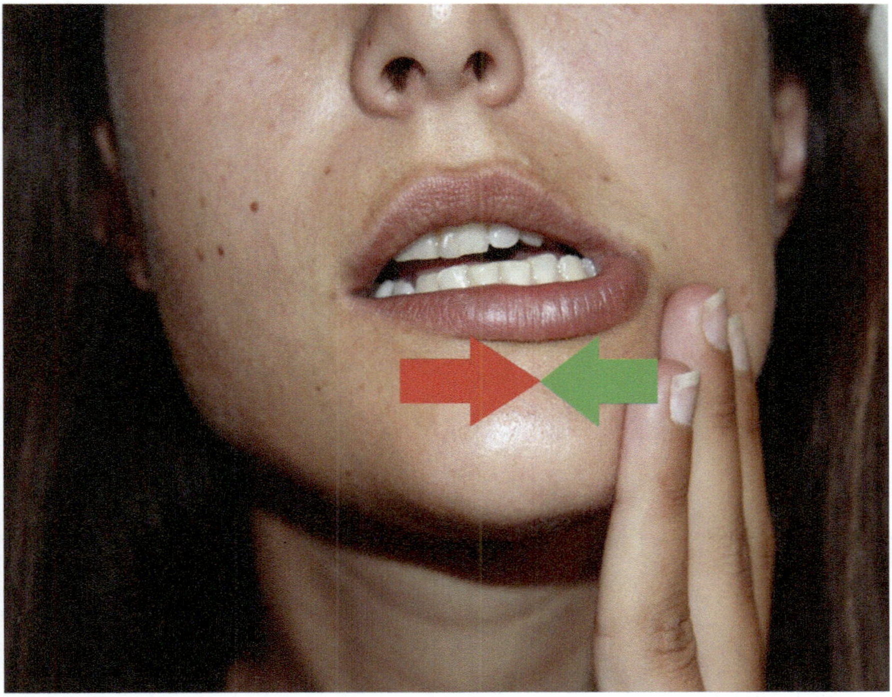

Fig. 14 Lateral movements on the left. Same protocol as previously: motor movement to the left side = *red arrow*; resistance = *green arrow*

- Take out the tongue and try to reach the left ear.
- Take out the tongue and try to reach the right ear.

So when considering possible pathological effects of atypical deglutition on respiratory, postural, or phonation spheres, rehabilitation of the swallowing function must be included in the therapeutic procedure [34, 39]. It may be necessary to call on a specialist such as a speech therapist, depending on the role of voice in human expression and social relation.

3 Clenching Self-Control: The *Lips Technique*

The awareness of the patient and his control of the parafunction is a key parameter of therapeutic success. The *lips technique* was empirically described by Dawson [22] and later explained neurophysiologically [49] based on evidence from fundamental research [9, 10]. It helps the patient fight efficiently against inappropriate parafunctional clenching.

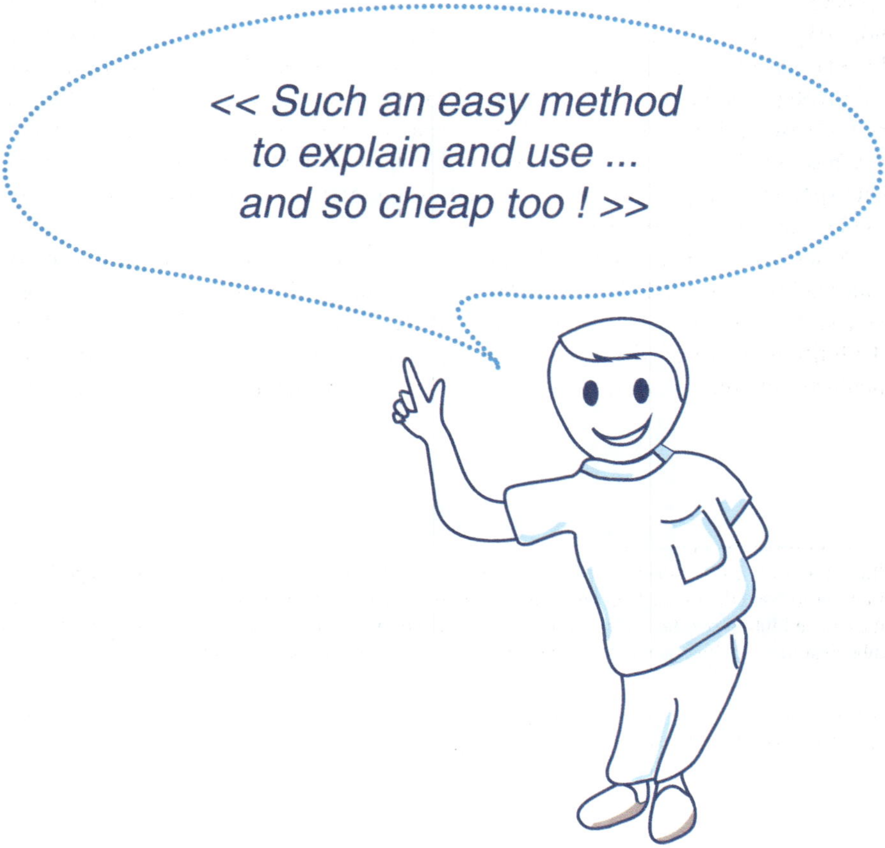

<< Such an easy method
to explain and use ...
and so cheap too ! >>

This stunning fact is as follows : somewhere in the brain, direct or indirect connections do exist between the facial nerves (VII) that control the lips' muscles (those activated during voluntary pinching) and the trigeminal nerves (V) that control the stomatognathic muscles particularly the jaw elevator muscles (used during teeth clenching). The voluntary motor action of the VII inhibits the automatic motor action of the V[9]. The patient must apply the technique throughout the day, for instance, every 30 mn during 3 mn, all the more when he realizes that he clenches his teeth. He must first open his mouth and then strongly press his lips together

[9]Current data do not allow to identify the nervous locus of this phenomenon: cortical suppressor area, brainstem, or other?

(Fig. 17). He must be careful not to bite his lips with his teeth! He must also make sure to open his mouth before he tightens his lips. The inhibiting action of the VII does not occur if the jaw elevator muscles are still contracted. When performed repeatedly[10], this method yields unexpected even astounding results. For instance, without the use of analgesics or anti-inflammatory drugs, calf cramps have reportedly disappeared as the patient gradually stopped clenching.

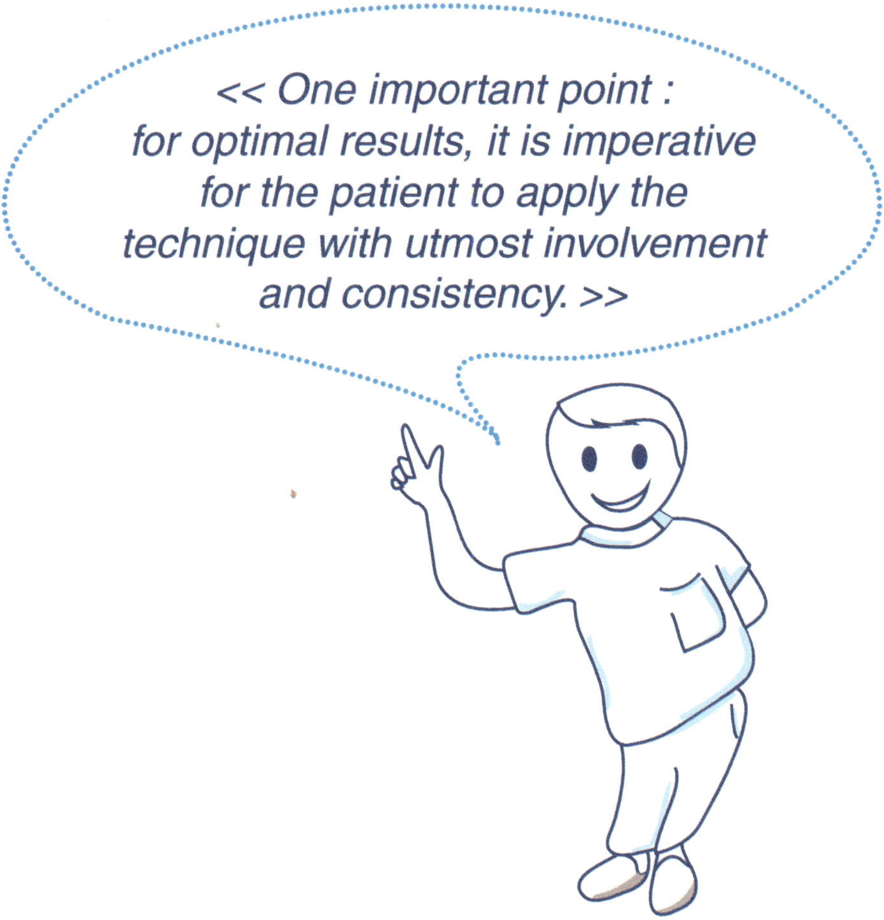

[10]For reinforcement, some dentists add an occlusal splint.

An easy way to remember to do the exercise consists in putting *small colored stickers* (any color the patient chooses) in familiar places, particularly in places where the patient's attention or concentration is maximal, such as the car dashboard, a computer or television screen, bathroom mirrors, a handbag, and a desk calendar. The perception, however, subliminal, of this *sign-signal* helps the patient remember instantly to use the *lips technique*. In this way, he relaxes his stomatognathic muscles and reduces his severe clenching habit. This is a good trick to make the patient aware of his clenching as soon as he notices the stickers.

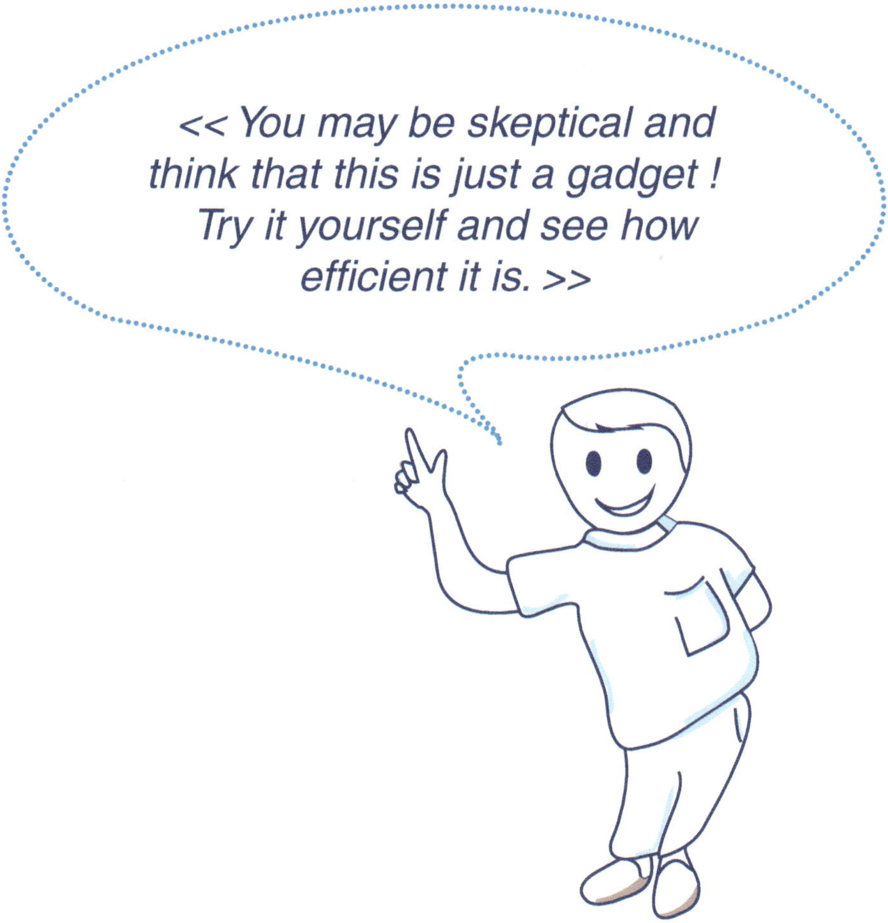
<< You may be skeptical and think that this is just a gadget ! Try it yourself and see how efficient it is. >>

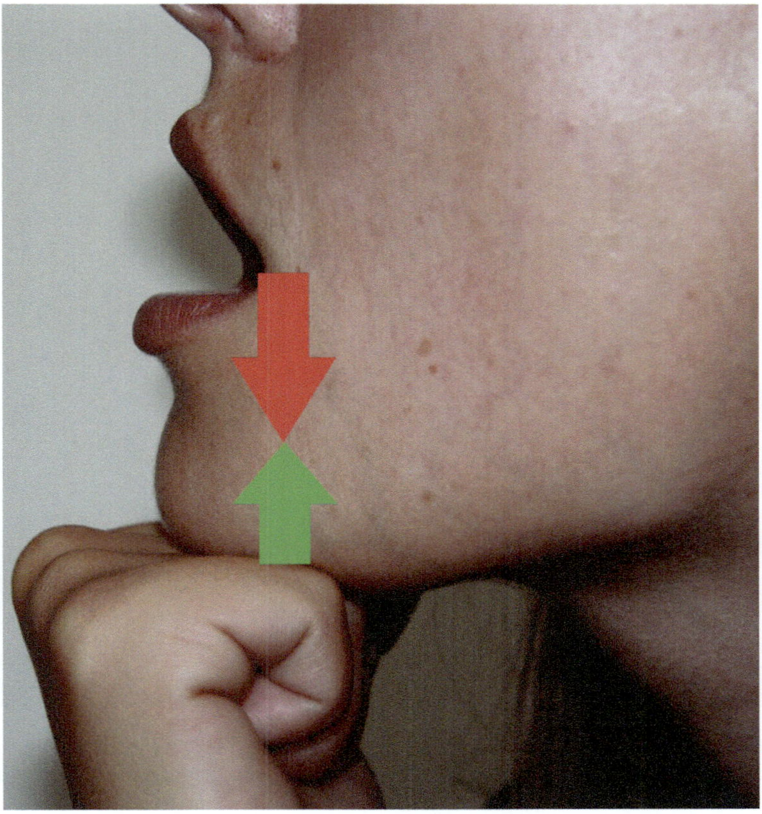

Fig. 15 Opening movements: the patient stands his or her fist under the jaw and opens the mouth (*red arrow*) against this resistance (*green arrow*). To be performed ten times

Finally, to prevent night clenching, here is another free piece of advice. Each evening while falling asleep, the patient should perform the *lips technique*, while thinking about a pleasant image, a sweet memory of the patient's choice. This has a positive influence on the quality of the sleep to come (Fig. 18). It may result in progressive reduction or even complete disappearance of a recurrent symptom: morning fatigue upon waking up (due to repeated episodes of severe nocturnal clenching). Some studies showed the highly aggravating effect of the parafunction on painful and dysfunctional symptoms [71, 72]. When it is prolonged, the parafunction aggravates the diagnosis and urges clinicians to increase or diversify drug prescription because of continuous patient's complaints [71]. Figure 19 shows the frequency per diem and a week that we recommend for some therapeutic tools.

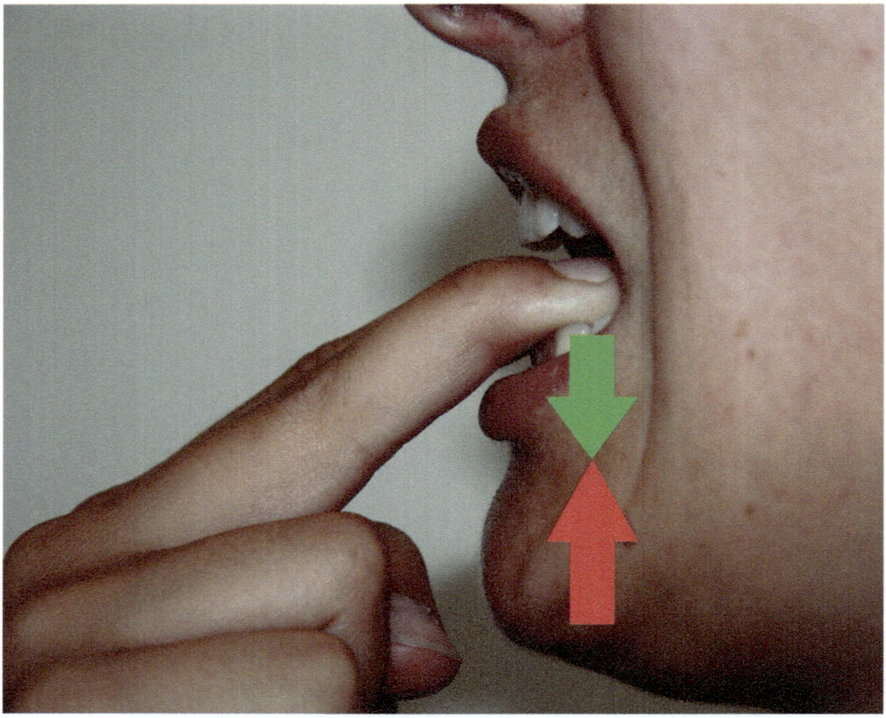

Fig. 16 Closing movements: the patient stands two fingers on the lower incisors as the mouth is opened and closes the mouth (*red arrow*) against this resistance (*green arrow*) until reaching a contact between fingers and upper incisors. To be performed ten times

4 Drug Prescription

Many cases of TMJ osteoarthritis or other rheumatoid diseases require anti-inflammatory drug treatments [23, 44]. To treat spasmed stomatognathic muscles, **myorelaxant drugs** may be used [46, 98]. They reduce neuromuscular overexcitability by decreasing central influences on hyper-reflexibility or through presynaptic inhibition of reflex circuits. Some authors recommended *gabapentin* for the management of oral parafunctions [11, 32]. The use of beta-adrenergic antagonist (propanolol) to treat nocturnal bruxism was also recommended [96]. Without any hypnotic drug, an etiological treatment based on the trigeminal RMT method can help patients recover a restorative physiological sleep. An adjuvant treatment based on *magnesium* may also contribute to relieve pain and fatigue [16]. More recently melatonin[11] has been suggested for its analgesic [2, 30, 103] and antioxidant effect [12, 82].

[11]Hormone synthesized in the pineal gland. Melatonin receptors are located in the thalamus, hypothalamus, dorsal horn of the spinal cord, spinal trigeminal tract, and trigeminal nucleus. A change from substance P to melatonin secretion has been revealed recently [75].

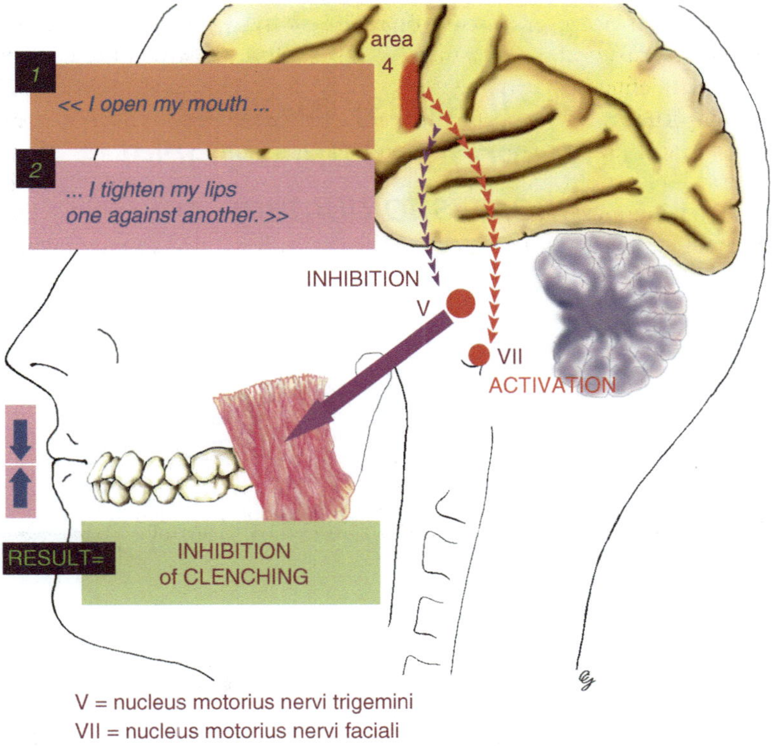

Fig. 17 The *Hartmann lips technique*

5 General Relaxation and Psychotherapy

In current literature, experts often support the concept that for a great number of patients, psychological and/or social problems stem from recurrent pain and ineffective treatments. Disappointment and health disorders surely contribute to frustration, hopelessness, a negative self-image, and even depression. Significant correlations between depression and TMD have definitely been observed but they still remain obscure [31, 35, 59, 76, 95, 101, 107].

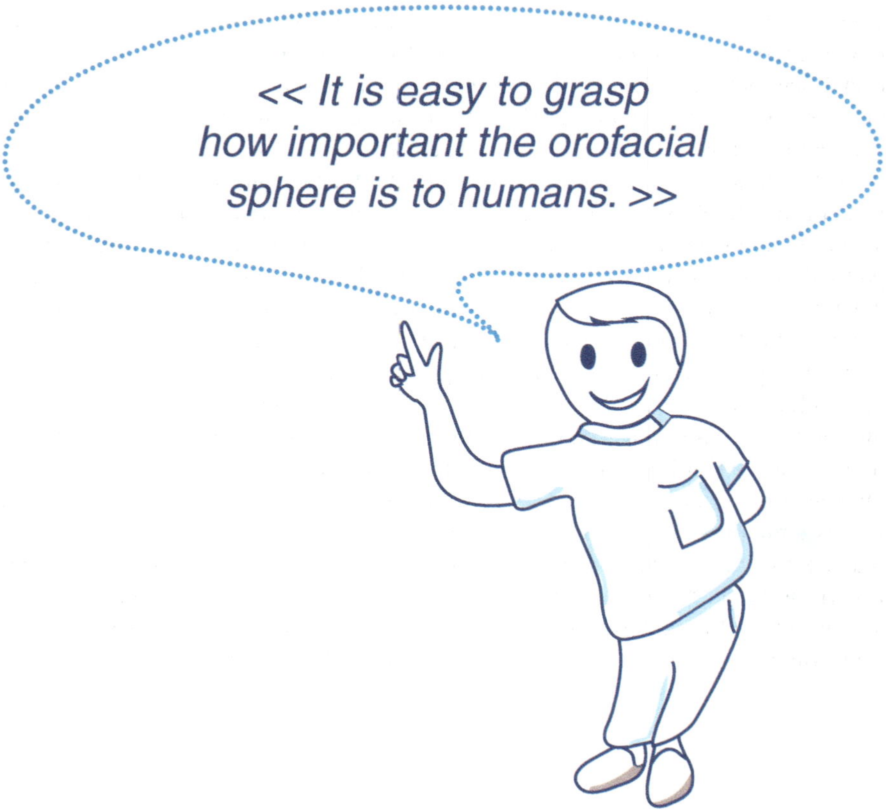

Humans have a great faculty for self-recovery against pain and dysfunctions originating from the oral sphere. This is where vegetative life (eating, breathing) meets with relational life (speaking, affection) where so many controlling nerve centers are involved in a sophisticated organization. This is why clinicians should also reflect on the sensitivity of patients to their own social, professional, and private surroundings. Among these factors, a leading cause of parafunctional habit such as severe clenching may be identified. Therefore, an etiological therapeutic protocol must also teach the patient to eliminate deleterious habits in disorders that could be benign yet need a multidisciplinary approach, such as reserving an appropriate place for relaxation and psychotherapy [40, 66, 89, 95, 107]. At any rate, behavioral methods seem to increase long-lasting benefits when compared to methods based on technique only [25, 33]. Awareness of a clenching tendency and efforts made to control it are such obvious factors in the reduction even in the relief of symptoms that informing the patient becomes essential [90]. As a result of non-adaptation,

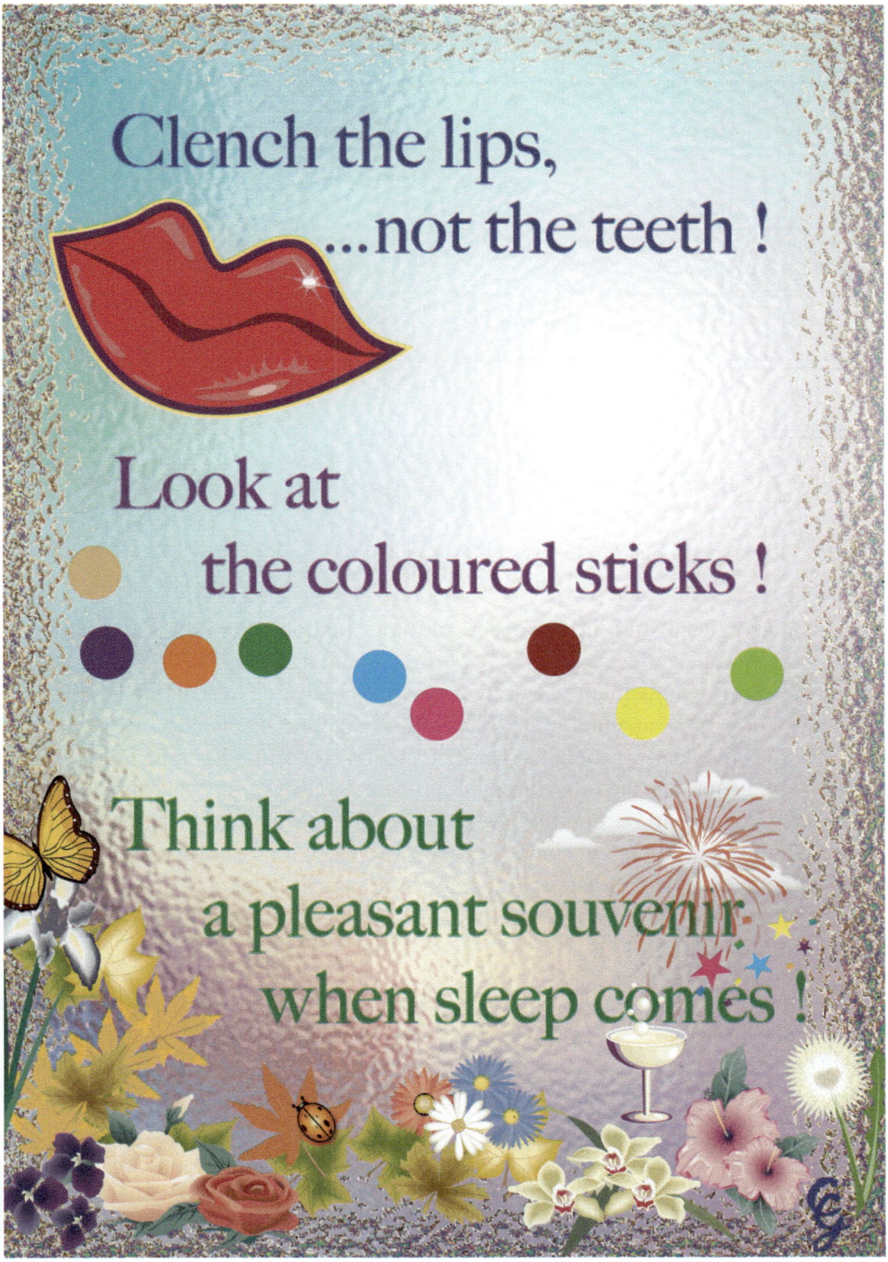

Fig. 18 Advice for self-controlling of parafunctional clenching

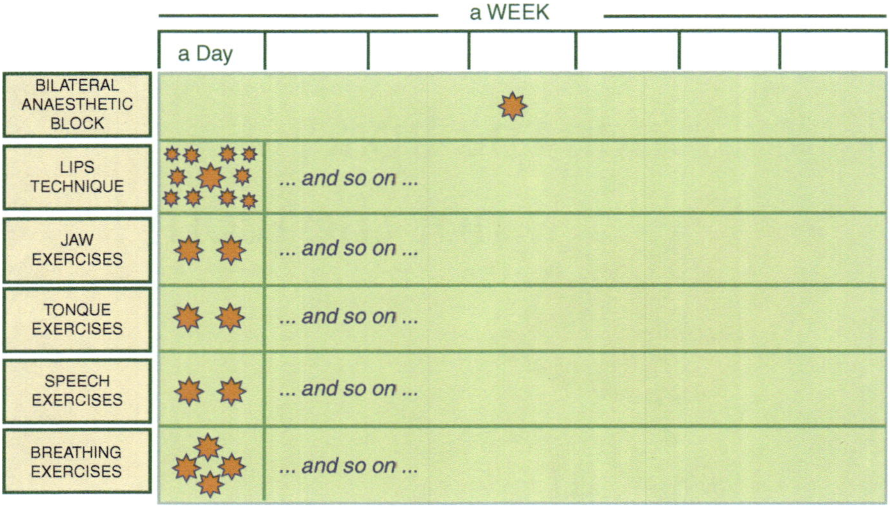

Fig. 19 Frequency per diem and a week of RMT tools

spastic tendencies justify the use of relaxation techniques. Methods based on relaxation therapy are a good option [17] and bring hopeful results [38, 77]. Some authors have revealed how this method can treat cases of syndrome of irritable bowel (SIB) [111]. It works by consolidating RMT results or by treating a central factor responsible for psychosomatic problems (spasticity). It is specially recommended for parafunction management and more largely for the treatment of emotional and behavioral disorders. Depending on the importance of conflicting factors in frustration, some cognitive physical treatments have a progressive effect on respiration [5, 19, 67]. It is possible to complement central relaxant actions with local actions on muscle tissues. The suggestion is to apply *warmth* to obtain local vasodilatation [45] by acting on vascular motor fibers.

References

1. Alvarez DJ, Rockwell PG (2002) Trigger points: diagnosis and management. Am Fam Physician 65(4):653–660
2. Ambriz-Tututi M, Rocha-Gonzàlez HI, Cruz SL, Granados-Soto V (2009) Melatonin: a hormone that modulates pain. Life Sci 84(15–16):489–498
3. Ash MM (1986) Current concepts in the aetiology, diagnosis and treatment of TMJ and muscle dysfunction. J Oral Rehabil 13:1–20
4. Bakke M, Moller E, Werdelin LM et al (2005) Treatment of severe temporomandibular joint clicking with botulinum toxin in the lateral pterygoid muscle in two cases of anterior disc displacement. Oral Surg Oral Med Oral Pathol Oral Radiol Endod 100(6):693–700
5. Barknowitz S (1996) La respiration, une fonction vivante. Ed Françaises du Graal (éd), Paris
6. Barriere P, Zink S, Riehm S et al (2009) Massage du muscle ptérygoïdien latéral dans le SADAM aigu. Rev Stomatol Chir Maxillofac 110:77–80

7. Bell WH (1985) Orofacial pains: classification, diagnosis, management, 3rd edn. Year Book Medical Pub Inc, Chicago
8. Blitzer A, Brin MF, Greene PE, Fahn S (1989) Botulinum toxin injection for the treatment of oromandibular dystonia. Ann Otol Rhinol Laryngol 98(2):93–97
9. Bratzlavski M (1972) Reflexes with intra-oral afferents in human lip musculature. Exp Neurol 37:179–187
10. Bratzlavski M (1976) Pauses in activity of human joint closing muscles. Exp Neurol 36:160–165
11. Brown ES, Hong SC (1999) Antidepressant-induced bruxism successfully treated with gabapentin. J Am Dent Assoc 130(10):1467–1469
12. Bubenik GA, Blask DE, Brown GM et al (1998) Prospects of the clinical utilization of melatonin. Biol Signals Recept 7(4):195–219
13. Clark GT (2003) The management of oromandibular motor disorders and facial spasms with injections of botulinum toxin. Phys Med Rehabil Clin N Am 14(4):727–748
14. Clark GT, Seligman DA, Solberg WK, Pullinger AG (1990) Guidelines for the treatment of temporomandibular disorders. J Craniomandib Disord 4:80–88
15. Couly G, Guilbertes F, Cernea P, Bertrand JC (1976) A propos de l'articulation temporomandibulaire du nouveau-né. Les relations oto-méniscales. Rev Stomatol 77:673
16. Cox IM, Campbell MJ, Dowson D (1991) Magnésium érythrocytaire et syndrome de fatigue chronique. Lancet (France) 337:757–760
17. Crasilneck M (1995) The use of the crasilneck bombardment technique in problems of intractable organic pain. Am J Clin Hypn 37(4):255–266
18. Cros PI, Freidel M, Borie J et al (1989) Quinze ans de traitements des syndromes algodysfonctionnels des articulations temporo-mandibulaires (SADAM). Rev Stomatol Chir Maxillo Fac 6:409–414
19. Cucchi G (1995) Alcyone: le souffle apaisé, chemin vers l'être. G Trédaniel (éd), Paris, 190p
20. Cyriac J (1977) Deep massage. Physiotherapy 63:60–61
21. Danzig W, May S, Mc Neill C, Miller A (1992) Effect of an anesthetic injected into the temporomandibular joint space in patients with TMD. J Craniomandib Disord 6:288–295
22. Dawson PE (1977) Les problèmes de l'occlusion. Evaluation diagnostique et traitement (Traduction: de Perelmuter S, Liger F) J Prélat (éd), Paris
23. Donaldson KW (1995) Rheumatoid diseases and the temporomandibular joint: a review. Cranio 13(4):264–269
24. Doual-Bisser A (1978) Rappel des notions fondamentales. Rapport 51è Congrès SFODF. SFODF (éd), Paris, pp 37–47
25. Dworkin SF (1997) Behavioral and educational modalities. Oral Surg Oral Med Oral Pathol Oral Radiol Endod 83(1):128–133
26. Eriksson PE (1989) Blood flow regulation in masticatory muscles. Proc Finn Dent Soc 85(4–5):273–277
27. Ferrante FM, Kaufman AG, Dunbar SA et al (1998) Sphenopalatine ganglion block for the treatment of myofascial pain of the head, neck and shoulders. Reg Anesth Pain Med 23:30–36
28. Freund B, Schwartz M, Symington JM (2000) Botulinum toxin: new treatment for temporomandibular disorders. Br J Oral Maxillofac Surg 38(5):466–471
29. Furto ES, Cleland JA, Whitman JM, Olson KA (2006) Manual physical therapy interventions and exercise for patients with temporomandibular disorders. Cranio 24(4):283–291
30. Gagnier JJ (2001) The therapeutic potential of melatonin in migraines and other headache types. Altern Med Rev 6(4):383–389
31. Gallagher RM, Marbach JJ, Raphael KG et al (1991) Is major depression comorbid with temporomandibular pain and dysfunction syndrome? A pilot study. Clin J Pain 7:219–225
32. Garcia-Borreguero D, Larrosa O, de la Llave Y et al (2002) Treatment of restless legs syndrome with gabapentin: a double-blind, cross-over study. Neurology 59(10):1573–1579
33. Gardea MA, Gatchel RJ, Mishra KD (2001) Long-term efficacy of biobehavioral treatment of temporomandibular disorders. J Behav Med 24(4):341–359

34. Garliner D (1976) Myofunctional therapy. Gen Dent 24(1):30–40
35. Gatchel RJ, Garofalo JP, Ellis E, Holt C (1996) Major psychological disorders in acute and chronic TMD: an initial examination. J Am Dent Assoc 127:1365–1374
36. Gaudy JF, Hadida A, Brunel G, Tavernier JC (1993) Les muscles masticateurs possédant une insertion méniscale au niveau de l' ATM. Inf Dent 39:3517–3521
37. Gelb H (1977) Clinical management of head, neck and TMJ pain and dysfunction: a multi-disciplinary approach to diagnosis and treatment. WB Saunders Co (ed), Philadelphia/London/Toronto
38. Gil IA, Rizzatti-Barbosa CM, Monteiro-Pedro V et al (1998) Multidisciplinary approach to chronic pain from myofascial pain dysfunction syndrome: a four-year experience at a Brazilian center. Cranio 16(1):17–25
39. Giuca MR, Pasini M, Pagano A et al (2008) Longitudinal study on a rehabilitative model for correction of atypical swallowing. Eur J Paediatr Dent 9(4):170–174
40. Green CS, Olson RE, Laskin DM (1982) Psychological factors in the etiology, progression and treatment of MPD syndrome. J Am Dent Assoc 105:443–448
41. Hagberg C, Agerberg G, Harberg M (1986) Discomfort and bite force in painful masseter muscles after intramuscular injections of local anesthetic and saline solution. J Prosthet Dent 56(3):354–358
42. Hall LJ (1984) Physical therapy treatment results for 178 patients with temporomandibular joint syndrome. Am J Otol 5(3):183–196
43. Hameroff SR, Crago BR, Blitt CD, Womble J, Kanel J (1981) Comparison of bupivacaine, etidocaine, and saline for trigger-point therapy. Anesth Analg 60(10):752–755
44. Hannequin JR (1987) Diclofenac et cartilage articulaire: études expérimentales. Conc Med Suppl 43:4207–4209
45. Hartmann F, Moheng P (1980) Sophrologie et vaso-motricité. L Quest Odont Stomatol 17:9–24
46. Hartmann F, Cucchi G (1986) Rôle du muscle ptérygoïdien latéral dans la phase de début du SADAM. Cah Proth 56:125–144
47. Hartmann F, Cucchi G (1987) Muscle ptérygoïdien lateral et SADAM: diagnostic précoce et traitement. Rev Odont Stomatol 16(3):209–218
48. Hartmann F, Sarrat P, Gaudy JF et al (1988) Muscle ptérygoïdien latéral, dissection anatomique et imagerie médicale. Perspectives dans le traitement du SADAM. Act Odont Stomatol 163:545–566
49. Hartmann F, Cucchi G (1993) Les dysfonctions cranio-mandibulaires (SADAM). Nouvelles perspectives médicales. Springer-Verlag (éd), Paris, 176p
50. Hendler N, Fink H, Long D (1983) Myofascial syndrome: response to trigger-point injections. Psychosomatics 24(11):990–999
51. Heylings DJA, Nielsen IL, Mc Neill C (1995) Lateral pterygoid muscle and the temporomandibular disc. J Orofac Pain 9(1):9–15
52. Ivanhoe CB, Lai JM, Francisco GE (1997) Bruxism after brain injury: successful treatment with botulinum toxin-A. Arch Phys Med Rehabil 78(11):1272–1273
53. Jankovic J, Schwartz K, Donovan DT (1990) Botulinum toxin treatment of cranial cervical dystonia, spasmodic dysphonia, other focal dystonias and hemifacial spasm. J Neurol Neurosurg Psychiatry 53(8):633–639
54. Jansen VD, Scudds R (1997) Sphenopalatine blocks in the treatment of pain in fibromyalgia and myofascial pain syndrome. Laryngoscope 107:1420–1422
55. Jolivet C, Nguyen Kim K, Klap P et al (1996) Apport de la toxine botulique dans la thérapeutique des dysfonctionnements cranio-mandibulaires. Act Odont Stomatol 195:483–493
56. Klein RN, Burk DT, Chase PF (2001) Anatomically and physiologically based guidelines for use of the sphenopalatine ganglion block versus the stellate ganglion block to reduce atypical facial pain. Cranio 19(1):48–55
57. Komatsu K, Yamaguchi T, Sato K et al (2000) A new exercise device for rehabilitation of lateral mandibular movements. J Orofac Pain Abstract 14(3):3
58. Kopp S, Wenneberg B (1981) Effect of occlusal treatment and intraarticular injections on temporomandibular joint pain and dysfunction. Acta Odont Scand 39:87–96

59. Korszun A, Hinderstein B, Wong M, Arbor A (1996) Comorbidity of depression with chronic facial pain and temporomandibular disorders. Oral Surg Oral Med Oral Pathol 82:496–500
60. Lobo-Lobo S, Mehta N, Forgione AG et al (2004) Use of theraflex-TMJ topical cream for the treatment of temporomandibular joint and muscle pain. Cranio 22(2):137–144
61. Lynch ME, Elgeneidy AD (1996) The role of sympathetic activity in neuropathic orofacial pain. J Orofac Pain 10(4):297–305
62. Madrid C, Reynes P (1989) Les aponévroses de l'espace ptérygo-mandibulaire. Acta Anat 136:55–60
63. Magnusson T, Syren M (1999) Therapeutic jaw exercises and interocclusal appliance therapy. A comparison between two common treatments of temporomandibular disorders. Swed Dent J 23(1):27–37
64. Maixner W (1989) Autonomic and somatosensory interactions: physiological and pathophysiological implications. Proc Finn Dent Soc 85(4):395–407
65. Manns AE, Garcia C, Miralles R et al (1991) Blocking of periodontal afferents with anesthesia and its influence on elevator EMG activity. Cranio 9(3):212–219
66. Marbach JJ, Dworkin SF (1975) Chronic MPD, group therapy and psychodynamics. J Am Dent Assoc 90:827–833
67. Martenot M, Saïto C (1977) Se relaxer. A Michel/Opéra Mundi (éd), Paris
68. Martins-Junior RL, Palma AJ, Marquardt EJ et al (2010) Temporomandibular disorders: a report of 124 patients. J Contemp Dent Pract 11(5):71–78
69. Mc Millan AS (1996) The efficacy of procaine in the treatment of myofascial pain in the jaw muscles. J Orofac Pain 10(2):187
70. Michelotti A, de Wijer A, Steenks M, Farella M (2005) Home-exercise regimes for the management of non-specific temporomandibular disorders. J Oral Rehabil 32(11):779–785
71. Molina OF, dos Santos J, Nelson SJ, Nowlin T (2000) Profile of TMD and bruxer compared to TMD and nonbruxer patients regarding chief complaint, previous consultations, modes of therapy, and chronicity. Cranio 18(3):205–219
72. Molina OF, Dos Santos J, Mazzetto M et al (2001) Oral jaw behaviors in TMD and bruxism: a comparison study by severity of bruxism. Cranio 19(2):114–122
73. Monteiro AA, Kopp S (1989) The sufficiency of blood flow in human masseter muscle during endurance of biting in the intercuspal position and on a force transducer. Proc Finn Dent Soc 8(4–5):261–272
74. Morgan DH, Hall WP, Vanwas SJ (1977) Diseases of the temporomandibular apparatus. CV Mosby Co (ed), St Louis
75. Mukda S, Moller M, Ebadi M, Govitrapong P (2009) The modulatory effect of substance P on rat pineal norepinephrine release and melatonin secretion. Neurosci Lett 461(3):258–261
76. Murray H, Locker D, Mock D, Tenenbaum HC (1996) Pain and the quality of life in patients referred to a craniofacial pain unit. J Orofac Pain 10:316–323
77. Nicolakis P, Burak EC, Kollmitzer J et al (2001) An investigation of the effectiveness of exercise and manual therapy in treating symptoms of TMJ osteoarthritis. Cranio 19(1):26–32
78. Ogus HD, Toller PA (1981) Common disorders of temporomandibular joint. J Wright & Sons Limited (ed), Bristol
79. Okesson JP (1989) Management of temporomandibular disorders and occlusion. CV Mosby Co (ed), St Louis
80. Orlando B, Manfredini D, Bosco M (2006) Efficacy of physical therapy in the treatment of masticatory myofascial pain: a literature review. Minerva Stomatol 55(6):355–366
81. Padamsee M, Mehta N, White GE (1987) Trigger point injection a neglected modality in the treatment of TMJ dysfunction. J Pedod 12:72–92
82. Peres MF (2005) Melatonin, the pineal gland and their implications for headache disorders. Cephalalgia 25(6):403–411
83. Petersen AM, Pedersen BK (2005) The anti-inflammatory effect of exercise. J Appl Physiol 98(4):1154–1162
84. Peterson GN, Schames J, Schames M, King E (1995) Sphenopalatine ganglion block: a safe and easy method for the management of orofacial pain. Cranio 13(3):177–181

85. Pogrel MA, Erbez G, Taylor RC, Dodson TB (1989) Liquid crystal thermography as a diagnostic aid and objective monitor for TMJ dysfunction and myogenic facial pain. J Craniomandib Disord 3:65–70
86. Quinn JH (1995) Mandibular exercises to control bruxism and deviation problems. Cranio 13(1):30–34
87. Ren K, Dubner R (1999) Central nervous system plasticity and persistent pain. J Orofac Pain 13(3):155–163
88. Riley JL 3rd, Myers CD, Currie TP et al (2007) Self-care behaviors associated with myofascial temporomandibular disorder pain. J Orofac Pain 21(3):194–202
89. Rudy TE, Turk DC, Kubinski JA, Zaki HS (1995) Differential treatment responses of TMD patients as a function of psychological characteristics. Pain 61:103–112
90. Rugh JD (1988) Behavioral therapy. In: Mohl ND, Zarb A, Carlsson GE, Rugh JDA (eds) Textbook of occlusion. Quintes Pub Co In, Chicago, p 329
91. Rugh JD, Solberg WK (1976) Psychological implications in temporal pain and dysfunction. Oral Sci Rev 7:3
92. Schwartz HC, Kendrick RW (1984) Internal derangements of the temporomandibular joint: description of clinical syndromes. Oral Surg Oral Med 58(1):24–29
93. Schwartz M, Freund B (2002) Treatment of temporomandibular disorders with botulinum toxin. Clin J Pain 18(6 Suppl):198–203
94. Silberstein S (2000) Botulinum toxin type A as a migraine preventive treatment. Headache 40(6):445–450
95. Sipilä K, Veijola J, Jokelainen J et al (2001) Association between symptoms of temporomandibular disorders and depression: an epidemiological study of the Northern Finland 1966 Birth Cohort. Cranio 19(3):183–187
96. Sjoholm TT, Lehtinen I, Piha SJ (1996) The effect of propranolol on sleep bruxism: hypothetical considerations based on a case study. Clin Auton Res 6(1):37–40
97. Song P, Schwartz J, Blitzer A (2007) The emerging role of botulinum toxin in the treatment of temporomandibular disorders. Oral Dis 13(3):253–260
98. Stanko J (1990) A review of oral skeletal muscles relaxants for the craniomandibular disorders (CMD) practitioner. Cranio 8:234–243
99. Steigerwald D, Verne SV, Young D (1996) A retrospective evaluation of the impact of TMJ arthroscopy on the symptoms of headache, neck pain, shoulder pain, dizziness and tinnitus. Cranio 14(1):46–54
100. Ström D, Holm S, Carlsson GE (1989) Blood-flow and metabolic response in a contracting canine masticatory muscle. Proc Finn Dent Soc 85(4–5):251–260
101. Suvinen TI, Hanes KR, Gerschman JA, Reade PC (1997) Psychophysical subtypes of temporomandibular disorders. J Orofac Pain 11(3):200–205
102. Tan EK, Jankovic J (1999) Botulinum toxin A in patients with oromandibular dystonia: long-term follow-up. Neurology 53(9):2102–2107
103. Tom B, De Vries P, Heiligers JP et al (2001) The lack of vasoconstrictor effect of the pineal hormone melatonin in an animal model predictive of antimigraine activity. Cephalalgia 21(6):656–663
104. Travell JG (1949) Basis of the multiple uses of local block of somatic trigger areas procaine infiltration of ethyl chloride spray. Miss Valley Med J 71:13–22
105. Travell JG, Simons DG (1983) Myofascial pain and dysfunction. The trigger-point manual. Williams & Wilkins (ed), Baltimore
106. Vazquez-Delgado E, Okeson JP (2004) Treatment of inferior lateral pterygoid muscle dystonia with zolpidem tartrate, botulinum toxin injections, and physical self-regulation procedures: a case report. Cranio 22(4):325–329
107. Vimpari SS, Knuuttia ML, Sakki TK, Kivela SL (1995) Depressive symptoms associated with symptoms of the temporomandibular joint pain and dysfunction syndrome. Psychosom Med 57:439–444

108. Von Lindern JJ, Niederhagen B, Bergé S, Appel T (2003) Type A botulinum toxin in the treatment of chronic facial pain associated with masticatory hyperactivity. J Oral Maxillofac Surg 61(7):774–778
109. Watts MW, Tan EK, Jankovic J (1999) Bruxism and cranial-cervical dystonia: is there a relationship? Cranio 17(3):196–201
110. Wenneberg B, Kopp S, Grönhald HG (1991) Long-term effect of intra-articular injections of a glucocorticosteroid into the TMJ: a clinical and radiographic 8-year follow-up. J Craniomandib Disord 5:11–18
111. Whorwell PJ, Prior A, Faragher EB (1984) Controlled trial of hypnotherapy in the treatment of severe refractory irritable bowel syndrome. Lancet 2:1232–1234
112. Wright EF (2000) Referred craniofacial pain patterns in patients with temporomandibular disorder. J Am Dent Assoc 131(9):1307–1315
113. Zeno E, Griffin J, Boyd C et al (2001) The effects of a home exercise program on pain and perceived dysfunction in a woman with TMD: a case study. Cranio 19(4):279–288

Part III
In Conclusion

Eliminating *stomatognathic muscle spasticity* and consecutive *trigeminal proprioceptive overstimulation and nociception* are the main objectives of RMT. This is true for TMD but clinicians should look for the presence of a spastic condition in clinical forms of other diseases (migraine, fibromyalgia, chronic fatigue, etc.) in stressed introverted patients with **severe clenching habits**. This would contribute to an improvement of symptomatology and a clearer evaluation of strong causal factors. The second phase of treatment must tend to eliminate these factors, based on a mostly multidisciplinary vision. All procedures must be considered to return a patient to his own physiological condition. A major key to success is the identification and elimination of the oral parafunctional habit referred to as clenching. For the patient as well as for the therapist, the first therapeutic results will help shed light on the connection between the implication of the oral parafunction and the multiple upsetting aspects of the observed pain and discomforts. The elimination of this parafunction will result in the reduction even the sedation of some signs and symptoms. But these results depend on one underlying condition: the subject must be committed on a daily basis without restriction to control (*lip method*) his **severe parafunctional clenching**. If not, the RMT could prove disappointing and even completely inefficient. If he clenches again, signs and symptoms will come back. Therefore, the patient must be continuously aware of his condition to put a quick stop to his inadequate response to individual or environmental stressors.

Part IV
Medical Prospects

Medical Prospects

1 The Trigeminal Nerve Is Wellknown For Its "Tic douloureux" But Largely Underestimated For Its Non-algic Sensory Role

> *"There is no greater sensory experience for the brain to manage than unremitting pain in trigeminally mediated areas"*. Carlson CR [20]

While their various peripheral sets and rich central nervous projections have been known for many years (see Part II), the clinical implications of the trigeminal paired V nerves continue to be underestimated. The medical world, like the dental world, has mainly focused on the algic aspects of V pathologies (neuralgia, dental pain, TMJ pain, etc.): in the twenty-first century, such view is very restrictive of clinical reality. While the *human oral sphere* plays an important role in physiological functions and adaptation, the V nerves participate in most sensitive and motor circuits in the stomatognathic area. Does the oral sphere play a special part in patients suffering from severe uncompensated stress? The nature of the paired V is admittedly highly reflexogenic: do the trigeminal sensory-motor territories serve as a sounding board to stress if we consider the importance of the oral sphere in human beings? These questions follow. Setting up a clear classification of signs and symptoms in TMD is quite a difficult task. For example, the Headache Classification is based on several structures of orofacial sphere including classic sets such as migraine, facial vascular algia, trigeminal neuralgia, and so on (see Part II).

Literature reviews on concepts relating to TMD reveal the difficulty that clinicians have been facing over the years since the famous Costen syndrome in unraveling the inextricable puzzle presented by this disconcerting entity[1], known as the *great impostor*. Today would it be helpful to make this pathological entity part of a larger syndrome, for instance, a *postural deficiency syndrome* [29] or a *dental distress syndrome* [37] or

[1]The link between TMJ disorders and occlusal or vertical dimension defects as factors contributing to pain and disorders of the stomatognathic system has been discussed for many years. A number of EMG studies seem to confirm this role, while others fail to show any such correlation.

F. Hartmann, G. Cucchi, *Stress and Orality*,
DOI 10.1007/978-2-8178-0271-8_16, © Springer-Verlag France 2014

central sensitivity syndromes (CSS) [157]? At any rate, a new approach sheds some light on the possible distant body alterations caused by pathophysiological processes in the oral sphere. Failure to recognize the importance of insidious chronic factors, especially with regard to the role of recurring microtraumas, may be due to the importance of acute factors, that is, sudden and violent muscle strain [150]. For instance, many clinicians are not inclined to consider the TMJ when confronted by a patient with neck symptoms, specially after a *whiplash injury* [8, 13, 14, 17, 55, 69, 72, 87, 121, 148, 151]. Otherwise, some experts took attention to early behavioral factors [23, 30, 109]: tendency to cut off bosom suckling, too soft food, oral breathing, and unilateral mastication, which break off growing physiological laws [106, 107]. Over and above craniofacial disproportion, outcome such as TMD and even respiratory, postural, and behavioral problems can appear.

It must be reminded that all any peripheral information takes a meaning when regarding how the central nervous system deals with it. So the individual psychological condition remains as a main element in self-adaptation towards any possible TMD generating or aggravating factor. Moreover, the famous Selye's works about stress led to an increasing realization of importance of psychophysiological factors as a possible cause for neuromuscular disorders. Thus Laskin [74] defined the *myofascial pain and dysfunction syndrome* (MPDS)[2]. Today, patients' psychological state and their social surroundings are best evaluated. This new approach may explicit clinicians' attention about adaptive behaviors towards previous factors. The MPDS has been considered as a psychosomatic disorder which placed the stomatognathic muscle as one of chosen targets of various *stressful psycho-socio-physiological factors* and itself as a predominant factor in the origin of symptoms. The resulting symptomatology appeared just as much to demonstrate the existence of an oral parafunctional activity [11, 32, 51, 52, 80, 94, 111] enlightening a **misunderstood teeth clenching** towards the well-known grinding, as a major pathogenic element [89, 93, 145]. When considered as a disease of maladaptation which may involve several individual levels (biomechanical, neuromuscular, endocrinal, immune, metabolic, psychological, social, etc.), TMD could be labeled as an oral one, owing to a major implication of this sphere in human interactive relation and adaptation [22]. Now, one has a better understanding of neurophysiologic mechanisms which arise as a result of many stressors, both with regard to skeletal muscles and also to nervous and endocrine systems. Central factors (psycho-emotional) are strongly working to the same pathological outcome because of reticular influence towards all motor neurons. For a long time, limited issues linking this

---

The bio-mechanistic approach gave preferential importance to "TMJ internal derangement" and influenced the design of articulators [26, 35, 75]. Some etiological factors related with dental occlusion were considered to be relevant: loss of posterior tooth and supporting zone [42, 43, 155, 156], maxillomandibular disproportion [113], abnormality of VDO [42, 60, 71], interposition of tongue between dental arches [60], infantile swallowing, and general abrasion of teeth caused by grinding. Another recurring theme is the consideration of postural and traumatic factors, not only at the level of the stomatognathic system but also as part of the global postural body system [37, 47, 96, 124].

[2]Many studies gave recognition to prevalence of central and psychosocial stressful factors in orofacial disorders [4, 15, 16, 21, 28, 31, 36, 42, 45, 51, 57, 62, 64, 67, 76, 79, 82, 83, 91, 98, 99, 102, 114, 115, 123, 125, 127, 129, 131, 133, 134, 141, 146, 152–154] in which frustration [53], even more than anxiety, seemed to be predisposing factors [138].

pain to TMD might originate from the amazing and disconcerting aspect of these painful topographies. In effect, in this type of pain without evident anatomical lesion, *trigeminal neuromuscular overexcitability and nociception* appear as major pathophysiological components. Sometimes as initiating factors, sometimes as promoting factors, and sometimes as aggravating factors, they all overlap in a pathophysiology which remains complex. But scientific data had led to a clearer appreciation of the role of trigeminal receptors in functional regulation of oral sphere: abnormal peripheral inputs should affect the stomatognathic muscles and consequently the corresponding articular structures. About functional troubles, it could only be possible to distinguish light to severe forms, if considering gravity; starting to advanced forms, if considering evolution and history; and local to extensive forms, if considering topography of symptoms. Every clinical case results from a combination between these parameters and patient's own reaction towards varied stressors. According to Bertrand (personal com.), "TM disorders are distinct but interrelated entities with complex etiology that involves the full extent of the Trigeminal Nervous System." Now, there is an evidence in clearly separating TMD with pure general articular diseases such as rheumatoid or viral forms when they involve TMJ or tumorous forms. The current mixed concept of TMD gives a key role to pathophysiological factors in neuromuscular dysfunction which usually resulted from a *combination of central and peripheral factors* [3, 6, 19, 24, 27, 31, 33, 34, 44, 47, 48, 53, 56, 61, 66, 85, 86, 90, 92, 97, 100, 104, 126, 135, 136, 147, 159] with an individual predisposition and a psychological dependence to bio-psychosocial factors [118]. Some complex interactions can take place between these different factors as evidenced by resulting symptoms which stem from many different causes; as it is true for any disease, these factors can be divided into activating, local, and general one. A similar approach distinguished between predisposing, initiating, and aggravating factors [85].

One of the most important scientific facts is the various and numerous *connections between trigeminal nervous centers and non-trigeminal one* (see Part II). So if considering all the major functions it participates to, that is, digestion, breathing, communication, posture, etc., is the oral sphere a particularly sensible target towards stressful mechanisms? If it is, any clinician must be mindful of spastic conditions of oral sphere such as *severe clenching in stressed patients*. Thus, to diagnose this deleterious parafunctional habit mainly appears as an absolute need. This is specially true in front of painful and discomforted patients, some of those diagnosed as migrainous, fibromyalgic of chronic fatigued, when previous classical therapies remained ineffective. A more holistic approach allows to put forward certain elements as follows. The first one is the importance of psychological failure to cope with stress. It can be responsible for a neuromuscular spasticity, particularly into oral sphere (stomatognathic spasticity). The second is oral parafunctions which are often responsible for perpetuate spastic states and consequently *referred pain and discomforts*. The third is the physiological nervous importance of paired V. These trigeminal neurons can extend towards non-trigeminal structures any sensitive overstimulation and/or nociception (parafunctional clenching). This is a possible main factor for intensifying pathological effect when severe and/or chronic stress goes on. In front of persistent symptoms, the patient logically asks himself: "What am I hurted by?" (Fig. 1). Several pathologies may be evoked. Here we choose three major famous diseases: migraine, fibromyalgia, and chronic fatigue.

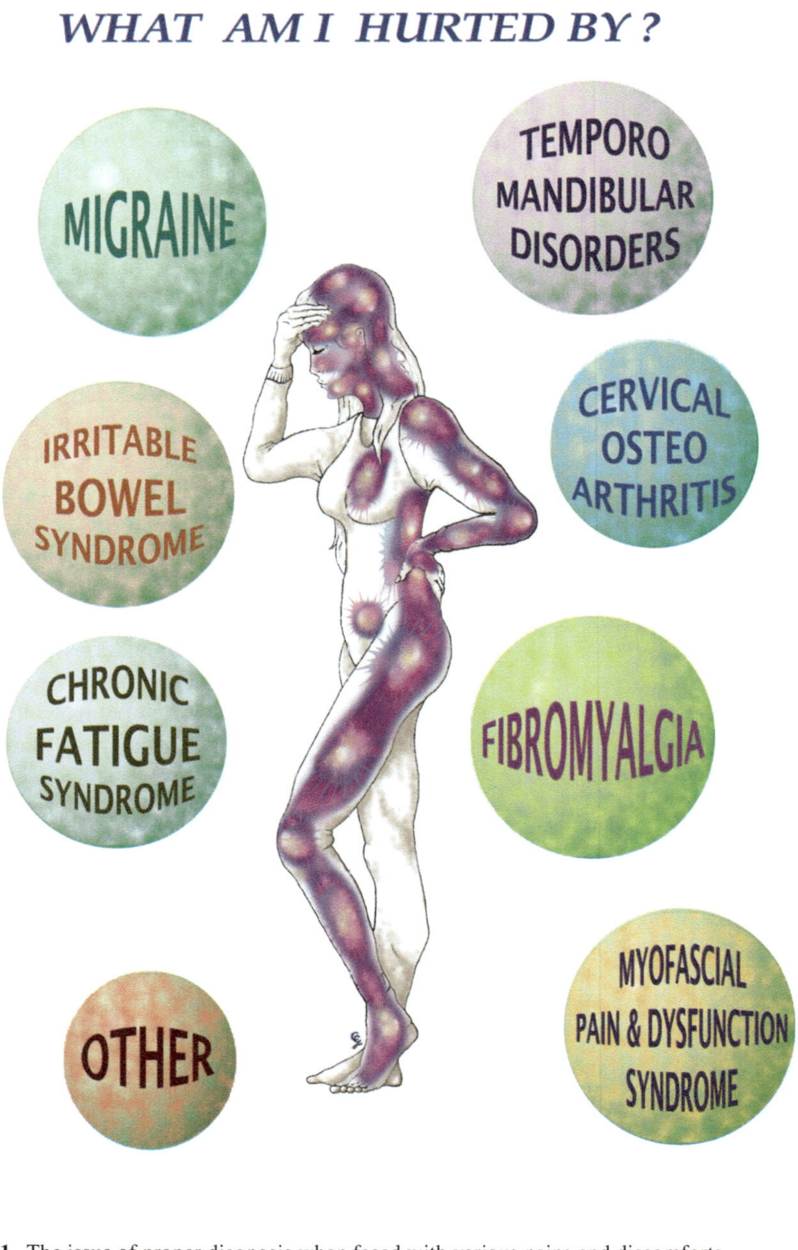

Fig. 1 The issue of proper diagnosis when faced with various pains and discomforts

2 Migraine

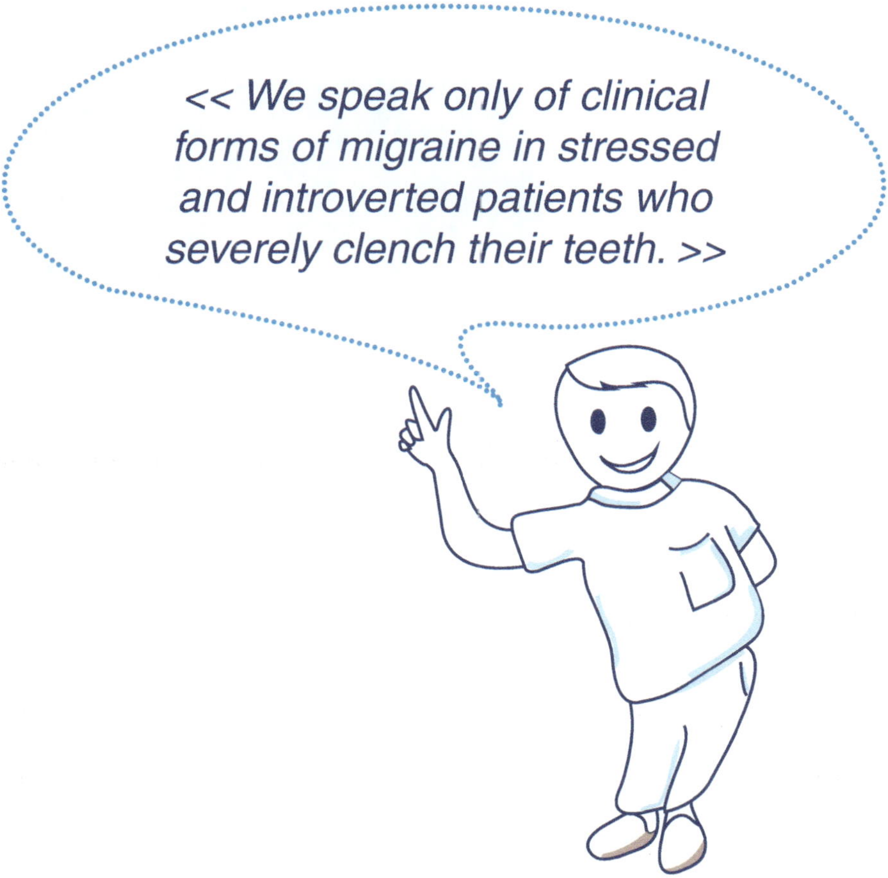
<< We speak only of clinical forms of migraine in stressed and introverted patients who severely clench their teeth. >>

Today, TMD is often paralleled with others clinical pathologies. For instance, some issues evoked the role of trigeminal overstimulation and of a lack in trigeminal ways controlling into starting of migrainous attacks [49]. Some issues recognized the responsible involvement of the V into headache, but by considering only its autonomic structures in regard to mechanism of cluster headache. According to Bartsch and Goasby [9, 10], "…a considerable population of neurons show convergent inputs from both dura as well as cervical cutaneous and muscle territories, which supports the view of a functional continuum between the caudal trigeminal nucleus and upper cervical segments involved in cranial nociception (…) This mechanism can be important in pain referral from cervical structures to the head and therefore have

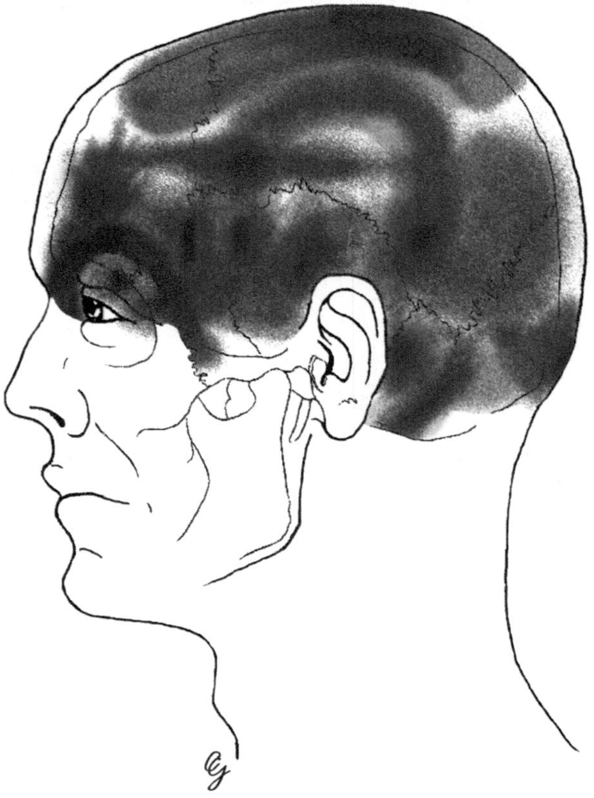

Fig. 2 Superimposed referred pain from different stomatognathic referred inputs; head posture and facial muscles mimicking migraine in the cranial and orbital areas: temporalis, sternocleidomastoideus, trapezius, suboccipiti, semispinalis capitis, semispinalis cervicis, splenius capitis, splenius cervicis, occipitofrontalis, and zygomaticus major

implications for most forms of primary headache." It is known as the presence of trigeminal SP neurons, of 5-HT neurons in the raphe dorsal nucleus, and of NorA neurons in the locus coeruleus. All these neurons, via fibers of cranial parasympathetic system (facial nerve, sphenopalatine ganglion, and otic ganglion), would elicit variations in intra- and extracranial blood flowing, which variations are responsible in migraine [49]. The central sensitization from primary trigeminal afferents could explain intracranial brain signs [18]. More recently, data enlightened that estrogen receptors in trigeminal neurons modulated nociceptive responses [110]. It has been also described in patients with painful palpated stomatognathic muscles, a concomitant presence of tension-type headache and migraine [5, 95]. Please take a look at the Fig. 2 which adds the referred pain as previously shown in many figures of chapter "Symptoms". Other issues provided some clinical observations which for the limit between TMD and migraine may appear as rather blurred [12, 38]. So it has been observed muscles painful palpation in some *atypical migrainous patients* [78]. Some clinicians noted a high migraine percentage in TMD patients [40, 122], when others found a higher rate of TMD signs [50, 88] or parafunctional habits [39] among migrainous patients. Otherwise, the link with stressful situations is now better admitted [120]. Some evoked the implication of nonvascular factors in some common migraines [116] in patients with parafunctional habits, as parafunction could constitute a trigger factor of migrainous attacks [73]. The parafunction is considered as

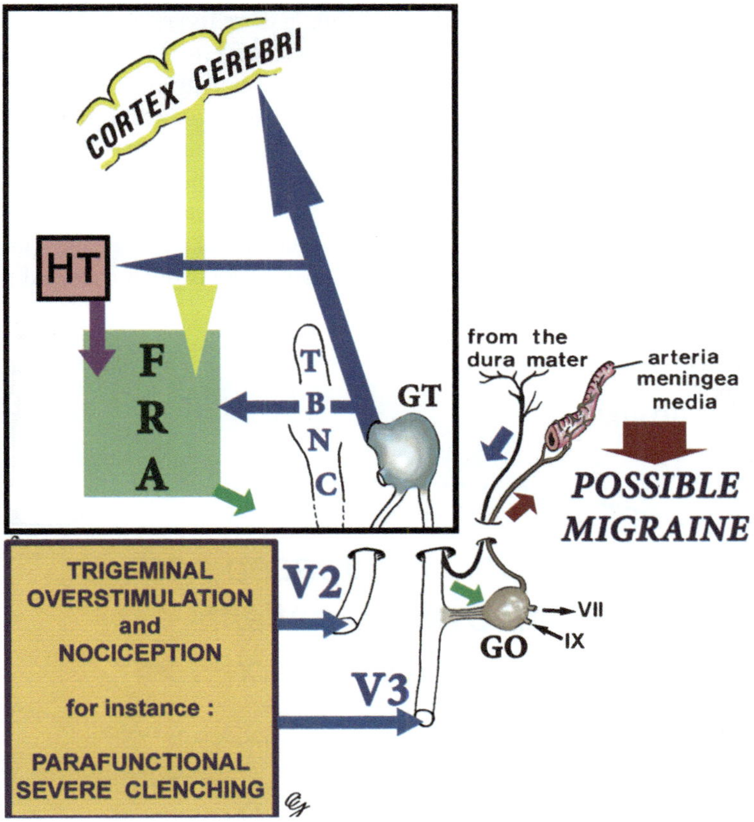

Fig. 3 Possible migraine in clenching patients. A pathophysiological model

one of the main factors to initiate migraine and tension-type headache [78]. It has been described a "functional continuum between the trigeminal SnC and upper cervical segments involved in cranial nociception" [9, 10, 18]. When confronted to an atypical migraine which for specific drug treatment failed, clinicians must repair a possible *stomatognathic muscle spasticity*. The successful trigeminal RMT will allow to confirm diagnosis in linking this disconcerting form of migraine to TMD[3]. More largely when a TMD treatment brings improvement, even sedation, in some *migraines*, *facial vascular algia* [143], or *trigeminal neuralgia*, the discussion stands about frequent connections between V and other central nervous structures (VII, IX, X, cervical roots, etc.) [108]. It has been shown that intracranial structures (such as the meninges and cerebral blood vessels) project their inputs towards the hypothalamus [81] as other trigeminal tissues do [139, 140]. That suggests that sensory and

[3]About local RMT, it can be evoked the situation of the otic gg. into infratemporal fossa, according to sedative effects on some migraines. The sympathetic root of otic gg., after entering into the skull, divides itself in a perivascular plexus to the arteria meningea medialis which is involved in migrainous phenomena. Figure 3 schematically presents anastomosis between V3 and otic gg. which of an efferent branch is distributed to the nervous plexus of arteria meningea medialis (branch of the arteria maxillaris).

nociceptive trigeminal informations originating in these tissues could be transferred to hypothalamus. So the overstimulated and nociceptive trigeminal afferents come over as a leitmotiv in most of the proposed pathophysiological models. Please refer to previous words in Part II about vascular reflex from nociceptive conditions. The trigeminal overstimulation and nociception during clenching might directly interfere on gg. oticus or indirectly after relaying in hypothalamus and cerebral cortex (Fig. 3). That enlarges the excitatory action which FR exerts on cranial sympathetic system. The local anesthetic injection into the fossa infratemporalis could have a local and/or central moderating effect on this neuronal racing and explicit observed progressive sedation on some migraines.

3 Fibromyalgia

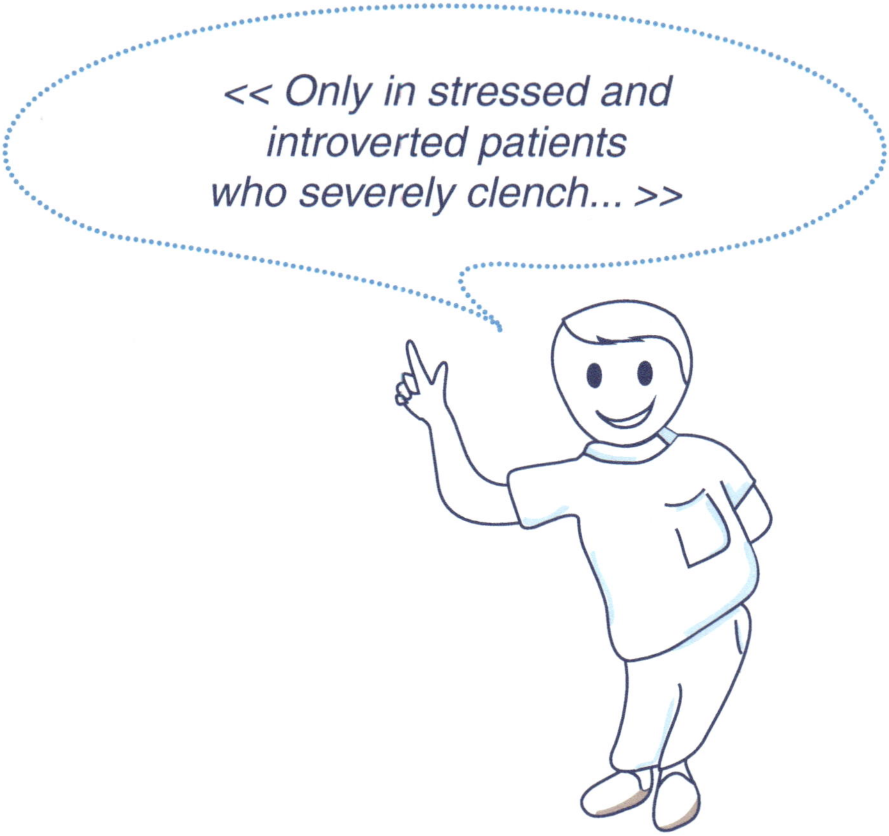

Fibromyalgia (FM) is mostly characterized by chronic widespread pain. The American College of Rheumatology (ACR) defined 18 points for establishing the right diagnosis, but they seem are modestly superior to sham points [54]. According to painful topographies which appear very far from oral sphere, it is interesting to compare this painful set to the classical description of FM as some searchers did [1, 7, 25, 41, 58, 105, 128, 149]. The real causes remain unknown, and the mechanisms unclear. That FM might be related to hypofunctional stress systems, particularly in the autonomic nervous system (ANS) and the hypothalamic-pituitary-adrenal (HPA) axis, is still discussed [59, 63, 101, 137], with rather hypothalamic alteration than pituitary [63]. The implication of female sexual hormones are also discussed [65, 117]. Some models propose that FM pain and some associated discomforts (fatigue, sleep disturbance, etc.) could themselves generate lowered neuroendocrine changes in the HPA axis [46]. The central sensitization state is often evoked in mechanisms of pain with fibromyalgic patients [132, 142, 158]. But central sensitization may be also induced by chronic nociceptive peripheral inputs [144] even by repeated non-nociceptive one. Thus, a recent hypothesis proposed the inflammation of intramuscular fascia [77] as source of sensitization. That might compare some aspects of FM to myofascial pain and dysfunction syndrome. Non-pharmacological, especially physical exercise, myofascial release and cognitive behavioral therapy are advised [77, 119]. The experts also described problems in memorizing, reasoning, concentrating, mood disturbances (depression), and some somatic symptoms: headaches, hepatic, intestinal troubles (irritation) and urinal troubles (urgency), eyes' watering, parched mouth, and limb numbness (pricking). Some FM symptoms (fatigue, awaking stiffness, sleeping disturbances, etc.) sometimes appear in TMD patients [41] but are still modestly linked with FM [158]. However, another important analogy between TMD and FM has been found: painful muscular palpation [25, 149]. When confronted to clenchers, the clinician may parallel TMD with FM as the both pathologies could have a same pathophysiological basis. It should be desirable to develop more clinical investigating procedures for validating this hopeful new approach. So experts and clinicians are invited in *firmly researching the snaky clenching in FM patients*. In any way, when confronted to such a case, the reader and clinician may legitimately wonder about the following questions: "Is my preliminary diagnosis of fibromyalgia so valid whereas I observe unexpected and amazing therapeutic results with this patient since he stopped clenching his teeth? Isn't it a question of TMD?"

4 Chronic Fatigue

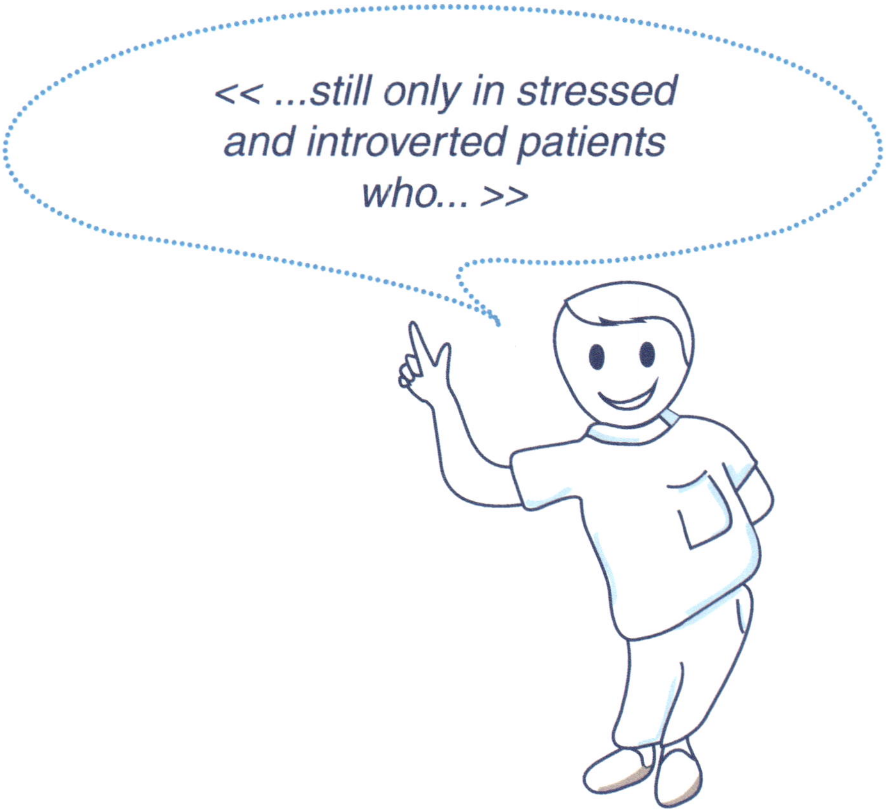

Described since 1750, chronic fatigue (CF) has only been received in acceptation in 1988. The patient complains about more than 6 months of fatigue attended to muscular and articular symptoms such as pain and often starting by a psychological shock. The gender discrepancy reports a major female ratio which is two to four more than male subjects. They are between 25- and 40-year-old-white women which often show depressive symptoms, frustration, and feeling of being confined. Experts are agreeing to accept that CF is one of the most mysterious diseases, without well-known cause. They just evoke three possible causes: genetic, viral, and neurological. The viral cause has been recently given up[4]. Even though the genetic lead cannot today be rejected, according to our personal clinical experience, we think that the main cause must be searched among the neurological factors. A larger number of observational studies and of clinical trials are needed to confirm the neuromuscular theory. It appears that many patients refute a possible psychological background of their illness. In reality fatigue keeps some links with "lack of motivation, failing interest for relationships, lack of pleasure for activities, desire to rest, to abstain from thinking, and heaviness and weakness" [2]. Otherwise, some experts have linked CF and TMD in stressed patients and evoked a shared underlying pathophysiological basis about the HPA axis [70]. Others described a nearby neurasthenia called as *syndrome of young urban professional* ("YUPPIES"). Although considering the deleterious pressure of several environmental stressors, the human response to stress is largely defined by the individual's basic personality structure. The numerous medical tests show an important decrement of personal energy. Diagnosis of CF is based on requiring four among the following symptoms: problems in concentration, short-term memory, sleeping disturbances, unexplained muscular pain (such as in FM), articular pain, headache, pain in the throat, neck or armpit adenopathy, and intolerance towards physical exercise. CF has also been related to some limited cardiac and ventilatory disturbances [130]. But CF tends to be no longer considered as a real homogenous syndrome [2]. Today, it is maintained that there is no specific and effective treatment for this pathology; the experts just recommend to operate to the physical and psychological components[5]. Recently, it has been observed that "... oxidative stress due to excess free radical formation was associated with jaw muscle pain in CF patients and suggest that these symptoms were likely to be associated with a pathogen-associated etiology" [112]. The knowledge of neuroscientific data overvalues the neuromuscular etiologic hypothesis, owing to consider the role of *trigeminal overexcitability* (spasticity, overstimulation, nociception) in its possibly referred outcome far from stomatognathic system. Here also it should be receivable to include an adequate, that is, highly careful, clinical investigation about the presence of parafunctional habit (clenching) in all the persistent CF patients.

About migraine, fibromyalgia, chronic fatigue, and their relationships to TMD, specific questions arise (Fig. 4). Do the paired V play a special role in mechanisms of adaptation? If they do, are they particularly involved when these mechanisms failed? How? Are they emphasizing some impacts of maladaptation towards non-trigeminal areas and/or immune and endocrinal functions? Besides, does the oral sphere play a particular part, for example, the amplification of sensitive nervous signals (overstimulation and/or nociception), in the occurrence and the persistence of the above-mentioned signs with a stressed individual? Can a parafunctional motor activity of the oral sphere (severe parafunctional clenching) observed on

[4]References: Paprotka et al. [103] and Knox [68].

[5]Continuing psycho-emotional tension is known to generate local muscular tension and widespread insidious contractures. Many years ago, Martenot tried to focus the clinicians' attention on these pathophysiological conditions as a big source of metabolic disturbances: tissular acidosis, hypoxia, non-eliminated free radicals, etc. may be suspected to facilitate abnormal states of chronic fatigue. Relaxation methods seem greatly useful to prevent or improve this kind of psychosomatic tendency [84].

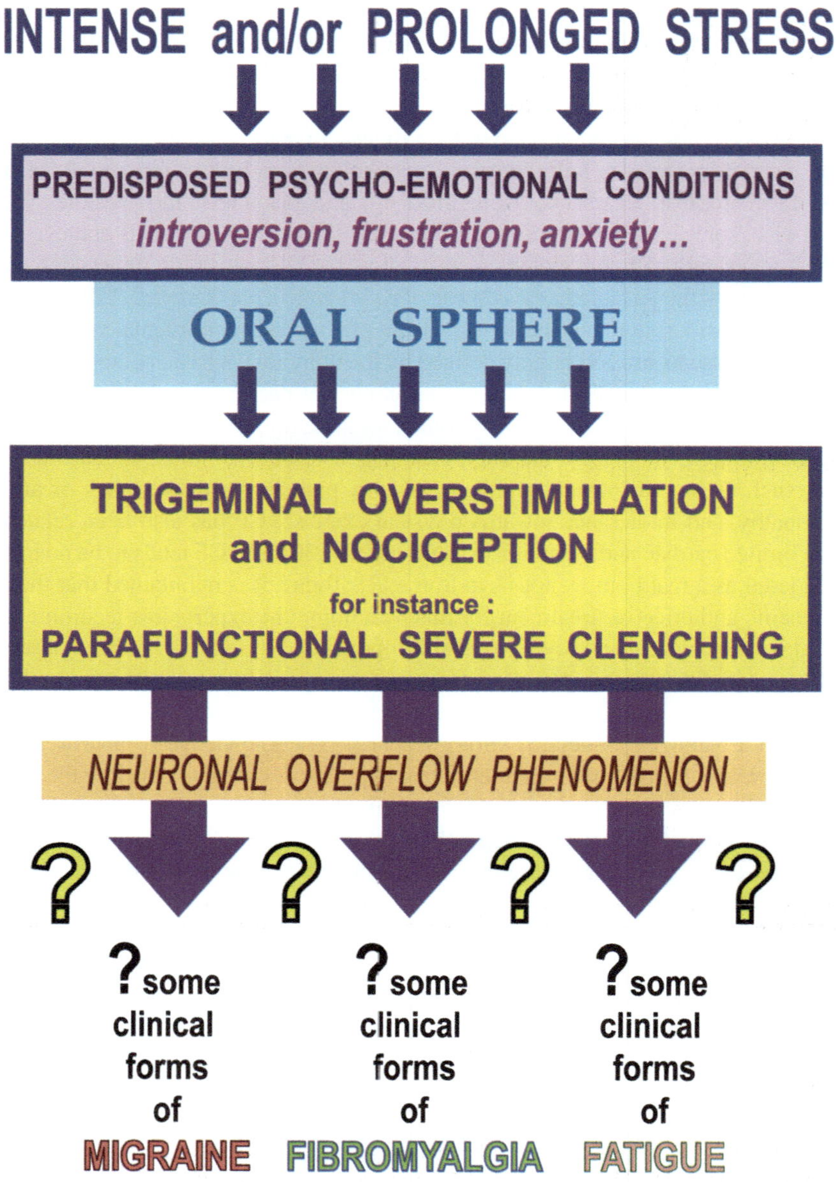

Fig. 4 Possible trigeminal implications in some clinical forms of migraine, fibromyalgia, and chronic fatigue. A model

many TMD diagnosed subjects in certain cases be implicated in the occurrence or the aggravation of painful symptoms and discomforts very remotely from that area? It is so curious to clinically observe in many cases the tight link between stopping the clenching and the release, even the complete sedation of several signs like pain or chronic fatigue. In the same way, clenching is likely to cause the return of signs

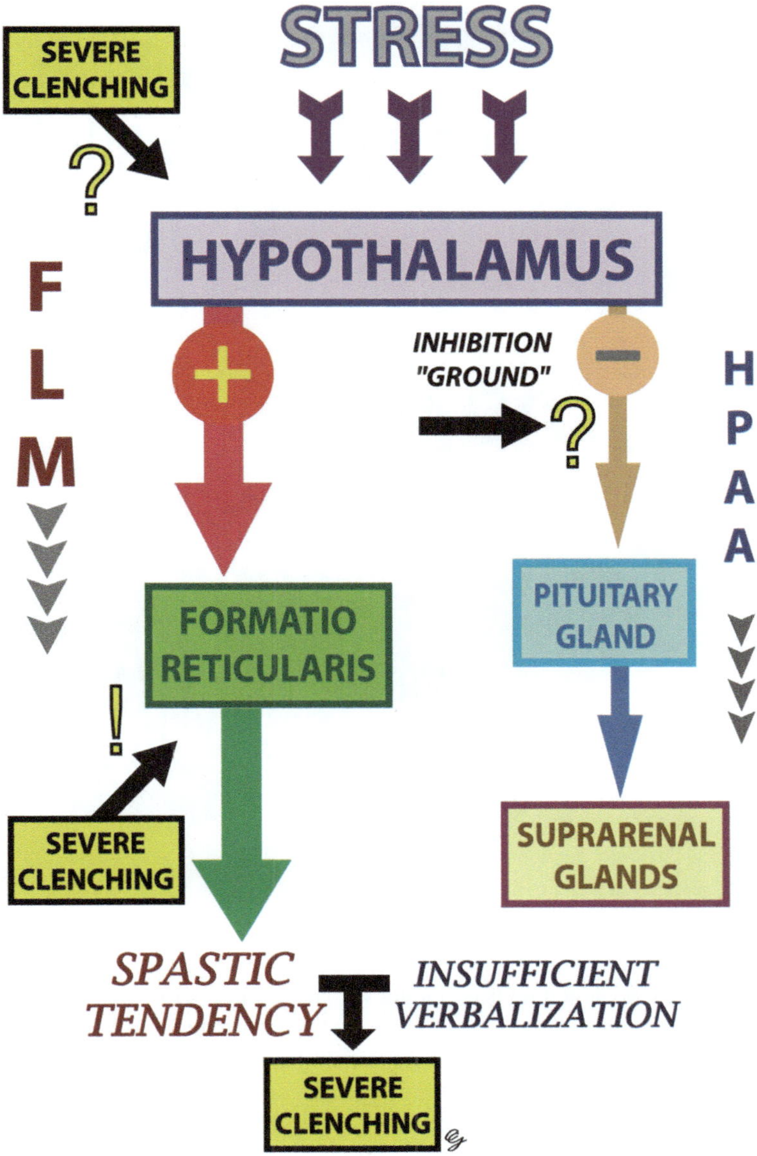

Fig. 5 Theory of depressed HPA axis and amplified FLM in stressed and introverted *clenchers*. A model

and symptoms in an aggravated form. According to our pathophysiological model (see Part II), patients with severe clenching are subject to a kind of *inhibition of action* (lack in verbalization). So are they unconsciously diminishing the normal HPA axis response towards stress? By the way, do they increase other circuits like the fasciculus longitudinalis medialis (Fig. 5) and tend to keep up the spastic condi-

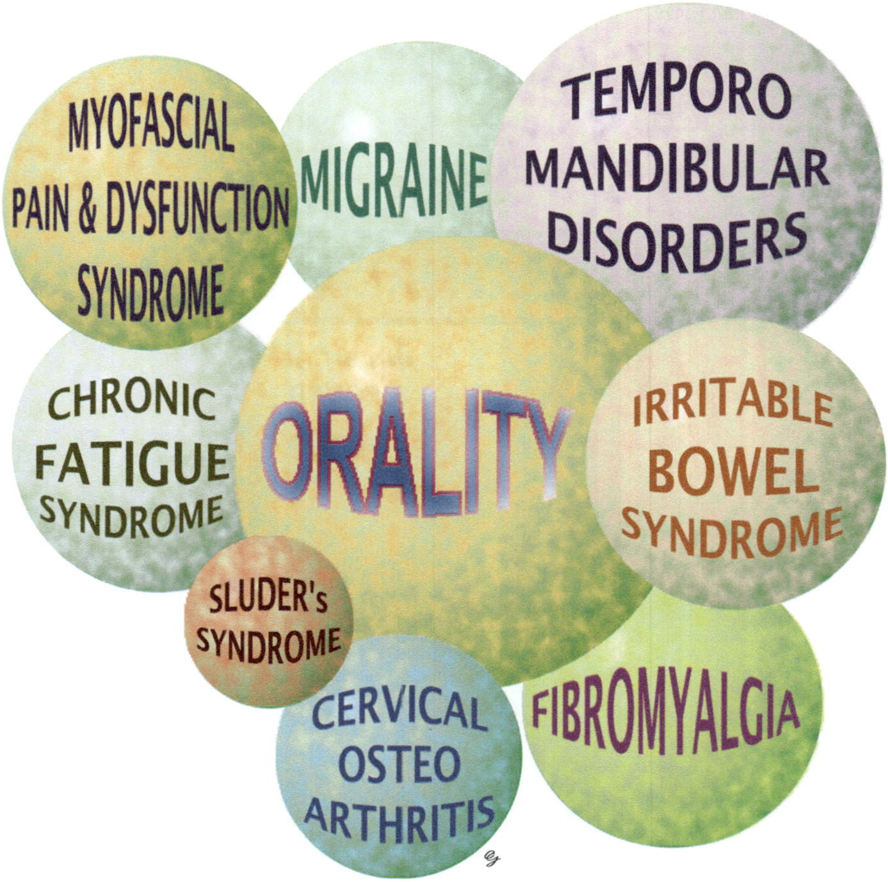

Fig. 6 Oral sphere and pain-causing diseases

tions? When severe clenching is replacing verbalization, does this kind of palliative inhibition take a main role in pathophysiology? What are the links between the oral sphere and apparently different diseases which generate remote pain and discomforts (Fig. 6)? Can this severe clenching be held responsible for painful complaints that the clinicians may meet with certain diagnosed M or FM or CF subjects? Are TMD, some M, some FM, some CF, and MPDS strictly different pathological entities (Fig. 7)? Or with a same etiologic basis in maladaptive conditions (Fig. 8)? Are there some forms with one or many common clinical components (Fig. 9)? Clinicians had better to collect their findings to progress in a better understanding of these often mysterious and recalcitrant pathologies towards usual therapies. In any case, the screening of the severe parafunctional clenching would deserve the

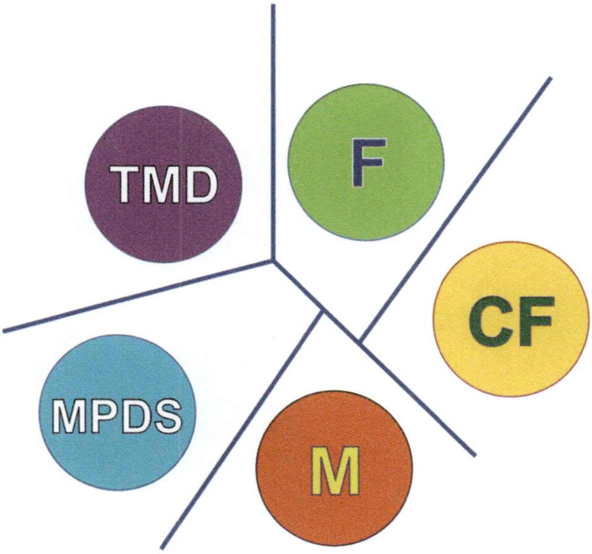

Fig. 7 Theory of clearly separate diseases

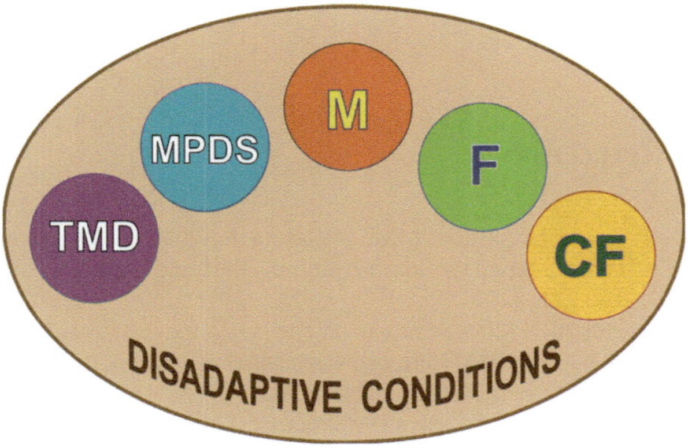

Fig. 8 Theory of different clinical forms caused by common global maladaptation

greatest attention of therapists, whatever their specialty is. When its presence is evidenced, the various related pathologies, that is, M, FM, CF, TMD, and MPDS, probably constitute different clinical aspects of a same wider mechanism of loss of adaptability when implying the oral sphere. Any time stress conditions meet a favorable psychological ground (anxiety, frustration, introversion), these are susceptible to nest deeply. Thus, it could be better understood that the failures recorded by some therapeutic protocols persist in ignoring the noxious role of the severe clenching within certain forms of pathologies.

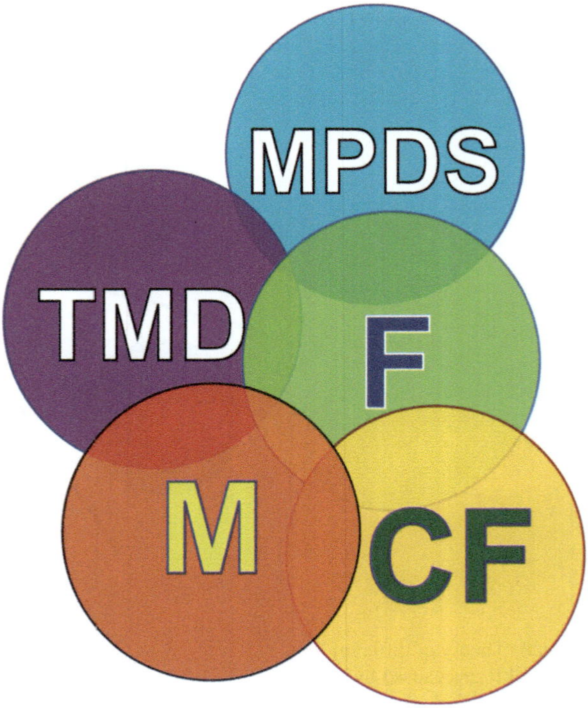

Fig. 9 Theory of common zones between closely related diseases

References

1. Aaron LA, Burke MM, Buchwald D (2000) Overlapping conditions among patients with chronic fatigue syndrome, fibromyalgia and temporomandibular disorder. Arch Intern Med 160:221–227
2. Adler RH (2004) Chronic fatigue syndrome (cfs). Swiss Med Wkly 134:268–276
3. Ash MM (1986) Current concepts in the aetiology, diagnosis and treatment of TMJ and muscle dysfunction. J Oral Rehabil 13:1–20
4. Auerbach SM, Laskin DM, Frantsve LM, Orr T (2001) Depression, pain, exposure to stressful life events, and long-term outcomes in temporomandibular disorder patients. J Oral Maxillofac Surg 59(6):628–633
5. Bakal DA, Kaganov JA (1977) Muscle contraction and migraine headache: psycho-physiologic comparison. Headache 17:208–215
6. Bakland LK, Christiansen EL, Strutz JM (1988) Frequency of dental in traumatic events in the etiology of temporomandibular disorders. Endod Dent Traumatol 4(4):182–185
7. Balasubramaniam R, de Leeuw R, Zhu H et al (2007) Prevalence of temporomandibular disorders in fibromyalgia and failed back syndrome patients: a blinded prospective comparison study. Oral Surg Oral Med Oral Pathol Oral Radiol Endod 104(2):204–216
8. Balla J (1989) The late whiplash syndrome. Aust N Z J Surg 50:610–614
9. Bartsch T, Goadsby PJ (2003) Increased responses in trigeminocervical nociceptive neurons to cervical input after stimulation of the dura mater. Brain 126(8):1801–1813
10. Bartsch T, Goasby PJ (2002) Stimulation of the greater occipital nerve induced increase central excitability of dural afferent input. Brain 125(7):1496–1509
11. Bessette R, Bishop B, Mohl N (1971) Duration of masseteric silent period in patients with TMJ syndrome. J Appl Physiol 30:864

12. Bevilaqua Grossi D, Lipton RB, Gigal ME (2009) Temporomandibular disorders and migraine chronification. Curr Med Group 13(4):249–331
13. Bezuur JN, Hansson TL, Wilkinson TM (1989) The recognition of craniomandibular disorders: an evaluation of the most reliable signs and symptoms when screening for CMD. J Oral Rehabil 16(4):367–372.
14. Bocchi L, Orso C (1983) Whiplash injury of the cervical spine. Ital J Orthop Traumatol 9:171–181
15. Bonjardim LR, Gaviao MB, Pereira LJ, Castelo PM (2005) Anxiety and depression in adolescents and their relationship with signs and symptoms of temporomandibular disorders. Int J Prosthodont 18(4):347–352
16. Brown FF, Robinson ME, Riley JL, Gremillion HA (1996) Pain severity, negative affect, and microstressors as predictors of life interference in TMD patients. Cranio 14(1):63–70
17. Burgess J (1991) Symptom characteristics in TMD patients reporting blunt trauma and/or whiplash injury. J Craniomandib Disord 5:251–257
18. Burstein R, Yamamura H, Malick A, Strassman AM (1998) Chemical stimulation of the intracranial dura induces enhanced responses to facial stimulation in brain stem trigeminal neurons. J Neurophysiol 79(2):964–982
19. Buyle-Bodin Y (1979) Neurophysiologie de l'articulation temporo-mandibulaire. Inf Dent 61(37):3403–3414
20. Carlson CR (2007) Psychological factors associated with orofacial pains. Dent Clin North Am 51(1):145–160
21. Celic R, Panduric J, Dulcic N (2006) Psychologic status in patients with temporomandibular disorders. Int J Prosthodont 19(1):28–29
22. Chase PF, Rosenoer L (1999) Parameters of odontostomatognathic disability: guidelines for evaluation of impaired simple and complex human functions involving the odontostomatognathic functional system. Cranio 17(1):70–76
23. Chateau M (1993) Orthopédie dento-faciale (T1). Cah Proth (éd), Paris. 346p
24. Chun D, Koskinen M, Moffett L (1990) Distress, jaw habits, and connective tissue laxity as predisposing factors to TMJ send in adolescent. J Craniomandib Disord 4:165–167
25. Cimino R, Michelotti A, Stradi R, Farinaro C (1998) Comparison of clinical and psychologic features of fibromyalgia and masticatory myofascial pain. J Orofac Pain 12:35–41
26. Clauzade M, Cardonnet M (1987) Diagnostic différentiel des dysfonctions de l'ATM. Cah Proth 58:125–169
27. Cohet M (1985) Concept neurophysiologique de la douleur dans le syndrome algo-dysfonctionnel de l'articulation temporo-mandibulaire. Acta Odont Stomatol 151:623–633.
28. Crews DA, Warfield CA (1985) Facial pain. Hosp Pract 15:171–179
29. Da Cunha MH, Da Silva A (1986) Le syndrome de déficience posturale. Son intérêt en ophtalmologie. J Franç Ophtalmol 9(II):747–755
30. Delaire J (1988) Plan d'occlusion et chirurgie maxillo-faciale. Orthod Franç 59:811–891
31. Devlin CV, Rothwell PS (1981) An investigation of TMJ disorders and bruxism in 500 regular attenders. J Dent Res 60 B:1162
32. Dohrmann RJ, Laskin DM (1978) An evaluation of electromyographic biofeedback in the treatment of myofascial pain-dysfunction syndrome. J Am Dent Assoc 96:656–662
33. Egermark-Eriksson I, Carlsson GE, Magnusson T (1987) A long-term epidemiologic study of the relationship between occlusal factors and mandibular dysfunction in children and adolescents. J Dent Res 66(1):67–71
34. Eversole L, Stone CE, Matheson D, Kaplan H (1985) Psychometric profiles and facial pain. Oral Surg 60(3):269–274
35. Farrar WB, Mc Carthy W (1982) A clinical outline of TMJ: diagnosis and treatment. Normandy Study Group for TMJ Dysfunction, 7th edn. Walker Co (ed), Montgomery
36. Fine E (1971) Psychological factors associated with non-organic temporomandibular joint pain-dysfunction syndrome. Br Dent J 131:402–404
37. Fonder AC (1980) The dental distress syndrome. Stress 1(1):10–17
38. Forsell H, Kanganiesmi I (1984) Mandibular dysfunction in patients with migraine. Proc Finn Dent Soc 80:217–222

39. Fragoso YD, Alves HH, Garcia SO, Finkelsztejn A (2010) Prevalence of parafunctional habits and temporomandibular dysfunction symptoms in patients attending a tertiary headache clinic. Arq Neuropsiquiatr 68(3):377–380
40. Franco AL, Gonçalves DA, Castanharo SM et al (2010) Migraine is the most prevalent primary headache in individuals with temporomandibular disorders. J Orofac Pain 24(3):287–292
41. Fricton JR, Sheldon GG (1995) Muscle disorders. In: Pertes RA, Sheldon GG (eds) Temporal mandibular disorders and orofacial pain. Quintessence, Chicago, p91
42. Friedman MH, Weisberg J (1985) Temporomandibular joint disorders. Quintes Pub Co, Inc, Chicago
43. Gambade S, Marteau JM, Caix P (2006) Rôle du muscle ptérygoïdien médial dans les dysfonctions cranio-mandibulaires. Méd Bucc Chir Bucc 12(2):73–82
44. Gaspard M (1979) L'appareil manducateur et la manducation (2 t). J Prélat (éd), Paris
45. Gatchel RJ, Stowell AW, Buschang P (2006) The relationships among depression, pain, and masticatory functioning in temporomandibular disorder patients. J Orofac Pain 20(4):288–296
46. Geenen R, Bijlsma JW (2010) Deviations in the endocrine system and brain of patients with fibromyalgia: cause or consequence of pain and associated features? Ann N Y Acad Sci 1193(1):98–110
47. Gelb H (1977) Clinical management of head, neck and TMJ pain and dysfunction: a multidisciplinary approach to diagnosis and treatment. WB Saunders Co (ed), Philadelphia/London/Toronto, 547p
48. Gil IA, Rizzatti-Barbosa CM, Monteiro-Pedro V et al (1998) Multidisciplinary approach to chronic pain from myofascial pain dysfunction syndrome: a four-year experience at a Brazilian center. Cranio 16(1):17–25
49. Goadsby PJ, Lance JW (1990) Physiopathologie de la migraine. Rev Prat 40(5):390–393
50. Gonçalves DA, Bigal ME, Jales LC et al (2010) Headache and symptoms of temporomandibular disorder: an epidemiological study. Headache 50(2):231–241
51. Green CS, Laskin DM (1983) Long-term evaluation of treatment for myofascial pain-dysfunction syndrome: a comparative analysis. J Am Dent Assoc 107(2):253–258
52. Green CS, Olson RE, Laskin DM (1982) Psychological factors in the etiology, progression and treatment of MPD syndrome. J Am Dent Assoc 105:443–448
53. Hampf G (1992) A new clinical approach to the treatment of temporomandibular dysfunction and orofacial dysesthesia: natural history and comparison with similar chronic pain conditions. J Craniomandib Disord 6(1):56–63
54. Harden RN, Revivo G, Song S et al (2007) A critical analysis of the tender points in fibromyalgia. Pain Med 8(2):147–156
55. Harkins S, Marteney J (1985) Extrinsic trauma: a significant precipitation factor in temporomandibular dysfunction. J Prosthet Dent 54:271–272
56. Hartmann F, Cucchi G (1987) Muscle ptérygoïdien lateral et SADAM: diagnostic précoce et traitement. Rev Odont Stomatol 16(3):209–218
57. Hendler N, Fink H, Long D (1983) Myofascial syndrome: response to trigger-point injections. Psychosomatics 24(11):990–999
58. Hsu MC, Clauw DJ (2007) Update on fibromyalgia and chronic widespread pain: translating recent findings into clinical practice. Adv Pain Manag 1(2):38–45
59. Iqbal R, Mughal MS, Arshad N, Arshad M (2010) Pathophysiology and antioxidant status of patients with fibromyalgia. Rheumatol Int 31(2):149–152
60. Jeanmonod A (1988) Occlusodontie. Applications cliniques. Cah Proth (éd), Paris
61. Jensen R, Olesen J (1996) Initiating mechanisms of experimentally induced tension-type headache. Cephalalgia 16(3):175–182
62. Johansson-Cahlin B, Samuelsson N, Dahlstrom L (2006) Utilization of pharmaceuticals among patients with temporomandibular disorders: a controlled study. Acta Odontol Scand 64(3):187–192
63. Jones KD, Deodhar P, Lozentzen A et al (2007) Growth hormone perturbations in fibromyalgia: a review. Semin Arthritis Rheum 36(6):657–679
64. Kafas P, Leeson R (2006) Assessment of pain in temporomandibular disorders: the bio-psychosocial complexity. Int J Oral Maxillofac Surg 35(2):145–149.

65. Kajantie E, Phillips DI (2006) The effects of sex and hormonal status on the physiological response to acute psychosocial stress. Psychoneuroendocrinology 31(2):151–178
66. Kampe T, Hannerz H, Strom P (1991) Five-year follow-up of mandibular dysfunction in adolescents with intact and restored dentitions: a comparative anamnestic and clinical study. J Craniomandib Disord 5:121–128.
67. Kight M, Gatchel RJ, Wesley L (1999) Temporomandibular disorders: evidence for significant overlap with psychopathology. Health Psychol 18(2):177–182
68. Knox K, Carrigan D, Simmons G et al (2011) No evidence of Murine-like gammaretroviruses in CFS patients previously identified as XMRV-infected. Science. doi:10.1126/science.1204963
69. Kolbinson DA, Epstein JB, Burgess JA, Senthilselvan A (1997) Temporomandibular disorders, headaches, and neck pain after motor vehicle accidents: a pilot investigation of persistence and litigation effects. J Prosthet Dent 77:46–53
70. Korszun A, Papadopoulos E, Demitrack M et al (1998) The relationship between temporomandibular disorders and stress-associated syndromes. Oral Surg Oral Med Oral Pathol Oral Radiol Endod 86(4):416–420
71. Kreisberg MK (1986) Headache as a symptom of craniomandibular disorders I: pathophysiology. Cranio 4(2):135–142
72. Krogstad BS, Jokstad A, Dahl BL, Soboleva U (1998) Somatic complaints, psychologic distress and treatment outcome in two groups of TMD patients, one previously subjected to whiplash injury. J Orofac Pain 12(2):136–143.
73. Lamey PJ (1988) Splint therapy in classical migraine. J Dent Res Abstract 67, (4):115
74. Laskin D (1969) Etiology of the pain-dysfunction syndrome. J Am Dent Assoc 79:147–153
75. Lauret JF (1988) Etude expérimentale de la "phase initiale" de la diduction mandibulaire. Thèse Doct Univ Nantes
76. Lindroth JE, Schmidt JE, Carlson CR (2002) A comparison between masticatory muscle pain patients and intracapsular pain patients on behavioral and psychosocial domains. J Orofac Pain 16(4):277–283
77. Liptan GL (2010) Fascia: a missing link in our understanding of the pathology of fibromyalgia. J Bodyw Mov Ther 14(1):3–12
78. Lous I, Olensen J (1982) Evaluation of pericranial tenderness and oral function in patients with common migraine, muscle contraction headache and "combination headache". Pain 12:385–393
79. Lupton DA, Johnson DL (1973) Myofascial pain-dysfunction syndrome: attitudes and other personality characteristics related to tolerance for pain. J Prosthet Dent 29:323–329
80. Magnusson T, Carlsson GE (1980) A 2 1/2 year follow up of changes in headache and mandibular dysfunction after stomatognathic treatment. J Prosthet Dent 49:398–402
81. Malick A, Burstein R (1998) Cells of origin of the trigeminohypothalamic tract in the rat. J Comp Neurol 400:125–144
82. Manfredini D, Bandettini di Poggio A, Cantini E et al (2004) Mood and anxiety psychopathology and temporomandibular disorder: a spectrum approach. J Oral Rehabil 31(10):933–940
83. Marbach JJ, Dworkin SF (1975) Chronic MPD, group therapy and psychodynamics. J Am Dent Assoc 90:827–833
84. Martenot M, Saïto C (1977) Se relaxer. Ed. A Michel/Opéra Mundi, Paris
85. Mc Neill C (1990) Craniomandibular disorders: guidelines for evaluation, diagnosis and management. Am Acad Craniomandib Disord. Quintes Pub (ed), Chicago, pp 13–53
86. Metha N, Forgione AS, Rosenbaum RS, Holmerg R (1984) "TMJ" triad dysfunction: a biologic basis of diagnosis and treatment. J Mass Dent Soc 33(4):173–217.
87. Miller DB (1998) Low velocity impact, vehicle damage and passenger injury. Cranio 16(4):226–229
88. Molina OF, Dos Santos J, Nelson SJ, Grossman E (1997) Prevalence of modalities of headaches and bruxism among patients with craniomandibular disorder. Cranio 15(4):314–325
89. Molina OF, Dos Santos J, Nelson SJ, Nowlin T (2000) Profile of TMD and bruxer compared to TMD and nonbruxer patients regarding chief complaint, previous consultations, modes of therapy, and chronicity. Cranio 18(3):205–218
90. Mongini F (1996) Headache and facial pain. Pathophysiology and treatment. IEA (ed), St. Louis

91. Moody PM, Kemper JT, Okesson JP et al (1982) Recent life changes and myofascial pain syndrome. J Prosthet Dent 48(3):328–330
92. Morgan DH, Hall WP, Vanwas SJ (1977) Diseases of the temporomandibular apparatus. A multidisciplinary approach. CV Mosby Co (ed), St Louis, 481p
93. Moss RA, Lombardo TW, Villarosa GA et al (1995) Oral habits and TMJ dysfunction in facial pain and non-pain subjects. J Oral Rehabil 22(1):79–81
94. Munro RR (1972) Electromyography of the masseter and anterior temporalis muscles in subjects with potential temporomandibular joint dysfunction. Aust Dent J 17:209
95. Myers DDE, Mc Call WD Jr (1983) Head pain as a result of experimental ischemic exercise of the temporalis muscle. Headache 23:113–116
96. Nahmani L, Amie M, Casteyde JP, et al. (1990) Kinésiologie, Théorie et Pratique. Comedent (éd), Paris
97. Nassif NJ, Talic YF (2001) Classic symptoms in temporomandibular disorder patients: a comparative study. Cranio 19(1):33–41
98. Nicholson RA, Lakatos CA, Gramling SE (1999) EMG reactivity and oral habits among facial pain patients in a scheduled-waiting competitive task. Appl Psychophysiol Biofeedback 24(4):235–247
99. Niemi PM, Le Bell Y, Kylmala M et al (2006) Psychological factors and responses to artificial interferences in subjects with and without a history of temporomandibular disorders. Acta Odontol Scand 64(5):300–305
100. Ogus HD, Toller PA (1981) Common disorders of temporomandibular joint. J Wright & Sons Limited (ed), Bristol
101. Okifuji A, Turk DC (2002) Stress and psychophysiological dysregulation in patients with fibromyalgia syndrome. Appl Psychophysiol Biofeedback 27(2):129–141
102. Ong KS, Keng SB (2003) The biological, social, and psychological relationship between depression and chronic pain. Cranio 21(4):286–294
103. Paprotka T, Delviks-Frankenberry KD, Cingöz O et al (2011) Recombinant origin of the retrovirus XMRV. Science. doi:10.1126/science.1205292
104. Parker MW, Kemper J (1982) Temporomandibular joint dysfunction and headache. Panminerva Med 24:107–112
105. Pennacchio EA, Borgstein J, Keith DA (1998) The incidence of pain in the muscles of mastication in patients with fibromyalgia. J Orofac Pain 12(2):abstract n° 29
106. Petrovic AG (1977) L'ajustement occlusal: son rôle dans les processus physiologiques de contrôle de la croissance du cartilage condylien. Orthod Franç 48:2–7
107. Petrovic AG, Stuzmann J (1979) Contrôle de la croissance post-natale du squelette facial: données expérimentales et modèle cybernétique. Act Odont Stomatol 128:811–841
108. Piovesan EJ MD, Kowacs PA MD, Oshinsky ML (2003) Convergence of cervical and trigeminal sensory afferents. Curr Pain Headache Rep 7:377–383.
109. Planas P (1992) La réhabilitation occlusale. (Traduction: Chateau M et Kolf J.) Masson (éd), Paris
110. Puri V, Cui L, Liverman CS, Roby KF et al (2005) Ovarian steroids regulate neuropeptides in the trigeminal ganglion. Neuropeptides 39(4):409–417
111. Rao SM, Glaros AG (1979) Electromyographic correlates of experimentally induced stress in diurnal bruxists and normals. J Dent Res 58:1872–1878
112. Richards RS, McGregor NR, Roberts TK (2005) Association between oxidative damage markers and self-reported temporomandibular dysfunction symptoms in patients with chronic fatigue syndrome. J Chron Fatig Syndr 12:3
113. Ricketts RM (1976) Essai de classification des troubles de l'articulation temporo-mandibulaire. Rev Odont Stomatol 114:253–273.
114. Rollman GB, Gillespie JM (2000) The role of psychosocial factors in temporomandibular disorders. Curr Rev Pain 4(1):71–81
115. Rudy TE, Turk DC, Kubinski JA, Zaki HS (1995) Differential treatment responses of TMD patients as a function of psychological characteristics. Pain 61:103–112
116. Ruff GA, Moss RA, Lombardo TW (1986) Common migraine: a review and proposal for a non-vascular aetiology. J Oral Rehabil 13:499–508

117. Samborski W, Sobieska M, Pieta P et al (2005) Normal profile of sex hormones in women with primary fibromyalgia. Ann Acad Med Stetin 51(2):23–26
118. Sarlani E, Grace EG, Reynolds MA, Greenspan JD (2004) Evidence for up-regulated central nociceptive processing in patients with masticatory myofascial pain. J Orofac Pain 18(1): 41–55
119. Sarzi-Puttini P, Atzeni F, Cazzola M (2010) Neuroendocrine therapy of fibromyalgia syndrome: an update. Ann N Y Acad Sci 1193(1):91–97.
120. Sauro KM, Becker WJ (2009) The stress and migraine interaction. Headache 49(9): 1378–1386
121. Schneider K, Zernicke R, Clark G (1989) Modeling of jaw-head-neck dynamics during whiplash. J Dent Res 68:1360–1365
122. Schokker RP, Hanson TL, Ansink BJJ (1990) Craniomandibular disorders in patients with different types of headache. J Craniomandib Disord 4:47–51
123. Selaimen CM, Jeronymo JC, Brilhante DP, Grossi ML (2006) Sleep and depression as risk indicators for temporomandibular disorders in a cross-cultural perspective: a case–control study. Int J Prosthodont 19(2):154–161
124. Servière F (1989) L'examen postural en exodontie quotidienne. Cah Proth 65:36–42
125. Sherman JJ, LeResche L, Huggins KH et al (2004) The relationship of somatization and depression to experimental pain response in women with temporomandibular disorders. Psychosom Med 66(6):852–860
126. Shimshak DG, DeFuria MC (1998) Health care utilization by patients with temporomandibular joint disorders. Cranio 16(3):185–193.
127. Shipman WG, Green CS, Laskin DM (1974) Correlation of placebo responses and personality characteristics in myofascial pain-dysfunction (MPD) patients. J Psychosom Res 18:475–483.
128. Simons DG (1990) Familial fibromyalgia and/or myofascial pain syndrome. Arch Phys Med Rehabil 71:258–259
129. Sipilä K, Veijola J, Jokelainen J et al (2001) Association between symptoms of temporomandibular disorders and depression: an epidemiological study of the Northern Finland 1966 Birth Cohort. Cranio 19(3):183–187
130. Soetekouw PM, Lenders JW, Bleijenberg G et al (1999) Autonomic function in patients with chronic fatigue syndrome. Clin Auton Res 9(6):334–340
131. Southwell J, Deary IJ, Geisler P (1990) Personality and anxiety in temporomandibular joint syndrome. J Oral Rehabil 17:239–243
132. Staud R, Spaeth M (2008) Psychophysical and neurochemical abnormalities of pain processing in fibromyalgia. CNS Spectr 13(3 suppl 5):12–17
133. Stockstill JW, Callahan CD (1991) Personality hardiness, anxiety, and depression as constructs of interest in the study of temporomandibular disorders. J Craniomandib Disord 5: 129–134
134. Stowell AW, Gatchel RJ, Wildenstein L (2007) Cost-effectiveness of treatments for temporomandibular disorders: biopsychosocial intervention versus treatment as usual. J Am Dent Assoc 138(2):202–208
135. Suvinen TI, Reade PC, Kemppainen P et al (2005) Review of aetiological concepts of temporomandibular pain disorders: towards a biopsychosocial model for integration of physical disorder factors with psychological and psychosocial illness impact factors. Eur J Pain 9(6): 613–633
136. Tanaka TT (1984) Recognition of the pain formula for head, neck and TMJ disorders: the general physical examination. Calif Dent Assoc J 12(5):43–49
137. Tanriverdi F, Karaca Z, Unluhizarci K, Kelestimur F (2007) The hypothalamo-pituitary-adrenal axis in chronic fatigue syndrome and fibromyalgia syndrome. Stress 10(1):13–25
138. Thomass LJ, Tiber N, Schireson S (1973) The effects of anxiety and frustration on muscular tension related to the temporomandibular joint syndrome. J Dent Res 36(5):763–768
139. Trub M, Mei N, Orofino J (1996) Periodontal and gastric convergences within the hypothalamic ventromedial nucleus area – single unit study on anesthetized rats. Behav Brain Res 72:33–37.

140. Trub M, Mei N, Orsini JC (1991) Macro and micro-electrode study of hypothalamic projections of periodontal afferents in the rat and cat. Brain Res Bull 27:29–34.
141. Turk DC, Rudy TE, Kubinski A et al (1996) Dysfunctional patients with temporomandibular disorders: evaluating the efficacy of a tailored treatment protocol. J Consult Clin Psychol 64(1):139–146
142. Valença MM, Medeiros FL, Martins HA et al (2009) Neuroendocrine dysfunction in fibromyalgia and migraine. Curr Pain Headache Rep 13(5):358–364
143. Vargo CP, Hickman DM (1997) Cluster-like signs and symptoms respond to myofascial/craniomandibular treatment: a report of two cases. Cranio 15(1):89–93
144. Vierck CJ Jr (2006) Mechanisms underlying development of spatially distributed chronic pain (fibromyalgia). Pain 124(3):242–263
145. Wänman A (1995) The relationship between muscle tenderness and craniomandibular disorders: a study of 35 years old from the general population. J Orofac Pain 9(3):235–243
146. Watanabe Y, Ishikawa T, Kino K et al (2005) Relationship between oral sensory thresholds and depressive moods. J Med Dent Sci 52(1):73–80
147. Weed ND (1983) When shoulder pain isn't bursitis. The myofascial pain syndrome. Postgrad Med 74(3):97–104, Should pain
148. Weinberg S, Lapointe H (1987) Cervical extension-flexion injury (whiplash) and internal derangement of the temporomandibular joint. J Oral Maxillofac Surg 45(8):653–656
149. Wolfe F, Katz RS, Michaud K (2005) Jaw pain: its prevalence and meaning in patients with rheumatoid arthritis, osteoarthritis and fibromyalgia. J Rheumatol 32:2421–2428
150. Wright WJ (1986) Temporomandibular disorders: occurrence of specific diagnoses and response to conservative management. Cranio 42:150–155
151. Wright EF, Domenech MA, Fischer JR (2000) Usefulness of posture training for patients with temporomandibular disorders. J Am Dent Assoc 131(2):202–210
152. Wright AR, Gatchel RJ, Wildenstein L et al (2004) Biopsychosocial differences between high-risk and low-risk patients with acute TMD-related pain. J Am Dent Assoc 135(4):474–483
153. Yap AU, Chua EK, Tan KB, Chan YH (2004) Relationships between depression/somatization and self-reports of pain and disability. J Orofac Pain 18(3):220–225
154. Yap AU, Tan KB, Chua EK, Tan HH (2002) Depression and somatization in patients with temporomandibular disorders. J Prosthet Dent 88(5):479–484
155. Yoshino G, Higashi K, Nakamura T (2003) Changes in head position due to occlusal supporting zone loss during clenching. Cranio 21(4):89–98
156. Yoshino G, Higashi K, Nakamura T (2003) Changes in weight distribution at the feet due to occlusal supporting zone loss during clenching. Cranio 21(4):271–278
157. Yunus MB (2007) Role of central sensitization in symptoms beyond muscle pain, and the evaluation of a patient with widespread pain. Best Pract Res Clin Rheumatol 21(3):481–497
158. Yunus MB (2007) Fibromyalgia and overlapping disorders: the unifying concept of central sensitivity syndromes. Semin Arthritis Rheum 36:339–356
159. Zhang ZK, Ma XC, Gao S et al (1999) Studies on contributing factors in temporomandibular disorders. Chin J Dent Res 2(3–4):7–20

General Synthesis

Experts have recently studied the possible correlation between TMD and other pathologies with symptoms similar to those of some clinical forms of migraine, fibromyalgia, and chronic fatigue. All oral structures play a role in the adaptation of human life mechanisms and respond to daily stressors such as eating or communicating. In all cases, muscles are buffer elements that try to maintain analgesic and proper functional conditions; their failure to do so generates referred pain and/or discomforts. The symptomatology varies with each patient's sensitivity to personal conditions of maladaptation: some suffer from TMJ troubles, others mainly complain of headaches, while others experience sleeping disorders and fatigue, etc. Each patient's mixed clinical setting can be a source of confusion in the clinician's diagnosis. Anglo-Saxon authors refer to TMD as the *great impostor*. In the face of such obscure pathology, neuroscience has contributed to a better and more rational understanding of the impostor and reduced the risk of wrong diagnoses and wrong therapeutic investigation. Scientific studies on stomatognathic structures yield interesting data for a clearer interpretation of these surprising clinical phenomena. It must be kept in mind that **trigeminal information can reach various non-trigeminal areas of the central nervous system** (CNS) such as the *hypothalamus, cerebellum, reticular formation, and superior colliculus*. When trigeminal afferents become excessive and/or nociceptive, they can be involved in generating some unexpected symptoms without any evident link with the oral sphere. This is particularly true in *stressed and introverted patients with oral parafunctional habits* such as **severe teeth clenching**. Clinical experiences comfort this view based on the deleterious consequences of clenching on somatic and psychic health. In spite of its polymorphous aspect dependent on patients, the over-volatility of the stomatognathic muscles results from convergent abnormal conditions in peripheral and central fields. Peripheral factors include occlusal disturbances, lingual dysfunction, dysfunctional posture or locomotion, acute injuries, iatrogenic treatments, etc. More intimate, psycho-emotional and social factors tend to hamper the patient's expression and often contribute to TMD. In any case, stomatognathic muscle spasticity is the *Gordian knot* in TMD and perhaps also in some atypical clinical forms of migraine, fibromyalgia, and chronic fatigue in clenching patients, which justifies using a trigeminal **Relaxing and**

F. Hartmann, G. Cucchi, *Stress and Orality*,
DOI 10.1007/978-2-8178-0271-8, © Springer-Verlag France 2014

Moderating Treatment (RMT) as the primary therapeutic protocol. The main purpose is to make allowance for the autonomous pathophysiological mechanism which experiences neuromuscular dysfunction. If not caught, this sort of *closed circle* situation is misleading and causes most therapeutic procedures to abort. Inversely the management of neuromuscular over-volatility and nociception is helpful in decreasing even suppressing pain and discomforts on the one hand and in facilitating a more accurate and adequate evaluation of the real factors of the disease involved, on the other hand. So the second phase is one of the investigations and treatments of the referenced etiological factors in order to minimize the risks of recurrence while keeping focus on the patient. Treatment procedures may vary depending on the case and sometimes on the practitioners' experience. Comprehensive continued therapeutic accompaniment should systematically involve multidisciplinary methods by specialists to ensure a proper and safe practice: psychological and social care, functional rehabilitation (deglutition, phonetics, etc.), occlusal rehabilitation (equilibration, prosthetics, orthodontics, etc.), skeletal rehabilitation (postural, physical, chiropractic and osteopathic treatments, orthopedics, etc.), and so on.

With the help of palpation for muscle pain, a misunderstood **teeth clenching** occurrence can emerge as the hidden part of an *oral parafunctional iceberg*. It can be the true revealer of stomatognathic muscle spasticity and pain. It can only happen however when the clinician pays close attention and conducts an exhaustive investigation because the patient himself is not always aware of his clenching. In the oral sphere, diurnal and/or nocturnal clenching triggers abnormal sensory stimulation in intensity, frequency, and/or durability and nociception. As long as they are both sensory and motor cranial nerves, the paired V are known to participate actively in the human adaptation process. Therefore, stomatognathic muscle spasticity, via the paired V, reacts to central nervous circuits. Otherwise, these abnormal nociceptive inputs could oversensitize the trigeminal nervous centers. This could stimulate some physiological reflexes, including those controlled by other cranial nerves. It could also stimulate spinal motor neurons all the way to the sacral cord. Based on scientific data, the reader can understand how such inputs may disturb the nervous centers just as a *virus* could disturb a computer program. When global adaptation to stress fails, the oral sphere seems to be a major zone of disturbances. Depending on how strong their connection is with *non-trigeminal nerve structures*, various painful signs and discomforts may also be felt very far for their anatomical area. Clinicians should no longer be puzzled by unexplained irregular heart rate, digestive problems, dizziness, lumbar pain, or painful calf spasms in stressed and introverted patients who clench their teeth tightly and/or durably and/or frequently. There can also be cases of atypical clinical forms classified as *migraine, fibromyalgia, chronic fatigue*, etc. The patient himself, when he becomes conscious of his severe clenching, usually asks the key question – "Doctor, why do I clench my teeth?" – leading to clear apprehension of the deep behavioral responsible factors.

The purpose of our book is not to evaluate the many psycho-emotional factors leading to individual attitudes such as severe parafunctional clenching. However, these complex phenomena involve the functional structures of an essential sphere of interhuman communication. They definitely need more consideration in the process of diagnosing and treating a serious health problem. The problem is invalidating to the patient. Clenching may be considered as an inadequate individual response (i.e., inhibition) to stress conditions which affect mainly the stomatognathic musculature but it is more significant.

Henceforth, it is evident that the oral sphere and its neuroanatomical components, especially the paired V, have long been underestimated by international medicine. Neuroscientific data has set two facts straight. One, the *paired V* (right and left) have a *great reflexogenous reactive ability*. Two, the trigeminal territories are richly connected to various central, cranial, and spinal nervous areas. Consequently, under stressful conditions, a sensory-motor trigeminal over-excitation (resulting from intensity and/or duration and/or frequency) may trigger dysfunctions and pathologies **well beyond the limits of the oral sphere** and may generate or aggravate signs and symptoms that are disconcerting to the clinician. Hence, the question is does this complex sensory-motor apparatus, largely involved in human adaptation, lead to a kind of magnifying

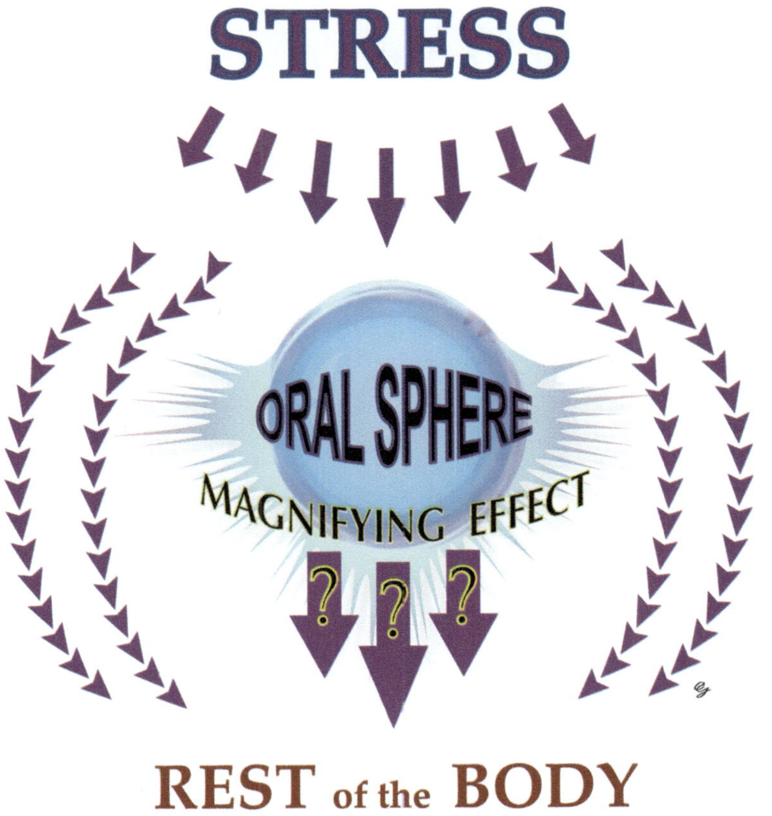

Fig. 1 The oral sphere: a possible magnifier for maladaptive stress mechanisms?

pathophysiological effect on the rest of the body (Fig. 1)? Now RMT sheds light on unresolved clinical cases of migraine, fibromyalgia, chronic fatigue, and so on.[1]

"Child! Clench your teeth and keep going" may be a popular saying in the western world, but it is a useful advice only when the clenching is short. **Durable parafunctional forms of teeth clenching are clinical disasters!**

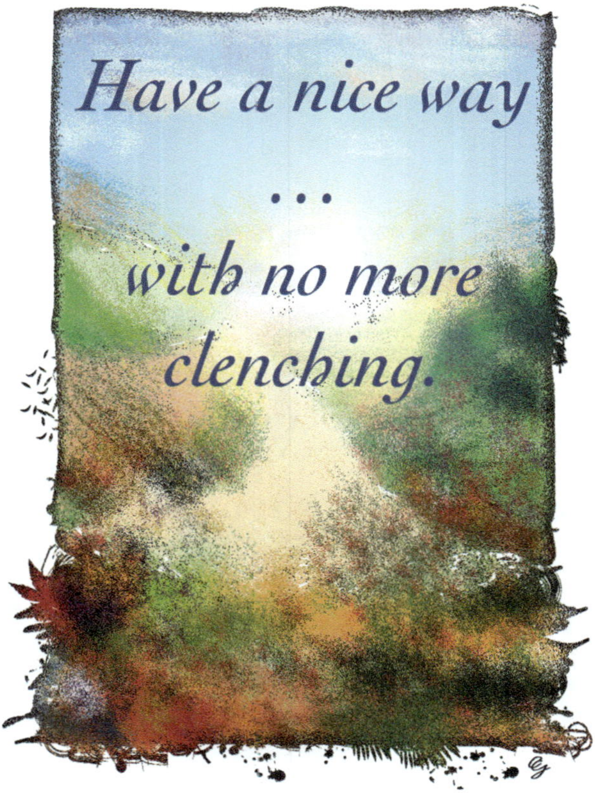

[1]You may refer your patients to the following website (available in English): http://tmd-dentalmedical.com/. They will find accurate information about parafunctional clenching and its outcome in the simplified adapted presentation we created for non-practitioners.

GPSR Compliance

The European Union's (EU) General Product Safety Regulation (GPSR) is a set of rules that requires consumer products to be safe and our obligations to ensure this.

If you have any concerns about our products, you can contact us on ProductSafety@springernature.com

In case Publisher is established outside the EU, the EU authorized representative is:

Springer Nature Customer Service Center GmbH
Europaplatz 3
69115 Heidelberg, Germany

Batch number: 10682471

Printed by Printforce, the Netherlands